The Behavioral Health Specialist in Primary Care

Mary Ann Burg, PhD, MSW, LCSW, is a Professor in the School of Social Work at the University of Central Florida, where she teaches courses on Behavioral Health, Social Work in Health Care, and Social Work Research. She also participates in teaching Interprofessional Education for the University of Central Florida, College of Medicine. She received her PhD in Sociology (with a concentration in Medical Sociology) from the University of Florida, and her MSW from Florida State University. For over 20 years, she has been active in research, scholarship, and publications on topics in behavioral medicine and in evaluating models for training interdisciplinary health professions on working in teams, especially in the primary care setting. She has 15 years of social work practice experience as a member of an interdisciplinary team in a family medical setting. She is a member of the National Association of Social Workers (NASW), American Public Health Association (APHA), Council for Social Work Education (CSWE), Association of Oncology Social Work (AOSW), and Society for Social Work Research (SSWR).

Oliver Oyama, PhD, ABPP, PA-C, CAQ-PSY, is Affiliate Associate Professor at the University of South Florida/Morsani College of Medicine and Associate Director of the University of South Florida Family Medicine Residency Program at Morton Plant Mease Healthcare where he teaches, practices, and coordinates the Behavioral Health Curriculum. He received his PhD in Clinical Psychology (with an interest in health psychology) from Indiana University and a Master of Health Sciences/Physician Assistant Certificate from Duke University. He is board-certified through the American Board of Professional Psychology in Clinical Psychology and in Clinical Health Psychology and is clinically active in both. He also practices as a certified Physician Assistant in family medicine with a Certificate of Added Qualifications in Psychiatry.

The Behavioral Health Specialist in Primary Care

SKILLS FOR INTEGRATED PRACTICE

Mary Ann Burg, PhD, MSW, LCSW

Oliver Oyama, PhD, ABPP, PA-C, CAQ-PSY

SPRINGER PUBLISHING COMPANY
NEW YORK

Springer Publishing Company, LLC
11 West 42nd Street
New York, NY 10036
www.springerpub.com

Acquisitions Editor: Stephanie Drew
Production Editor: Michael O'Connor
Composition: MPS Limited

ISBN: 978-0-8261-2987-1
e-book ISBN: 978-0-8261-2988-8

15 16 17 18 19 / 5 4 3 2 1

Library of Congress Cataloging-in-Publication Data

The behavioral health specialist in primary care : skills for integrated practice / [edited by] Mary Ann Burg, Oliver Oyama.
p. ; cm.
Includes bibliographical references and index.
ISBN 978-0-8261-2987-1 — ISBN 978-0-8261-2988-8 (e-book)
I. Burg, Mary Ann, editor. II. Oyama, Oliver N., 1959- , editor.
[DNLM: 1. Delivery of Health Care, Integrated—methods. 2. Mental Health Services. 3. Behavioral Medicine. 4. Mental Health. 5. Primary Health Care—methods. WM 30.1]
RA790.5
326.1—dc23

2015016249

Printed in the United States of America by McNaughton & Gunn.

CONTENTS

CONTRIBUTORS

Eileen Mazur Abel, PhD, MSW Clinical Professor, University of Southern California, School of Social Work, Virtual Academic Center, Los Angeles, California

Gail Adorno, PhD, LCSW, ACSW Assistant Professor, University of Texas at Arlington, School of Social Work, Arlington, Texas

Beth A. Bailey, PhD Director of Primary Care Research, Professor of Family Medicine, Quillen College of Medicine, East Tennessee State University, Johnson City, Tennessee

Thomas W. Bishop, PsyD, HSP Assistant Professor, Director of Behavioral Medicine, Department of Family Medicine, Quillen College of Medicine, East Tennessee State University, ETSU Family Physicians of Johnson City, Johnson City, Tennessee

Mary Ann Burg, PhD, MSW, LCSW Professor, School of Social Work, College of Health and Public Affairs, University of Central Florida, Orlando, Florida

Elise Butkiewicz, MD Medical Director, Overlook Family Medicine, Associate Director and Clinical Faculty, Atlantic Health System, Overlook Family Medicine Residency, Summit, New Jersey

James S. Campbell, MD Associate Professor and Program Director, Louisiana State University Health Sciences Center, Department of Family Medicine, Kenner, Louisiana

Antonia Carbone, PharmD, BCPS, BCACP Clinical Assistant Professor of Pharmacy Practice, Fairleigh Dickinson University School of Pharmacy/ Overlook Family Medicine, Florham Park, New Jersey

Candace Coleman, MD Resident Physician, Family Medicine, Northwestern Feinberg School of Medicine and Erie Family Health Center, Chicago, Illinois

Amy B. Dailey, PhD, MPH Associate Professor, Department of Health Sciences, Gettysburg College, Gettysburg, Pennsylvania

Ruth DeBusk, PhD, RD Faculty, Tallahassee Memorial HealthCare, Family Medicine Residency Program, Tallahassee, Florida

Deborah Edberg, MD Assistant Professor, Family Medicine, Northwestern Feinberg School of Medicine, Program Director, McGaw Northwestern Family Medicine Residency Program, Erie Family Health Center, Chicago, Illinois

Michael Floyd, EdD Professor Emeritus, Department of Family Medicine, Quillen College of Medicine, East Tennessee State University, Johnson City, Tennessee

Denise Gammonley, PhD, LCSW Associate Professor, School of Social Work, University of Central Florida, Orlando, Florida

Paul W. Goetz, PhD Assistant Professor, Surgery and Psychiatry, Cardiac Behavioral Medicine, Bluhm Cardiovascular Institute of Northwestern, Chicago, Illinois

Stuart Green, DMH, MA, LCSW Behavioral Scientist, Atlantic Health System, Associate Director, Overlook Family Medicine Residency Program, Summit, New Jersey

Chris Herndon, PharmD, BCPS Associate Professor, Department of Pharmacy Practice, Southern Illinois University, Edwardsville, Illinois and Clinical Associate Professor, Department of Community and Family Medicine, St. Louis University School of Medicine, St. Louis, Missouri

Michele M. Larzelere, PhD Associate Professor, Louisiana State University Health Sciences Center, Department of Family Medicine, Kenner, Louisiana

Shawn A. Lawrence, PhD, LCSW Associate Professor, MSW Program Coordinator, School of Social Work, University of Central Florida, Orlando, Florida

Amy Miano, MSW, LCSW Social Worker, Overlook Medical Center, Atlantic Health System, Summit, New Jersey

Vicki J. Michels, PhD Chairperson and Professor, Department of Addiction Studies, Psychology, and Social Work, Minot State University, Minot, North Dakota

Oliver Oyama, PhD, ABPP, PA-C, CAQ-PSY Associate Director, Affiliate Associate Professor, University of South Florida/Morton Plant Mease Family Medicine Residency Program, Clearwater, Florida

Julie Lewis Rickert, PsyD Associate Director, Associate Professor, University of North Dakota School of Medicine and Health Sciences Center for Family Medicine – Minot, Minot, North Dakota

Katherine Sanchez, PhD, LCSW Assistant Professor, University of Texas at Arlington, School of Social Work, Arlington, Texas

Cathy Snapp, PhD Director of Behavioral Medicine, Tallahassee Memorial HealthCare, Family Medicine Residency Program, Tallahassee, Florida

Fred Tudiver, MD, FAAFP Professor, Department of Family Medicine, Quillen College of Medicine, East Tennessee State University, Johnson City, Tennessee

Timothy A. Urbin, PhD, MBA, HSP Assistant Professor, Director of Behavioral Medicine, Department of Family Medicine, Quillen College of Medicine, East Tennessee State University, ETSU Family Physicians of Bristol, Bristol, Tennessee

Elfie Wegner, APN Atlantic Health System Family Medicine, Summit, New Jersey

Tracy Wharton, PhD, LCSW Assistant Professor, School of Social Work, University of Central Florida, Orlando, Florida

Santina Wheat, MD Assistant Professor, Family Medicine, Northwestern Feinberg School of Medicine and Erie Family Health Center, Chicago, Illinois

Jack Woodside, MD Professor, Quillen College of Medicine, East Tennessee State University, Johnson City, Tennessee

PREFACE

Our conceptualization of health and illness has changed dramatically since the time of Hippocrates, the Greek physician who lived in 400 BCE and who first established medicine as a discipline. Nonetheless, Hippocrates cleverly observed that, "*Healing is a matter of time, but it is sometimes also a matter of opportunity.*" In most parts of the globe, the major causes of mortality have changed from acute illness and communicable diseases to chronic diseases attributable to behavioral and dietary risk factors. Thus, the chances for living a long and healthy life are more dependent than ever on how an individual behaves and the opportunities individuals have to engage in healthy behaviors. The medical community has come to understand that patient-centered health care, especially provided within the primary care setting, is needed in order to improve population health. Optimally, patient-centered health care engages an interdisciplinary health care team and is built on clinical opportunities to work closely with patients to support their healthy behaviors and encourage healthy lifestyle changes.

The opportunity for making huge improvements in population health and longevity is here, but it requires a trained health workforce including behavioral health specialists. All members of the primary care team ideally should be trained in the essentials of behavioral health care including the physician, physician assistant, nurse practitioner, nursing staff, pharmacy personnel, nutritionist, psychologist, social worker, and rehabilitation and mental health counselor. This book is designed to provide essential knowledge and skills in behavioral health for all members of the primary care health team.

The book begins with a short history of the development of evidence for the value of the biopsychosocial model in primary care and an overview of the role of the behavioral health specialist in the primary care team. In order to provide context for the practice of behavioral health care, we review the theoretical basis for understanding health behavior and the development of brief counseling methods for influencing patients to engage in healthier behaviors. Current epidemiological trends of some of the most common presenting conditions in primary care set the stage for moving into chapters on specific conditions, including diabetes, cardiovascular conditions, chronic pain, sleep disorders, geriatric conditions, cancer-related conditions, substance abuse, and obesity. Each of these chapters begins with a typical referral note from a primary care provider requesting a behavioral health assessment or intervention and concludes with a sample of how the behavioral health specialist might respond to the referral. These sample referrals and consultation notes are intended to provide a practical example of how the behavioral health specialist might function on a primary care team and how our patients might navigate an integrated health care system within the patient-centered medical home. The book concludes with a chapter on systems medicine, which will provide readers with a vision of the future of health care engaging the developing science of brain function and how the brain can be modified to improve our experience of health and wellness.

The reader will see that the authors of these chapters represent many of the professional disciplines included in the primary care team. These contributors have significant experience in the practice of behavioral health and the interdisciplinary provision of health care. The contributors also enrich the chapters with their own research and publication experience in the field of behavioral health care. Both of the editors have many years of experience working as behavioral health specialists in primary care and in collaborating in research on various behavioral health topics within the primary care setting.

It is our intent that this book provides a relevant, practical, and timely resource for all members of the integrated primary care team, but particularly those functioning as behavioral health specialists. Whether currently in training, new to their profession, transitioning onto a primary care team, or merely wishing to learn more about integrated behavioral health, it is our hope that this book encourages effective and efficient patient care that leads to positive changes in health behaviors and improvements in the health and well-being of our patients. Each chapter provides an extensive bibliographic review and the reader is encouraged to explore these and other resources as we optimize our "opportunity" to heal.

Mary Ann Burg and Oliver Oyama

ACKNOWLEDGMENTS

The motivation, encouragement, and ideas that have led to this book come from our patients, our colleagues, and the many influential writings on this topic. We acknowledge all those clinicians, academicians, scientists, and researchers who came before us to steer health care to where it is today. We are indebted to our contributing authors from across the country who gave of their time to this project. Each had other personal and professional responsibilities that had to be juggled and we sincerely thank you for your efforts.

Most importantly, heartfelt thanks from both of us to our dear family members and supportive friends who keep us balanced and grateful.

ONE

INTRODUCTION TO THE INTEGRATED PRIMARY CARE TEAM

OLIVER OYAMA

The behavioral health specialist (BHS) is a distinctly new member of the primary care medical team. In this chapter, you learn how and why the BHS is now considered a critical component of primary care medicine. You also learn how the incorporation of behavioral health services into primary care medicine is part of a dynamically changing environment in U.S. medicine fueled by new ideas of whole-person and patient-centered health care and by research on how clinical attention to individual health behaviors can impact health care costs and health outcomes.

First it is valuable to start by defining terms. *Primary care* is defined as the "provision of integrated, accessible health care services by clinicians who are accountable for addressing a large majority of personal health care needs, developing a sustained partnership with patients, and practicing in the context of family and community" (Institute of Medicine [IOM], 1994). *Integrated primary care* involves the care of patients within the primary care setting by primary care providers (physicians, physician assistants, and advanced practice registered nurses—hereafter PCPs) and other disciplines to include the BHS (psychologist, social worker—hereafter BHS), dietician, pharmacist, or disease care manager, among others. The term *behavioral health* refers to the psychosocial care of patients that goes far beyond a focus on diagnosing mental or psychiatric illness. Coming from the field of behavioral medicine and using the biopsychosocial model (described in the following), behavioral health encompasses not only mental illness but also factors that contribute to mental well-being such as environmental forces (culture, family, economics), lifestyle factors (behaviors/habits, substance use, inactivity), and cognitions (thoughts, beliefs) that can lead to mental illness. The focus of behavioral health is not exclusively mental illness but more broadly includes problems traditionally under the realm of medical care (e.g., diabetes, hypertension, asthma). By understanding the behavioral underpinnings of these medical problems, the BHS can assist in the treatment of a broader range of biopsychosocial problems, thereby having a greater impact on whole person care. Finally, the move away from the "mental illness" terminology also addresses the cultural stigma of mental illness and brings mental wellness and its care into the mainstream of health care.

There are two general views of what is meant by integrating behavioral health into primary care. One view refers to the inclusion of primary care services in existing behavioral health care settings such as a mental health hospital or outpatient setting. Research suggests that the chronically mentally ill do not have similar access to primary care resources or utilize these resources to a lesser degree than those without chronic mental illness (Druss et al., 2010). It is believed that by providing these services in the context of primary mental health care the frequency, morbidity, and cost of common biomedical illnesses will be reduced. In fact, one element of the recent Patient Protection and Affordable Care Act of 2010 (ACA) emphasizes the expansion of pilot programs in which primary care services are brought into behavioral health settings (ACA, 2010).

Qualitatively different is another view of integrated primary care in which behavioral health providers or services are brought into traditional primary care medical settings such as the outpatient primary care clinic. Here the main focus of services is physical health with the addition of mental health services within the available services. In this model of integration, the dynamic interplay of behavior, mental health, and physical health is acknowledged and emphasized. The BHS addresses not only mental illness in this setting but also plays an essential role in maintaining the physical health of primary care patients. It is this second view or perspective that forms the focus of this chapter and this textbook.

BIOPSYCHOSOCIAL INTEGRATION IN PRIMARY CARE: A HISTORICAL PERSPECTIVE

The integration of behavioral or psychosocial care with biomedical care has a long history in the practice of medicine and specifically in the development and practice of primary care medicine. References of the interaction between mind and body date to the 10th century (Deuraseh & Talib, 2005). However, it is important to realize that the conceptualization of mental processes and human behavior as key factors in health and illness is an idea that has emerged, disappeared, and reemerged in the practice of medicine over the centuries. In the early years of "modern medicine," that is, the era we know as the beginning of a scientific and technologically sophisticated medicine that emerged in the beginning of the 20th century, mind–body dualism and reductionism dominated and shaped the definition of disease and medical response to treating disease. Heart disease, for example, was viewed as a failure of the heart muscle or a heart valve that required a technological fix (i.e., surgery), and little consideration was given to the role of the patient's mental health or lifestyle behaviors in the development of heart disease or the process of treating the heart defect.

Psychosomatic medicine, coming from the psychoanalytic medical tradition of the early 20th century, examined the relationships between psychology, the autonomic nervous system response, and emotions (Brown, 1986;

Deuraseh & Talib, 2005; National Institutes of Health [NIH], 2000). This new focus on systemic processes in health and illness helped pave the way in the 1970s for the emergence of the field of behavioral medicine, an organized psychology that formally conferred credibility to the mind–body relationship (Schwartz & Weiss, 1978a, 1978b). Roughly around the same time, family medicine was established as a medical specialty founded on the principles of continuous and comprehensive care and guided by Engel's biopsychosocial care model (American Board of Family Medicine, n.d.). In the 1980s, the field of health psychology was formed as a discipline within psychology to promote and maintain health through the prevention and treatment of illness, the identification of the causes of illness, and the analysis and improvement of the health care system and of health policy formation (Matarazzo, 1982).

In 1948, the World Health Organization (WHO) developed an expansive definition of health: "Health is a state of complete physical, mental and social well-being and not merely the absence of disease or infirmity" (WHO, 1948). Since this time, and spurred by the broader definition of health and illness, there has been interest from organized medicine (Baird, Blount, & Brungardt, 2014), organized psychology (Levant, 2005), and government (Hunter & Goodie, 2012; Substance Abuse and Mental Health Services Administration [SAMHSA], n.d.), in developing care models that incorporate wide-ranging biopsychosocial care. This interest is also echoed worldwide with both the WHO and the World Organization of Family Doctors (WONCA) noting that the "current provision of mental health in primary care is still globally insufficient and unsatisfactory" and that integration of mental health services into primary care can and should be an important priority (WHO/WONCA, 2008).

In 2001, the IOM's *Crossing the Quality Chasm: A New Health System for the 21st Century* and its subsequent *Health Professions Education: A Bridge to Quality* identified patient-centered care and utilizing interdisciplinary teams in caring for the medical needs of the population as critical for meeting the needs of the 21st century health system (Institute of Medicine, 2001; Knebel & Greiner, 2003). These interdisciplinary teams would be composed of members who possess a variety of skills, many not within the scope of the primary care physician (Grumbach & Bodenheimer, 2004). In 2002, the *Future of Family Medicine* project was developed from the medical home model of the 1960s and proffered a personal medical home for each American (Future of Family Medicine Project Leadership Committee, 2004; Palfrey, 2006). The Agency for Healthcare Research and Quality (AHRQ) then adopted the model as their guide to "revitalizing the Nation's primary care system" through five functions: comprehensive care, patient-centered care, coordinated care, accessible services, and quality and safety (AHRQ, n.d.). The first three of these functions highlight biopsychosocial, integrative, team-based care, and relationship-based whole person care spanning services from prevention and wellness to acute care to chronic care. This model and subsequent governmental policy is foundational to the development of integrated primary care teams.

EVIDENCE FOR INCORPORATING BIOPSYCHOSOCIAL CARE IN PRIMARY CARE

Mental Health Care in Primary Care

It is well recognized that behavioral and emotional disorders are common and among the most frequent diagnoses seen in primary care (Roca et al., 2009). While referral to specialty mental health providers for mental health care is the traditional approach used after identifying such disorders, the data suggest that these referrals are difficult to accomplish (Cunningham, 2009) and that many patients do not follow through with these referrals (Fisher & Ransom, 1997; Slay & McCleod, 1997). The majority of patients with mental health needs rely solely on receiving their mental health care from their primary care providers (Brody, Khaliq, & Thompson, 1997). While primary care providers are willing to provide these services (Oyama, Burg, Fraser, & Kosch, 2011), a number of factors such as skills preparation, clinical time demands, and reimbursement likely hinder this from occurring. There is clearly a gap between the identified mental health needs in primary care and the patient-centered, timely, and efficient services needed to meet these needs.

Health Behavior Change and Medical Illnesses

Up to 40% of each of the five leading causes of death in the United States (heart disease, cancer, unintentional injuries, cerebrovascular disease, chronic lower respiratory diseases) is preventable (Centers for Disease Control and Prevention [CDC], n.d.). Specific behaviors such as increasing exercise, reducing high fat diets, adhering to medical treatments, using personal safety devices such as car safety belts or motorcycle helmets, or using good stress management strategies are integral to reducing these preventable deaths. Primary care medicine is the ideal setting in which to address these behaviors with patients. Primary care providers, however, often have limited time and resources to spend more than brief moments discussing these with patients. BHSs are experts in behavioral change and are a viable solution to this health care dilemma.

LEGISLATING INTEGRATED HEALTH CARE

Two significant pieces of governmental legislation have influenced the recognition of and need for integrated health care in the United States from the biopsychosocial perspective. The Mental Health and Addiction Equity Act of 2007 required that there be no more restrictions to the insurance benefits for mental health or substance use/abuse treatment than there were for general medical/surgical treatments (Civic Impulse, 2015). This enhanced the recognition of behavioral health care at the funding level. The ACA followed and is the U.S. government's most recent attempt to reform health care by providing improved access to care and addressing expanding health care spending (ACA, 2010). The ACA includes provisions that potentially impact integrated primary care. The major provisions in the ACA involve increasing access to care, improving health care quality and health system performance, promoting care coordination, and improving workforce training and development. These provisions include specific language for integration of care and the preparation of health care providers who can function within an integrated health care system.

MODELS OF INTEGRATED PRIMARY CARE

Many models exist of the integration of primary medical and behavioral health care. One of the earliest models is mentioned in 1976 in the description of the development of primary care teams at a large health maintenance organizations (HMOs) (Collins & Fund, 2010). Interestingly, this was a year before Engel's influential paper delineating the "biopsychosocial model" and it was almost 20 years before further discussions of such models of integrated primary care are found in the literature. Blount and Bayona (1994) discuss possible explanations why these early writings did not impact overall health care delivery at the time. These descriptions of integrated models did not lead to health system changes as they failed to offer specifics of how care might be organized and did not clarify the interactions among team members and patients that would need to occur in order to bring the models to fruition. Newer models built on those from the 1970s provided greater specificity of theory and practice (Hunter, Goodie, Oordt, & Dobmeyer, 2009; O'Donohue, Byrd, Cumming, & Henderson, 2005; O'Donohue, Cummings, Cucciare, Runyan, & Cummings, 2006).

Foundational to the discussion of models of care are the types of relationships that might exist between medical and behavioral health service providers in primary care (Blount, 2003; Doherty, 1995; Doherty, McDaniel, & Baird, 1996). These relationships have been commonly categorized as *coordinated*, *colocated*, or *integrated*.

The *coordinated* care model is the oldest and most commonly used model in primary care. PCPs would refer patients identified as having mental health concerns to specialists in mental health (psychologists, social workers, psychiatrists, counselors/therapists). These patients would receive care from these mental health specialists, often located away from the primary care setting, and be referred back to the primary care provider after treatment concluded. These specialists were trained in and performed these functions on patients with common mental illnesses such as depression, anxiety, and substance abuse, to name a few. During their primary care clinic office visit, the patient might be given the contact information for a mental health specialist and asked to contact the specialist to make an appointment. In another process the primary care practice might relay the referral to the mental health specialist who would in turn contact the patient to schedule the appointment. There are benefits and drawbacks to both processes. There might also be prearranged agreements between both providers relative to the process of referral, communications, documentation, or other aspects of coordinating the patient's care.

Doherty (1995) and Doherty et al. (1996) distinguish between two levels of *coordinated care*, *minimal collaboration*, and *basic collaboration at a distance*. *Minimal collaboration* is the traditional private practice model described previously in which patients are referred to BHSs in separate facilities at separate sites, having separate systems and with rare communication between providers. *Basic collaboration at a distance* again involves providers at separate facilities at separate sites and having separate systems but providers communicate about shared patients by letter, phone, and so on. While this form of collaborative care sounds optimal it is this author's experience that in primary care it is rare that this type of communication occurs between PCPs and BHSs. Furthermore, both levels of care inherently communicate to the patient the division of services and the compartmentalizing of "mental health" or "behavioral" care as distinct and separate from primary "medical" care. The stigmatization is obvious and could be a reason for the poor follow-up rates of primary care patients attending the initial appointment with the BHS.

In the *colocated* model or Doherty's (1995) *basic collaboration on-site* model, the BHS is located in the same office, suite, or building as the PCP. Incident to this proximity is that the PCP and BHS have a greater opportunity to consult each other via brief phone calls or even face-to-face contacts and consults. Theoretically this may lead to higher rates of referral and coordination of care. Again, the patient would either make the appointment to see the BHS or a prearranged scheduling process might be utilized. *Colocated* care offers more efficient integration than *collaborative* care and may reduce some of the obstacles to *coordinated* behavioral health care. A related model is the *reverse colocated* model that has received attention more recently in the mental health community (Shackelford, Sirna, Mangurian, Dilley, & Shumway, 2013). In this model, PCPs are located in mental health settings (often a community mental health center or other mental health specific service agency) to provide non psychiatric primary medical care to the chronically mentally ill, a group with historically low utilization of primary care services.

Within this level of care also falls *care/case management*. Care/case management employs care managers, often medically trained personnel (medical assistants, nurses, health education specialists), who facilitate a patient's participation in a disease-specific (e.g., diabetes, depression, chronic pain) protocol of care (Ashburn & Staats, 1999; Sadur et al., 1999; Williams, Angstman, Johnson, & Katzelnick, 2011). The manager would coordinate the patient's care that typically involves various clinical providers (often including behavioral health providers), would ensure and document the patient's progress through a structured treatment protocol, and might even provide some aspect of the actual care to the patient. Managers trained in behavioral health or health education might also address the behavioral issues involved in the patient's health concerns (e.g., smoking cessation, weight loss, medication adherence). The manager could be located in a variety of settings and financially supported by the primary care clinic, a hospital department, an HMO, or even an accountable care organization.

As evidence for the biopsychosocial model and the influence of psychological and social factors on physical health grew, the fields of health psychology, medical social work, and psychiatry ultimately expanded their scope of care identifying broader targets for their interventions other than traditional mental illness. It has become generally accepted that the health of patients with hypertension, diabetes, or coronary artery disease requires consideration of psychosocial factors. The patient with hypertension may need specialty help to quit smoking and manage stress more effectively. Patients with diabetes might need an intensive intervention to assist with regularly checking their blood glucose levels and taking their insulin as prescribed. Patients with coronary artery disease may need to change their diet if losing weight was recommended. PCPs recognize the importance of these psychosocial factors and the role BHSs play in the care of their patients. This broader scope of care calls for a new and closer model of communication between PCP and BHS.

The *integrated care* model involves this greater level of communication and contact among patient, PCP, and BHS. In this model, the PCP and BHS would share the same medical record, might occasionally see the patient at the same visit, and would develop and work toward mutually agreed upon treatment plans and goals. This is the highest level of integration. Doherty further divides this level into two separate levels: *close collaboration in a partly integrated system* and *close collaboration in a fully integrated system* (Doherty, 1995, 1996). The difference in these two levels is the degree to which both parties are committed to the "biopsychosocial/systems paradigm," regularly meet to collaborate, have a balance of power and influence among the providers relative to their roles and areas of expertise, and are operationally cohesive.

A further refinement of the integrated care model moves the BHS from *multidisciplinary* involvement in the care of primary care patients to the *interdisciplinary* care of patients. Kirkpatrick, Vogel, and Nyman (2011) describe how in this model the BHS not only shares information, sees patients with the PCP, and works toward mutually agreed upon treatment plans and goals, but also is involved in what they describe as *boundary blurring between disciplines and cross-training (within the limits of professional scope of practice)* to achieve those treatment plans and goals. BHSs would step outside of their traditional discipline-specific roles to address whatever the patient needs at the moment. The PCP might contribute by providing some behavioral health interventions themselves as they interact with a patient, and similarly the BHS might identify a need for a follow-up appointment with the PCP to discuss a new physical symptom and proactively schedule the care with the PCP. This describes what may be the practice ideal in integrated primary care—all members of the integrated primary care team fluidly responding to the identified need(s) of the patient.

Research support for integration of behavioral health care in the primary care setting is rapidly growing. Recent reviews find that integration in primary care improves patient access, patient adherence to treatment regimens, clinical outcomes, financial viability, patient satisfaction, and provider satisfaction (Blount, 2003; Vogel, Malcore, Illes, & Kirkpatrick, 2014). Further research utilizing both traditional quantitative methodology as well as more descriptive qualitative designs will be necessary to fully elucidate the contributions made by integrated primary care teams. Peek, Cohen, and deGruy (2014) furthermore recommend development of a set of shared language and definitions in the field of integrated behavioral health to inform policymaking, business modeling, and future research.

EDUCATING HEALTH CARE PROVIDERS IN INTEGRATED HEALTH CARE

The IOM examined the current curriculum content, teaching techniques, and assessment methodologies used by U.S. medical schools to teach behavioral and social science content to medical students (Vanselow & Cuff, 2004). Because of very different curricular designs among the medical schools and limits to curricular databases, the study was not able to describe the current state of medical education in integrated health care. However, the authors recommended that all medical students receive instruction in integrated health care throughout their 4 years of education and offered recommendations for curricular content in the behavioral and social science domain, strategies to incentivize educators to work and develop curriculum in this area, and urged medical examination boards to include this content area in their assessment of medical professionals.

Since the inception of family medicine (the stereotypic primary care specialty) as a medical discipline, behavioral health has been a required component of postgraduate training. BHSs often teach and provide specialty consultation during the graduate and postgraduate training experience. In the family medicine residency program in which this author functions, similar to many other family medicine residency programs, faculty and residents refer patients for evaluation, consultation, and treatment for routine mental health problems (depression, anxiety, substance abuse) that present to family medicine. They also refer patients with traditional biomedical problems such as hypertension, diabetes, and chronic obstructive pulmonary disease (COPD) for assistance with treatment adherence, to help patients cope with their illness, or to manage the psychosocial sequelae of their illness (e.g., mood disorder, family disruption, illness worry).

Similar efforts at preparing nonphysician providers for integrated primary care, including psychologists, social workers, psychiatrists, marriage and family therapists, nurses, and pharmacists, demonstrate the efforts being placed on preparing a multidisciplinary workforce to function within the integrated primary care environment (Council on Social Work Education, n.d.; Cowley et al., 2014; McDaniel, Belar, Schroeder, Hargrove, & Freeman, 2002; McDaniel, Doherty, & Hepworth, 2014; Naylor & Kurtzman, 2010; Ratka, 2012). It is incumbent on educators of both medical and behavioral health professionals to identify the behavioral health competencies required for integrated care in order to design training programs that effectively and efficiently teach these core clinical competencies. In 2009, six national education associations of schools of the health professions formed the Interprofessional Education Collaborative® (IPEC) to promote learning experiences and competencies to help prepare future health professionals for enhanced team-based care of patients and improved population health outcomes (IPEC, 2015).

IPEC recommends that students in the health care professions be taught four basic competencies for integrated health care:

- Assert values and ethics of interprofessional practice by placing the interests, dignity, and respect of patients at the center of health care delivery, and embracing the cultural diversity and differences of health care teams.
- Leverage the unique roles and responsibilities of interprofessional partners to appropriately assess and address the health care needs of patients and populations served.
- Communicate with patients, families, communities, and other health professionals in support of a team approach to preventing disease and disability, maintaining health, and treating disease.
- Perform effectively in various team roles to deliver patient/population-centered care that is safe, timely, efficient, effective, and equitable.

Robinson and Reiter (2007) also describe core competencies in integrated care using six domains: (a) clinical practice skills, (b) practice management skills, (c) consultation skills, (d) documentation skills, (e) team performance skills, and (f) administrative skills. Each domain includes a number of attributes that can be used to guide the training and practice of the BHS.

Integration in primary care involves more than merely incorporating BHSs into primary care clinical teams. There are a number of themes consistent across each of the published sets of integrated care competencies and in the following we distilled these common themes into practical guidelines for practice for the BHS in the integrated care environment (Belar & Deardorff, 1995; O'Donohue et al., 2006; Robinson & Reiter, 2007).

A PRACTITIONER'S GUIDE TO SUCCESSFUL BEHAVIORAL HEALTH INTEGRATION IN PRIMARY CARE

- *In order to work as a team one must think like a team*

Behavioral health–trained professionals traditionally develop their knowledge and learn their craft within the training model of their discipline, be it psychology, social work, or mental health. Previously, within the traditional medical model behavioral health-trained professionals operated as *subspecialists* in behavioral health. As subspecialists, they waited for patients to self-refer or to be referred by other providers. Then they would provide services directly to patients seldom interacting or collaborating with other professionals involved in the care of the patient apart from possibly sharing a written evaluation or treatment report. This subspecialty model is obviously counter to what is ideal and is being promoted in this textbook.

The nature of being an interdisciplinary health care team involves considering and valuing the contributions of other team members and developing team goals of care that each member of the team work toward. This requires a shift in approach for many behavioral health trained professionals. The integrated

BHS will be aware of the importance of the dietician on the team, for example, and thus will assist the patient in achieving dietary goals in the context of the behavioral health interventions. This obviously works in the opposite direction as physician, dietician, pharmacist, and so on are aware of the skills and approaches of the BHS and work toward supporting the patient's behavioral health treatment goals. Identifying goals of care from other specialists on the team and assisting patients in attaining these goals is the true nature of team-based care (à la Kirkpatrick's "boundary blurring" described in the section "Models of Integrated Primary Care").

- *Do not lose sight of the BHS's expertise and the unique set of knowledge and skills that the BHS brings to the team*

While sounding contrary to the preceding section, it is an interesting phenomenon that occasionally one member of the integrated health care team may become so interested in or motivated by another specialty's focus for a particular patient that he or she inadvertently forgets what they have to offer in the patient's care. The mental health team member, for instance, may become interested in the psychopharmacology for the patient's major depressive disorder and undervalue or even fail to utilize counseling interventions to help the patient with the mental disorder. Each member of the team would ideally work to stay true to his or her specific discipline of training and practice while at the same time valuing and supporting the involvement and goals of the others.

- *Adapt one's practice style to the clinic context*

The medical profession including primary care typically involves a philosophical approach and workflow that is often contrary to the traditional training and practice of most BHSs. BHSs are trained to thoroughly assess patients often without regard to time or with lengthy time allowances as compared to the time spent in most primary care encounters. Psychologists, for instance, may spend 60 to 90 minutes in a new patient evaluation or even hours doing a neuropsychological assessment. In primary care, patient encounters are usually measured in quarter hours. When the BHS practices using traditional practice time standards, the other primary care team members may view the BHS as being out of touch with the practical demands of a busy primary care practice. This could have the unintended consequence of alienating the BHS from others in the team, ultimately affecting the BHS's perceived value to the team and future referrals to the BHS.

In integrated primary care, patient interactions must be *briefer* and *more focused*, targeting more manageable short-term goals than most BHSs have been taught. This could be limiting contacts with patients to 15- to 20-minute sessions, or teaching a relaxation exercise to a diabetic patient with anxiety and choosing not to focus on their troubled marriage, or even quickly seeing a patient in the examination room with the PCP to help support the provider in delivering a troubling diagnosis. Referrals can and should be made for more in-depth interventions such as psychotherapy or complicated psychopharmacology that may take longer than is feasible in the integrated care environment.

Day-to-day functioning of the BHS varies dramatically and typically involves multiple brief contacts with patients, community resources, outside providers, and those on the integrated team. This will be described in detail later in the chapter. The major point here is that the traditional model of hour-long patient sessions is contrary to the primary care setting and the integrated team agenda.

- *Maintain a broad perspective on targets for behavioral health interventions while staying focused on assessments and treatments (e.g., targeted, brief, realistic goals)*

The traditional targets for behavioral health interventions are mental illnesses such as depression, anxiety, or substance abuse. The BHS is particularly prepared to assess for and treat these disorders as part of the integrated primary care team. However, as mentioned earlier, there are behavioral factors that are not psychiatric that are involved in many or even most medical illnesses. Diabetics must optimize their diabetes management by using a strict insulin regimen. The hypertensive patient might need to adopt a new behavior of regular exercise to lose weight. Asthmatics might not be using their spacer device regularly with the metered dose inhaler. For each of these examples, there are behaviors that can lead to the success or failure in meeting health care goals. BHSs might work with diabetics to design a process by which they come to understand and remember their insulin regimen. They might, in collaboration with a physical therapist, develop a graded exercise program with cardiac patients and teach cognitive skills to combat thoughts that could lead to nonadherence. They might help the PCP work with asthmatics to identify obstacles to using their spacer device regularly and strategies to overcome them.

- *An important role for the BHS is educating others on the team about the role of the BHS and the broader application of behavioral principles in health and illness*

As mentioned previously, the integrated team consists of health care providers with varied training, clinical foci, and clinical backgrounds. Many will not have been exposed to the behavioral elements of health and illness to the degree the BHS has. While other providers on the team may value what the BHS can contribute to the care of patients, they may see what the BHS does as separate and distinct from what they do. Behavioral health as conceptualized and discussed in this chapter overlaps with most if not all disciplines of health care. There are behavioral elements involved when making a new diagnosis of diabetes and sharing that diagnosis with the patient. There are behavioral elements to working on dietary modifications, weight loss, or physical activity plans with the patient. There are behavioral elements in addressing adherence to a new medication regimen. There are certainly behavioral elements in assisting patients with comorbid mental illness. The BHS is clearly a crucial member of the team providing direct service to the patient in some of these areas but also, and possibly more importantly, to remind and educate other team members of these elements. By assisting other team members in conceptualizing these behavioral elements and empowering them to use behavioral health strategies and techniques themselves, the BHS is modeling true team function with common goals and shared intervention strategies. The other team members become extensions of the BHS within their medical disciplines. While this may seem a subtle or even insignificant goal, it is imperative to a successfully functioning integrated team for all members to not only value the contributions of the other team members but to take on some of the language and intervention strategies used by the others. If team members merely "refer" the patient to another specialist for the other specialist's perceived unique knowledge or skill, the team becomes merely a coordinated or collocated unit without realizing the benefits of full integration of care.

Educating others on the team on the broader applications of behavioral health can take many forms. Most commonly interdisciplinary team rounds provide an opportunity for each member of the team to discuss his or her assessment and conceptualization of the patient's presenting problem and treatment plan. As the BHS shares these with other team members, the BHS influences them in developing new understandings, language, and skills that will shape and cultivate the interdisciplinary team.

■ *Availability is crucial*

A key characteristic for the BHS to be relevant and useful to the integrated primary care team is availability. At a basic level this involves a clear, smooth, and efficient referral process such that patients are seen by the BHS as soon as possible. In optimized integrated behavioral health, the BHS would be available for face-to-face or phone consult within a very short period of time. For example, ideally when a PCP sees a patient with hypertension, obesity, and tobacco abuse, they may use motivational interviewing or another behavioral change strategy to get the patient to verbalize commitment to working on a specific behavioral change; it would then be ideal if the PCP could step out of the examination room to get the BHS to do a brief meet-and-greet with the patient. If the BHS were available to do more at that time, the BHS could extend the work of the PCP by continuing and reinforcing the brief motivational intervention and by scheduling the patient for a follow-up appointment. If not, the mere act of bringing in the BHS at the moment of care communicates to the patient several important values of integrated primary care. First, the patient is exposed to the concept of the integrated team by having the PCP introduce the BHS right then and there. The traditional model of the PCP telling the patient they will refer the patient to a subspecialist or tasking the patient with locating and scheduling an appointment with a subspecialist on his or her own is contrary to the integrated team model. By having the BHS on site and available communicates to the patient the closeness of the working relationship. Second, by introducing the BHS, the PCP shares the *mantle of importance* that patients often place on their PCP. This is not an insignificant part of team process as the patient is being asked to trust a new health care provider with whom they have no knowledge or experience. Ideally, patients develop trusting relationships with their PCPs so the "warm handoff," as it is often referred, allows the PCPs to communicate their value of, respect for, and expectation that the new provider will be helpful in the care of the patient.

How PCPs present the role of BHSs or introduce them to the patient often requires coaching (Belar & Deardorff, 1995). The author has found that when PCPs make a point of building up their relationship with the BHS, clearly articulating the expectation they have of how the BHS can help the patient with a particular health goal, and encouraging the patient to "give it a try," the patient is much more likely to participate and have a much better chance of a positive health impact. Finally, the more often the PCP involves the BHS in the care of their patients and gives the verbal explanation to the patient of the value of integrated care, the more the perspective and skills are reinforced and valued for the PCP. The positive relationship between belief and behavior (cognitive consonance) is reinforcing and can strengthen the behavior, allowing it to be more seamlessly performed.

Just-in-time or *curbside* interactions among the integrated team members are also significant for successful functioning within the integrated primary care team. These interactions serve to trigger referrals, support others in their care of patients, educate team members about shared patients, and educate and reinforce team members in their understanding of *the BHS's* contributions to the care of shared patients.

■ *Learn something about medicine (pathophysiology of illness and disease, pharmacology)*

Particularly in primary care it is incumbent on the new BHS to develop a rudimentary understanding of certain aspects of medicine and pharmacology. Many BHSs have trained in health care settings and may have had formal education in the pathophysiology of common illnesses as well as their medication management. For those who have not, the learning curve is steep but manageable. Various resources exist to help learn the fundamental aspects of the assessment, diagnosis, and treatment of the common illnesses and conditions seen by the BHS in primary care. Additionally, one advantage of a well-functioning integrated primary team is that the PCPs on the team are often very open to sharing their knowledge with others in the same way the BHSs share their knowledge and skills as mentioned previously. Basic, but more than a lay person's, understanding of medical terminology, disease processes, pharmacology, common laboratory and imaging tests, and treatment options go a long way to enhance the communication within the team. It is not practical to have the same level of medical knowledge as the PCP but a degree of knowledge positively correlates with ease of communication and possibly even successful integration within the integrated team. The BHS can be marginalized by others on the team for lacking basic professional level health care knowledge (O'Donohue et al., 2006)

■ *Practice evidence-based "medicine" as much as possible*

An evolving concept within the science and practice of medicine is "evidence-based medicine." Evidence-based medicine, similar to the field of psychology's scientist–practitioner model of the 1940s, involves using empirical evidence to guide clinical practice (Frank, 1984). It is encouraged that the practice of medicine (broadly defined here to include all the subspecialties included in the integrated primary care team), whenever possible, use established and proven techniques and strategies in the promotion of health and the assessment and treatment of illness and disease. To this end, the BHS should employ such techniques and strategies that have evidence for their use. Because of a number of factors (limits to funding, smaller sample sizes, use of qualitative research methods), behavioral health research may not be as available or seen as robust by non behavioral providers as, for example, a study exploring the clinical outcome of one pharmaceutical product compared to another in 5,000 patients. Regardless, the BHS should have a basic understanding of research methodology, skills in reviewing research, and where to locate relevant research to guide practice. The scientific method can also be useful in working with individual patients, developing hypotheses, implementing an intervention, and evaluating outcomes. The BHS should also be willing to share behavioral health research with those on the integrated team who may not have been exposed to this literature to inform their understanding of behavioral health.

■ *Communications with others on the team (written and verbal) should be brief*

Possibly one of the most crucial elements in the success of the BHS in the primary care setting is communication. We discussed earlier the importance of the availability of the BHS and the face-to-face or "curbside" consultations at the point of care. Not only should the BHS be rapidly available to engage the patient or other team members but the type and form of communication must be adapted to the primary care setting.

Most professionals who function as BHSs are trained to provide thorough, albeit it lengthy, written assessments and reports. This author recalls early psychological evaluations provided to PCPs of at least four pages in length (typed single spaced). While proud of the thoroughness and detail of the evaluation report, I quickly learned that length of communications (written or verbal) negatively correlated with length of time the PCP would spend reading my report and possibly even negatively related to the value they placed on my contributions to the care of their patient. The adage "When in Rome…." should be considered when documenting in the integrated primary care environment. A PCP is inundated daily with multiple forms of information and communications about patients, their practice, medicine, and health care in general. The busy PCP must learn to juggle all the demands placed on them by efficiently filtering information. This includes information from other health care providers. It is not uncommon for this author, a BHS also trained in the medical model and who practices family medicine, to receive reports from other specialists and to review only limited portions of a lengthy report. What is crucial to the PCP in reviewing reports is the chief complaint that sent the patient to the specialist, the diagnosis that was uncovered, and the recommended treatment plan. Understanding that this is a typical approach for reviewing reports by most PCPs the BHS should (a) limit the length of written documentation, (b) clearly identify the diagnosis(es) that are found or that the BHS will be targeting, and (c) succinctly and briefly articulate how these will be addressed.

A common format of medical documentation is the "SOAP note" with the acronym SOAP referring to the four sections of most medical notes: Subjective, Objective, Assessment, and Plan. The **Subjective** section of the note or report identifies the chief complaint; history of present illness including previous evaluations, treatments, and outcomes; relevant past medical, psychiatric, social, and family history; current allergies and medications; tobacco, alcohol, or drug use; assessment of other symptoms; and anything else pertinent to evaluating the chief complaint. The **Objective** section of the note presents observations of the patient to include results of the exam (physical, psychological, etc.), blood work, imaging, or any other process or test evaluating the various body systems (e.g., cardiovascular, pulmonary, neurological, psychiatric). The **Assessment** section identifies the diagnosis(es) found and possibly a list of other diagnoses that should be considered (differential diagnoses). Finally, the **Plan** section highlights the clinician's thinking in critically evaluating the other sections and offers the plan for future evaluation or treatment of the chief complaint. Typically these notes are brief and to the point. They often consist of the accumulation of incomplete sentences that stray from formal literary convention in order to communicate a large amount of information in as few words as possible. This can be very challenging for social science–trained health care professionals to emulate, as mentioned earlier.

Lastly, documentation by the BHS should be entered into a shared patient health record as quickly as possible as it is not uncommon for other health care decisions to be postponed dependent on receipt of the BHS's report. Each of the disease/disorder-specific chapters of this textbook will present examples of how behavioral health documentation might look. No one format is better than another but they all should be reviewed in light of the concepts recommended previously. As stated by Kirkpatrick et al. (2011), "theoretical discussions, speculative musing, or complicated case conceptualizations are not valued" in primary care.

The timing, format, and content of verbal communications should also be considered in the same light as written communications as already discussed. Brief and succinct communications with other team members should be the rule with longer or more in-depth conversations reserved for particularly involved or difficult cases, or in situations in which others on the team require a more conceptual framework to successfully care for a patient.

BHSs typically learn effective ways of communicating with patients in their unique training programs. When communicating with patients/clients BHSs learn to use good attending skills, open/closed-ended questions, reframing, summarizing, and so on. These skills should be considered and employed when working with others on the integrated team. They are, after all, individuals like ourselves who appreciate good eye contact, positive regard, honesty, and genuineness, among other things. As helping professionals, we occasionally turn on those skills when interacting with patients but forget to use them as well with colleagues.

Finally, with respect to specific terms used in behavioral health, consider limiting the use of specialty technical terms when conversing with other team members. Reaction formation, transference, cognitive restructuring, empathy may all be well-understood terms in the BHSs' professional community, but often not understood by others in the medical setting. Use of these terms could distance the BHS from others, can detract from the core of the intended communication, and at worst can be off-putting and hinder good collaboration with other team members. When communicating with others on the team, the BHS should tailor the communication to the receiver's knowledge, perspective, and position.

VIGNETTE OF A TYPICAL DAY FOR THE BHS ON THE INTEGRATED PRIMARY CARE TEAM

The daily activity and schedule of the BHS on the integrated primary care team will undoubtedly look very different when compared to what their activity might be in a behavioral health specialty clinic or private practice. Their activity will also vary depending on the primary care setting in which they work. The following is a vignette that includes an amalgam of the activities of the BHS in a stereotypical family medicine outpatient setting.

The BHS might start her day by connecting with each PCP in the outpatient family medicine clinic reviewing the patients scheduled for the day. She would not only identify patients to see briefly along with the PCP or another team member, but also might share what she knows about a particular patient in preparing the PCP for the patient. Afterward she might see two patients scheduled for 20-minute visits addressing progress on their treatment of depression and insomnia. She may then have a scheduled new patient and perform a 45-minute screening to determine what behavioral health factors led the PCP to refer the patient and to begin treatment planning. After the screening she documents her brief screening report in the shared electronic health record (EHR). She then receives a call from the Women's Health Clinic affiliated with the family medicine practice with the request for her to meet a patient who has a high score on the Edinburgh Postnatal Depression Scale to determine what screening, referral, or intervention might be indicated. She does so and based on the encounter suggests that the provider consider starting an antidepressant and schedule the patient for brief cognitive behavior therapy with the BHS. She again documents the encounter in the shared EHR.

After returning to her office she responds to several messages from patients and receives a page asking if she would see another patient in the family medicine clinic who is reporting anxiety in anticipation of an upcoming medical procedure. She sees the patient and delivers a brief coping intervention, provides follow-up reading resources on coping with the medical procedure, and offers to be available should the patient require further intervention. As she walks back to her office she is stopped in the hall by one of the family medicine physician assistants (PA) asking for her suggestion on a patient with whom he struggles. The patient is often emotional at appointments since the death of the patient's mother. After hearing more details she suggests the PA openly discuss with the patient the observed bereavement and identify any existing resources for support (family, friends, and religious affiliation) explaining that the patient may not be effectively utilizing available support resources. She also gives the PA the contact information for the local hospice bereavement service if more intensive intervention is deemed necessary.

Back in her office, the BHS completes the final details on a three-session smoking cessation program that she plans to offer to clinic patients over the next few months. At lunch she joins her medical colleagues at their monthly in-training session where they are discussing the management of patients presenting with headache. While she learns about the biomedical aspects of the evaluation and treatment of headache, she offers psychosocial factors that should be considered in the development, maintenance, and treatment of headache of which her medical colleagues are appreciative. After lunch she has two 30-minute counseling sessions with two separate patients. The first patient has illness worry and frequent emergency department and outpatient visits related to overuse of Internet healthcare resources. A second patient she sees along with the clinic dietician where the focus is assisting the diabetic patient in learning how to make good dietary choices and how to utilize behavioral strategies to maximize success.

Near the end of the session with the patient with diabetes she is called out of the session by a nurse reporting that one of the physicians is concerned about a patient who may need crisis mental health care. After a brief discussion with the physician and examination of the patient she concurs and helps facilitate the patient's voluntary admission to a local crisis mental health stabilization unit. After the patient leaves she debriefs with the physician who is appreciative that she was immediately available to help with the crisis. The physician notes that while he does not see these crisis mental health situations often, he feels more prepared now should he have another patient in a similar situation and would be better able to facilitate the referral if voluntary admission was deemed necessary. She documents the previous encounters in the shared EHR.

With a brief break in her schedule she notes that a female patient is scheduled to have an implantable contraceptive device placed in her upper arm shortly. The patient's PCP offers to have her sit in on the procedure if she would care to. She takes the opportunity to become informed about the procedure to broaden her medical knowledge and experience. At the same time she is able to provide the patient support throughout the procedure. Upon returning to her office she responds to calls from patients and from a community physical therapist who wants to share his experience with a chronic pain patient who was referred to him by the practice. He is aware that the patient's primary care practice has an integrated team and that she is the BHS at the practice. The physical therapist informs her that during his work with the patient he noted that the patient's pain is affecting the patient's relationship with his wife. He mentioned to the patient that their family practice has a BHS who might be able to help and obtains permission to notify the BHS so that someone might speak with the patient about chronic pain and its effect on families at his next visit. She thanks the physical therapist and notices while reviewing the patient's EHR that the patient is scheduled for an outpatient visit next week. She documents the information from the physical therapist in the EHR for the PCP to see and schedules a reminder to herself to touch base with the PCP that morning to see if he has any questions before seeing the patient.

The reader may see this vignette as a day of fairly fragmented activities with multiple brief encounters with patients, community providers, and other integrated team members. It is just this brief, solution-focused, didactic, patient-centered, and collaborative daily schedule that is at the heart of integrated care.

Other conceptualizations of how integrated primary care is practiced and the skills needed to impact the success of the BHS on integrated primary care teams have been documented elsewhere (Gatchel & Oordt, 2003; Hunter et al., 2009; O'Donohue et al., 2006). Ultimately the BHS appreciates that he or she has two different "customers" when working in integrated primary care, the patient and the team (Kirkpatrick et al., 2011). Keeping this understanding at the forefront of the BHS's perceived professional mission, practice and goals will maximize the likelihood of becoming a successful, satisfied, and valued member of the integrated primary care team.

REFERENCES

Agency for Healthcare Research and Quality, PCMH Resource Center. (n.d.). Retrieved from http://pcmh.ahrq.gov

American Board of Family Medicine. (n.d.). History of the specialty. Retrieved from www.theabfm.org/about/history.aspx

Ashburn, M. A., & Staats, P. S. (1999). Management of chronic pain. *The Lancet, 353*(9167), 1865–1869.

Baird, M., Blount, A., & Brungardt, S. (2014). The Working Party Group on Integrated Behavioral Healthcare. Joint principles: integrating behavioral health care into the patient-centered medical home. *Annals of Family Medicine, 12*(2), 183–185.

Belar, C. D., & Deardorff, W. W. (1995). *Clinical health psychology in medical settings: A practitioner's guidebook.* Washington, DC: American Psychological Association.

Blount, A. (2003). Integrated primary care: Organizing the evidence. *Families, Systems, & Health, 21*(2), 121.

Blount, A., & Bayona, J. (1994). Toward a system of integrated primary care. *Family Systems Medicine, 12*(2), 171.

Brody, D. S., Khaliq, A. A., & Thompson, T. L. (1997). Patients' perspectives on the management of emotional distress in primary care settings. *Journal of General Internal Medicine, 12*(7), 403–406.

Brown, T. M. (1986). Alan Gregg and the Rockefeller Foundation's support of Franz Alexander's psychosomatic research. *Bulletin of the History of Medicine, 61*(2), 155–182.

Centers for Disease Control and Prevention. (n.d.). Up to 40 percent of annual deaths from each of five leading US causes are preventable. Retrieved from www.cdc.gov/media/releases/2014/p0501-preventable-deaths.html

Civic Impulse. (2015). H.R. 1424—110th Congress: Paul Wellstone. *Mental Health and Addiction Equity Act of 2007.* Retrieved from https://www.govtrack.us/congress/bills/110/hr1424

Collins C., & Milbank Memorial Fund. (2010). *Evolving models of behavioral health integration in primary care.* New York, NY: Milbank Memorial Fund.

Council on Social Work Education. (n.d.). Social work and integrated behavioral healthcare project. Retrieved from www.cswe.org/CentersInitiatives/DataStatistics/IntegratedCare.aspx

Cowley, D., Dunaway, K., Forstein, M., Frosch, E., Han, J., Joseph, R., ... Unutzer, J. (2014). Teaching psychiatry residents to work at the interface of mental health and primary care. *Academic Psychiatry, 38*(4), 398–404.

Cunningham, P. J. (2009). Beyond parity: Primary care physicians' perspectives on access to mental health care. *Health Affairs, 28*(3), w490–w501.

Deuraseh, N., & Talib, M. A. (2005). Mental health in Islamic medical tradition. *International Medical Journal, 4*(2), 76–79.

Doherty, W. J. (1995). The why's and levels of collaborative family health care. *Family Systems Medicine, 13*(3–4), 275.

Doherty, W. J., McDaniel, S. H., & Baird, M. A. (1996). Five levels of primary care/behavioral healthcare collaboration. *Behavioral Healthcare Tomorrow, 5*(5), 25.

Donaldson, M. S., Yordy, K. D., & Vanselow, N. A., Institute of Medicine, Division of Health Care Services. Committee on the Future of Primary Care, Donaldson. (1994). *Defining primary care: an interim report.* Washington, DC: National Academy Press.

Druss, B. G., Silke, A., Compton, M. T., Rask, K. J., Zhao, L., & Parker, R. M. (2010). A randomized trial of medical care management for community mental health settings: The Primary Care Access, Referral, and Evaluation (PCARE) study. *American Journal of Psychiatry, 167*(2), 151–159.

Fisher, L., & Ransom, D. C. (1997). Developing a strategy for managing behavioral health care within the context of primary care. *Archives of Family Medicine, 6*(4), 324.

Frank, G. (1984). The Boulder Model: History, rationale, and critique. *Professional Psychology: Research and Practice, 15*(3), 417.

Future of Family Medicine Project Leadership Committee. (2004). The future of family medicine: A collaborative project of the family medicine community. *Annals of Family Medicine, 2* (Suppl. 1), S3–S32.

Gatchel, R. J., & Oordt, M. S. (2003). Clinical health psychology and *primary care*: Practical advice and clinical guidance for successful collaboration. Washington, DC: American Psychological Association.

Grumbach, K., & Bodenheimer, T. (2004). Can health care teams improve primary care practice? *JAMA, 291*(10), 1246–1251.

Hunter, C. L., & Goodie, J. L. (2012). Behavioral health in the Department of Defense Patient-Centered Medical Home: History, finance, policy, work force development, and evaluation. *Translational Behavioral Medicine,* 2(3), 355–363.

Hunter, C. L., Goodie, J. L., Oordt, M. S., & Dobmeyer, A. C. (2009). *Integrated behavioral health in primary care: Step-by-step guidance for assessment and intervention.* Washington, DC: American Psychological Association.

Institute of Medicine. (2001). *Crossing the quality chasm: A new health system for the 21st century.* Washington, DC: National Academy Press.

Interprofessional Education Collaborative®. (2015). What is interprofessional education (IPE)? Retrieved from https://ipecollaborative.org/About_IPEC.html

Kirkpatrick, H., Vogel, M. E., & Nyman, S. (2011). 5 changes psychologists must make to be successful in integrated primary care. *Register Report,* (Spring). http://www.nationalregister.org/pub/the-national-register-report-pub/the-register-report-spring-2011/5-changes-psychologists-must-make-to-be-successful-in-integrated-primary-care

Knebel, E., & Greiner, A. C. (Eds.). (2003). *Health professions education: A bridge to quality.* Washington, DC: National Academies Press.

Levant, R. F. (2005). Health care for the whole person. *Monitor on Psychology, 36*(5), 5.

Matarazzo, J. D. (1982). Behavioral health's challenge to academic, scientific, and professional psychology. *American Psychologist, 37*(1), 1.

McDaniel, S. H., Belar, C. D., Schroeder, C., Hargrove, D. S., & Freeman, E. L. (2002). A training curriculum for professional psychologists in primary care. *Professional Psychology: Research and Practice, 33*(1), 65.

McDaniel, S. H., Doherty, W. J., & Hepworth, J. (2014). *Medical family therapy and integrated care.* Washington, DC: American Psychological Association.

National Institutes of Health. (2000). Psychosomatic medicine: "The puzzling leap." Retrieved from www.nlm.nih.gov/exhibition/emotions/psychosomatic.html

Naylor, M. D., & Kurtzman, E. T. (2010). The role of nurse practitioners in reinventing primary care. *Health Affairs, 29*(5), 893–899.

O'Donohue, W. T., Byrd, M. R., Cummings, N. A., & Henderson, D. A. (Eds.). (2005). *Behavioral integrative care: Treatments that work in the primary care setting.* New York, NY: Routledge.

O'Donohue, W. T., Cummings, N. A., Cucciare, M. A., Runyan, C. N., & Cummings, J. L. (2006). *Integrated behavioral health care: A guide to effective intervention.* Amherst, NY: Humanity Books.

Oyama, O., Burg, M. A., Fraser, K., & Kosch, S. G. (2011). Mental health treatment by family physicians: current practices and preferences. *Family Medicine, 44*(10), 704–711.

Palfrey, J. (2006). *Child health in America: Making a difference through advocacy*. Baltimore, MD: Johns Hopkins University Press.

Patient Protection and Affordable Care Act, 42 U.S.C. § 18001. (2010). Retrieved from www.gpo.gov/fdsys/pkg/PLAW-111publ148/content-detail.html

Peek, C. J., Cohen, D. J., & deGruy III, F. V. (2014). Research and evaluation in the transformation of primary care. *American Psychologist*, *69*(4), 430.

Ratka, A. (2012). Integration as a paramount educational strategy in academic pharmacy. *American Journal of Pharmaceutical Education*, *76*(2), Article 19, 1–2.

Robinson, P., & Reiter, J. (2007). Behavioral consultation and primary care: A guide to integrating services. New York, NY: Springer Science + Media.

Roca, M., Gili, M., Garcia-Garcia, M., Salva, J., Vives, M., Garcia Campayo, J., & Comas, A. (2009). Prevalence and comorbidity of common mental disorders in primary care. *Journal of Affective Disorders*, *119*(1), 52–58.

Sadur, C. N., Moline, N., Costa, M., Michalik, D., Mendlowitz, D., Roller, S., ... Javorski, W. C. (1999). Diabetes management in a health maintenance organization. Efficacy of care management using cluster visits. *Diabetes Care*, *22*(12), 2011–2017.

Schwartz, G. E., & Weiss, S. M. (1978a). Yale conference on behavioral medicine: A proposed definition and statement of goals. *Journal of Behavioral Medicine*, *1*(1), 3–12.

Schwartz, G. E., & Weiss, S. M. (1978b). Behavioral medicine revisited: An amended definition. *Journal of Behavioral Medicine*, *1*(3), 249–251.

Shackelford, J. R., Sirna, M., Mangurian, C., Dilley, J. W., & Shumway, M. (2013). Descriptive analysis of a novel health care approach: Reverse colocation—Primary care in a community mental health "home." *The Primary Care Companion for CNS Disorders*, *15*(5), 1–11.

Slay, J. D., & McCleod, C. (1997). Evolving an integration model: The Healthcare partners experience. In Cummings, N. A., Cummings, J. L., & Johnson, J. N. (Eds.). *Behavioral Health in Primary Care: A Guide for Clinical Integration* (p. 139). Madison, CT: Psychosocial Press.

Substance Abuse and Mental Health Services Administration. (n.d.). Retrieved from www.integration.samhsa.gov

Vanselow, N., & Cuff, P. A. (Eds.). (2004). *Improving medical education: Enhancing the behavioral and social science content of medical school curricula*. Washington, DC: National Academies Press.

Vogel, M. E., Malcore, S. A., Illes, R. A. C., & Kirkpatrick, H. A. (2014). Integrated primary care: Why you should care and how to get started. *Journal of Mental Health Counseling*, *36*(2), 130–144.

Williams, M., Angstman, K., Johnson, I., & Katzelnick, D. (2011). Implementation of a care management model for depression at two primary care clinics. *The Journal of Ambulatory Care Management*, *34*(2), 163–173.

World Health Organization. (1948). Retrieved from http://who.int/about/definition/en/print.html

World Health Organization (WHO), World Organization of Family Doctors (WONCA). (2008). New report calls for mental health to be better integrated into primary care. Retrieved from www.who.int/mental_health/policy/services/PressReleaseWHO-WoncaReportLaunch_Melbourne.pdf?ua=1

TWO

TRENDS IN ILLNESS AND HEALTH CARE UTILIZATION

AMY B. DAILEY AND MARY ANN BURG

EPIDEMIOLOGIC TRANSITIONS—HISTORICAL TRENDS IN ILLNESS AND CAUSES OF DEATH

The term "epidemiology" refers to the study of the distribution, determinants, and possible control of diseases and other factors relating to health and illness. Chronic illness is the main focus of this book, and in this chapter you get an overview of current trends in chronic illness so that you can consider the work of the behavioral health specialist (BHS) in context. It is also useful to take a historical view of population trends in illness and death to understand why chronic illness has surpassed acute causes of mortality only in the past century and to consider how trends in health and illness may change in the future.

The term "epidemiologic transition," first used by the epidemiologist Abdel Omran in 1971, refers to three major historical and successive stages in the human experience of illness, population growth, and life span, and the determinants of these shifts (Omran, 2005). In Omran's theory, in the first stage, the "Age of Pestilence and Famine," mortality was high, and life spans were short—20 to 40 years. Epidemics, wars, and famine were the major causes of death. Huge and sudden population losses due to diseases such as tuberculosis and the Black Death in the 1300s killed one quarter of the European population (Barrett, Kuzawa, McDade, & Armelagos, 1988). The second stage, the "Age of Receding Pandemics," began with the Industrial Revolution. Improved sanitation and modernization of medicine resulted in a decline in infectious disease, a higher rate of population growth, and an increased life span. Improvements in biomedical interventions, including antimicrobial therapies and vaccinations, continued the extension of the life span. Throughout this transition, the major causes of mortality gradually shifted to chronic disease, including diabetes, cardiovascular disease (CVD), chronic obstructive pulmonary disease (COPD), and cancers. This culminates in Omran's third stage of the epidemiologic transition, the "Age of Degenerative and Man-Made Diseases," wherein chronic diseases, also referred to as the "diseases of civilization" and "sociobehavioral illnesses," surpass acute illness and infectious disease as the major source of mortality. And, for the most part, in most parts of the globe the major causes of mortality from communicable diseases have now been replaced by noncommunicable diseases attributable to behavioral and dietary risk factors (Ezzati & Riboli, 2013). In fact, it has been suggested that many countries have moved into a new phase of the epidemiologic transition, coined the "Age of Obesity and Inactivity," which is threatening the progress made in earlier stages of the transition (Gaziano, 2010).

Omran theorized that as modernization progressed in the different regions of the globe, developing countries would achieve similar rates and trends in mortality and similar life spans as the more modernized countries. However, epidemiologists now realize that Omran's theory did not account for the new pathogens that have emerged in recent decades, including human immunodeficiency virus (HIV) and Ebola virus. These new pandemics are creating spikes in mortality while the rates of chronic illnesses continue to climb in developing countries, especially in Africa and Eastern Europe. Across the globe, antibiotic-resistant pathogens are rapidly becoming another major threat to human health, including carbapenem-resistant *Enterobacteriaceae* (CRE), drug-resistant gonorrhea, *Clostridium difficile* (*C. diff*), fluconazole-resistant *Candida,* and methicillin-resistant *Staphylococcus aureus* (MRSA) (Centers for Disease Control and Prevention [CDC], 2013). *C. diff* alone causes 250,000 hospitalizations and 14,000 deaths per year in the United States. The major cause of these illnesses is the overuse of antibiotics: Every time an antibiotic is used bacteria develop resistance to the antibiotic. Furthermore, as much as 50% of antibiotic use is probably unwarranted. The CDC estimates that antibiotic-resistant illnesses add over $30 billion in direct health care costs and lost productivity. The CDC is alarmed at the rapid trend in antibiotic resistance and they have issued recommendations for responding to this new "epidemic" including reducing the use of antibiotics, immunization, heightened infection prevention actions, and the development of new antibiotics (CDC, 2013a).

CURRENT BURDEN OF DISEASE IN THE UNITED STATES

While these emerging pathogens and infections are harbingers of future trends in the burden of disease in the United States, according to a comprehensive report of U.S. health from 1990 to 2010, substantial progress has been made in improving population health (Murray et al., 2013). The gap in life expectancy between Blacks and Whites has substantially decreased (Figure 2.1; National Center for Health Statistics [NCHS] 2014). Life expectancy increased by approximately 3 years, and all-cause death rates across all ages decreased (Figure 2.2). Furthermore, age-adjusted death rates due to stroke have declined 37% in the past decade, rates for heart disease have decreased 30%, and cancer death rates have decreased 13% (NCHS, 2014). Preventable hospitalizations among the Medicare population have also declined in the past decade (United Health Foundation, 2013).

Meanwhile, the United States lags behind other countries on many health indicators; in fact, the United States ranked 28th out of 34 wealthy nations in years of life lost due to premature mortality (YLL). Americans may be living longer on average, but the number of residents living with chronic conditions and disabilities is on

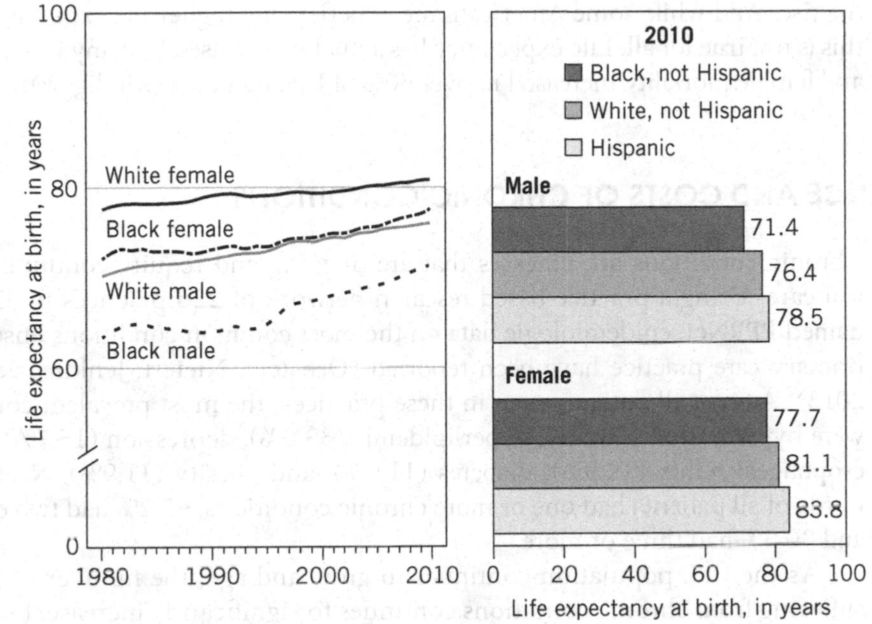

Figure 2.1 Life expectancy at birth, by selected characteristics: United States, 1980–2010.
Note: Life expectancy by Hispanic origin was available starting 2006.
Source: CDC/NCHS, *Health, United States, 2013*, Table 18. Data from the National Vital Statistics System (NVSS).

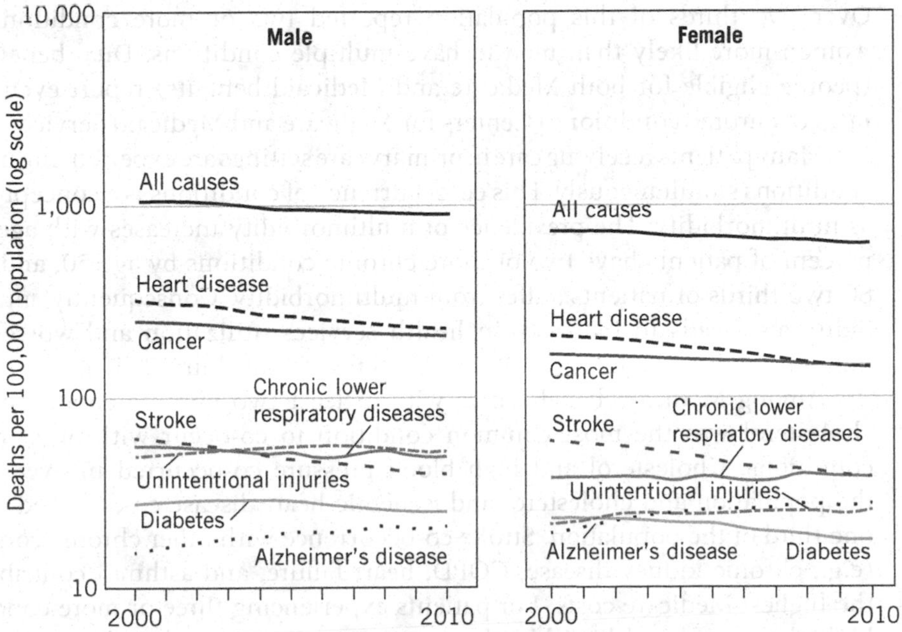

Figure 2.2 Age-adjusted death rates for selected causes of death for all ages, by sex: United States, 2000–2010.
Source: CDC/NCHS, Health, United States, 2013, Table 20. Data from the National Vital Statistics System (NVSS).

the rise. And while some Americans are experiencing higher life expectancy rates, this is not true for all. Life expectancy has actually decreased in many U.S. counties, and female mortality increased in over 40% of U.S. counties (Kindig, 2013).

PREVALENCE AND COSTS OF CHRONIC CONDITIONS

Chronic conditions are illnesses that are ongoing and require continuing medical care. Using a practice-based research network of 226 practices in 43 states, named PPRNet, epidemiologic data on the most common conditions observed in primary care practice have been reported (Ornstein, Nietert, Jenkins, & Litvin, 2013). Among all patients seen in these practices, the most prevalent conditions were hypertension (33.5%), hyperlipidemia (33.0%), depression (18.7%), gastroesophageal reflux (14.9%), diabetes (11.9%), and obesity (11.9%). Nearly two-thirds of all patients had one or more chronic conditions, 45.2% had two or more, and 30.3% had three or more.

As the U.S. population continues to grow and age, the number of patients suffering from chronic conditions continues to significantly increase. For example, in 2014 there were nearly 14.5 million cancer survivors, with that number expected to climb to an estimated 19 million survivors (DeSantis et al., 2014). Medicare beneficiaries make up a significant portion of the U.S. population experiencing chronic conditions. Examining over 31 million beneficiaries, the most common conditions experienced were high blood pressure (58%), high cholesterol (45%), heart disease (31%), arthritis (29%), and diabetes (28%). Over two thirds of this population reported two or more conditions, with women more likely than men to have multiple conditions. Dual beneficiaries (people eligible for both Medicare and Medicaid benefits) report even higher rates of chronic conditions (Centers for Medicare and Medicaid Services, 2013).

Many patients receiving care in primary care settings are experiencing multiple conditions simultaneously. This co-occurrence of conditions is a concept known as multimorbidity. The prevalence of multimorbidity increases with age. Forty percent of patients have two or more chronic conditions by age 50, and by age 80 two thirds of patients suffer from multimorbidity. Consequently, multimorbidity also leads to increases in health services utilization and worse health outcomes (Huntley, Johnson, Purdy, Valderas, & Salisbury, 2012).

Among Medicare beneficiaries with at least two chronic conditions, high cholesterol was the most common condition to co-occur with other chronic conditions. Cholesterol and high blood pressure co-occurred in over 50% of the population and cholesterol and ischemic heart disease co-occurred on over one third of the population. Stroke co-occurrence with other chronic conditions (e.g., chronic kidney disease, COPD, heart failure, and asthma) contributes to the highest Medicare costs. For patients experiencing three or more conditions, high cholesterol and high blood pressure co-occurred with ischemic heart disease in over one third of the population, followed by co-occurrence with diabetes and arthritis. Stroke paired with chronic kidney disease and one of the following conditions—asthma, COPD, depression, or heart failure—are the costliest triad comorbidities (Centers for Medicare & Medicaid Services [CMS], 2013).

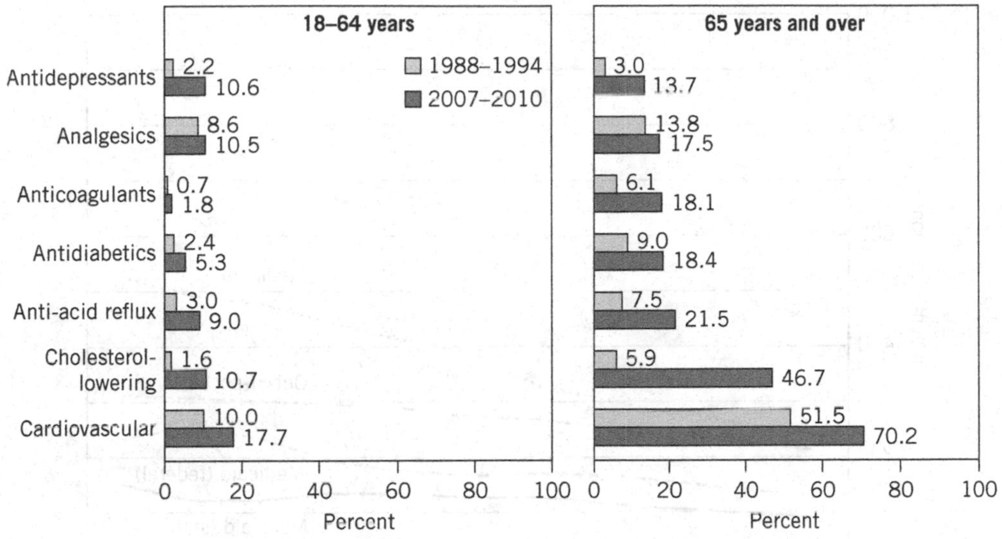

Figure 2.3 Prescription drug use in the past 30 days among adults aged 18 and over, by age and selected drug class: United States, 1988–1994 and 2007–2010.

Notes: Cardiovascular agents include drug classes such as angiotensin-converting enzyme (ACE) inhibitors, beta blockers, calcium channel blockers, and diuretics.

Source: CDC/NCHS, National Health and Nutrition Examination Survey. See Appendix I, National Health and Nutrition Examination Survey (NHANES).

Utilization

In 2012, nearly 85% of the population had at least one health care visit, which includes visits for illness, injury, or preventive care (NCHS, 2014, p. 5). Preventive medical care services remain less than optimal. Among children 19 to 35 months of age, 68% had completed a combined series of childhood vaccinations. Less than 38% of adults had received an influenza vaccination in the past year. Rates of influenza vaccination increased with age, with approximately two thirds of adults 65 and over reported receiving the influenza vaccine in the past year (NCHS, 2014).

As the number of Americans living with chronic conditions rises, so does the number of Americans taking prescription medications. Nearly half (47.5%) of the population has been prescribed at least one medication, over 20% (20.8%) has been prescribed three medications, and over 10% has been prescribed five or more medications. Drugs prescribed for chronic conditions including hypertension, high cholesterol, diabetes, cardiovascular conditions, depression, and acid reflux are on the rise for all ages. Over 70% of adults aged 65 and over took at least one cardiovascular drug, and there has been a dramatic increase in the use of cholesterol-lowering drugs in this age group (Figure 2.3; NCHS, 2014).

Unfortunately, the number of adults aged 18 to 64 reported not receiving or delayed seeking needed medical care, not receiving needed prescription drugs, or not receiving needed dental care due rising costs. Lack of insurance continues to be a major contributor to this trend (NCHS, 2014).

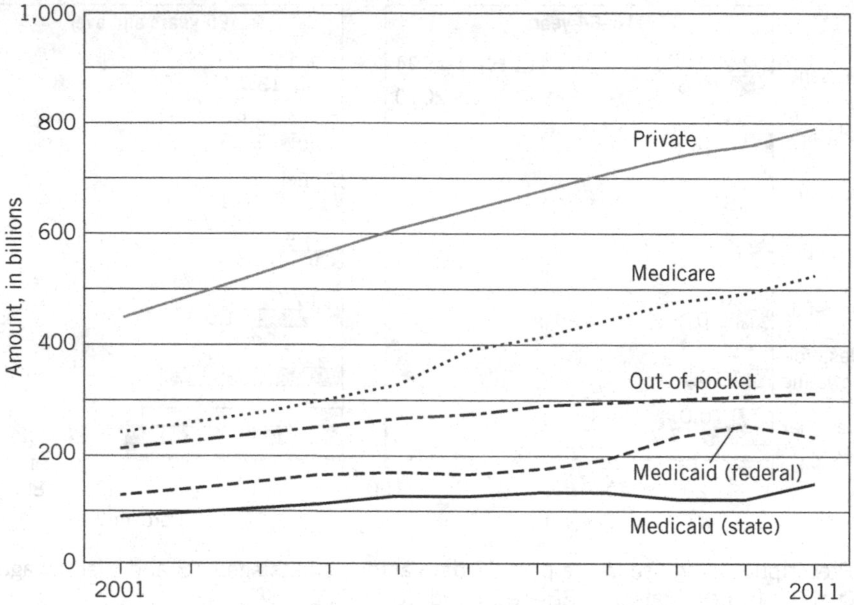

Figure 2.4 Personal health care expenditures, by source of funds: United States, 2001–2011.
Source: CDC/NCHS, Health, United States, 2013, Table 115. Data from the Centers for Medicare & Medicaid Services, National Health Expenditure Accounts (NHEA).

Economic Burden

More than two trillion dollars are spent on personal health care expenditures in the United States, with a per capita expenditure of $7,326 (2011), and this number continues to increase (Figure 2.4; NCHS, 2014). Hospital care accounted for 31.5% of national health care expenditures, physician and clinical services accounted for 20%, and prescription drugs accounted for nearly 10% (NCHS, 2014). The largest percentage of expenditures was paid by private health insurance (34.5%), 22.9% by Medicare, and 16.4% by Medicaid (NCHS, 2014). Given these percentages, it is concerning that the percentage of the population under the age of 65 receiving private health insurance through their employers has significantly decreased in the past decade (NCHS, 2014). While over 20% of the population reported having no health insurance (2012), the percentage of young adults (ages 19–25) without insurance decreased from 33.8% in 2010 to 26.3% in 2012 (NCHS, 2014). With fewer individuals covered by private insurance, more and more of health care costs are being covered through state and national public funds, largely through Medicare, Medicaid, and other publicly funded programs (Council of State Governments, 2006).

More than one trillion dollars are spent annually on chronic conditions (Devol & Bedroussian, 2007). The increasing incidence and prevalence of chronic disease is a significant factor in the continued growth of medical expenditures. The good news is that, according to a study by the Milken Institute (DeVol & Bedroussian, 2007), if reasonable improvements in health-related behaviors were achieved, millions of new cases of disease could be avoided and billions, and even trillions, of dollars in treatment costs and lost labor productivity could be saved. The two most important behavioral factors that would influence these disease and cost reductions are obesity and smoking.

The Milken Institute estimated $218 billion in annual savings in treatment costs could be achieved with significant changes in behavior, preventive measures, and innovation (DeVol & Bedroussian, 2007).

Health care costs for patients with behavioral health disorders and mental health disorders are higher, largely because of high utilization of behavioral health services and medical services. In a study of Maine Medicaid data, it was found that having multiple chronic conditions significantly influences behavioral health costs regardless of the behavioral health condition, suggesting that improved integration of behavioral and medical services would yield economic benefits (Freeman, McGuire, Thomas, & Thayer, 2014).

Predictably, Medicare beneficiaries with multiple chronic conditions are the heaviest users of the health care system. While much of the costs associated with these users can be attributed to hospitalizations, postacute care services, home health visits, and primary care visits have increased steadily, particularly for those with multiple chronic conditions. As the number of chronic conditions increases per patient, per-capita Medicare spending increases dramatically. For example, in 2010 of the $300 billion spent on Medicare, nearly half ($140 billion) was attributable to the 14% of the Medicare population that was experiencing six or more chronic conditions (CMS, 2013).

HEALTH-RELATED QUALITY OF LIFE

Identifying morbidity and mortality of chronic conditions is important to our understanding trends in outpatient care. However, health-related quality of life (HRQOL) is also important to assess the management of chronic conditions, the prevention of further complications, and the enhancement of functional abilities of patients experiencing chronic conditions. Patients who report living with a chronic condition experience poorer quality of life than those without chronic conditions, and those who report multiple chronic conditions are at even higher risk (Chen, Baumgardner, & Rice, 2011). While arthritis, obesity, and hypertension are some of the most prevalent chronic conditions in the United States, CVD and diabetes appear to influence HRQOL the most. Those who report these conditions have seven to eight times the odds of reporting fair or poor health than people with no chronic conditions.

TRENDS IN SPECIFIC CHRONIC ILLNESSES

Diabetes

Over 29 million Americans are estimated to be living with diabetes; 21 million have been diagnosed, and over 8 million likely have the disease but have not been diagnosed (CDC, 2014). While the prevalence of diabetes continues to increase, the proportion of cases that are estimated to be undiagnosed has decreased. This suggests that significant improvements in screening and diagnosis are occurring (Selvin, Parrinello, Sacks, & Coresh, 2014).

There are substantial racial/ethnic disparities in diabetes prevalence with a 2010 to 2012 prevalence of 15.9% for American Indians/Alaska Natives, 13.2% for non-Hispanic Blacks, 12.8% for Hispanics, 9.0% for Asian Americans, and 7.6% for non-Hispanic Whites. The rate of new cases of diabetes is highest for individuals 45 to 64 years of age (12.0 cases per 1,000 population). According to data for underlying causes of death, diabetes ranks seventh in leading causes of death in the United States. Thousands more deaths in the United States have diabetes listed as a contributing cause of mortality (CDC, 2014).

Patients with diabetes often have diseases that co-occur with diabetes because of shared risk factors, but diabetes can also cause serious complications. Some of these complications include heart disease, stroke, blindness, kidney failure, and lower-limb amputation. According to data from 2009 to 2012, over 70% of diabetics reported hypertension or being prescribed antihypertensive medications (CDC, 2014). Approximately 65% reported high cholesterol or taking cholesterol-lowering prescription drugs. Heart disease and stroke are significantly more likely to occur in diabetes patients (CDC, 2014). Over 4 million people have been diagnosed with diabetic retinopathy, which can lead to severe vision losses. Kidney failure is also significantly associated with diabetes. In fact, 44% of all new cases of kidney disease in 2011 were caused by diabetes (CDC, 2014). Furthermore, approximately 60% of non traumatic lower-limb amputations among adults occur in people with diabetes (CDC, 2014). Additional diseases that tend to co-occur with diabetes include nerve damage, nonalcoholic fatty liver disease, periodontal disease, hearing loss, erectile dysfunction, depression, and complications of pregnancy.

Control of risk factors is important in the prevention of vascular diseases and mortality in the diabetes population. According to a review of national data by Ali et al. (2013), significant changes in behaviors have been observed from 1999 to 2010 among individuals living with diabetes. The percentage of diabetes patients that meets recommended guidelines for glycemic control, blood pressure, and lipid levels has significantly improved. Despite these improvements nearly half of diabetes patients did not meet these recommended levels for basic diabetes care. Diabetes patients without health insurance were significantly less likely to meet recommended guidelines. Additional measures of diabetes care also showed improvement over the past decade. Daily glucose monitoring, annual lipid-level measurements, food examinations, annual influenza vaccination, and receipt of pneumococcal vaccinations were all on the rise. Yet little progress was made in terms of tobacco use or annual eye and dental examinations. Given the link between tobacco and cardiovascular conditions, and the link between diabetes and cardiovascular conditions, it is alarming that over 20% of diabetes patients continue to smoke. However, there is good news about cardiovascular risk for diabetics; the 10-year probability of coronary heart disease (CHD) decreased by several percentage points (Ali et al., 2013).

According to the American Diabetes Association (2013), about $245 billion (direct and indirect costs) were spent on diabetes in the United States in 2012.

Diabetes-related costs continue to rise; costs have been estimated to have increased over 40% from 2007 to 2012. On average, individuals with diabetes incur nearly $14,000 in medical expenditures per year, with over half of those costs directly attributed to diabetes care. These amounts are more than twice that for those living without diabetes. More than one out of five health care dollars spent in the United States is spent on diabetes-related expenditures. Over 40% of diabetes costs are due to inpatient hospital care, followed by prescription drug costs (18% of expenditures). While direct costs make up the bulk of the $245 billion, there are nearly $70 billion of indirect costs that are primarily due to absenteeism, reduced productivity, inability to work due to diabetes-related disability, and lost work due to early mortality (American Diabetes Association, 2013).

Cardiovascular Conditions

Modest improvements in CHD and CVD trends have been observed since 1999 to 2000. Examining data from the National Health and Nutrition Examination Survey, Go et al. (2014) predicted the 10-year risk for CHD significantly decreased from 7.2% in 1999 to 2000 to 6.5% in 2009 to 2010. While CVD risk has also decreased over time, this trend was not statistically significant. Decreasing risk for CHD and CVD was particularly apparent for women. Notably, decreases in CHD and CVD risk were not observed for all racial/ethnic groups. Increases in CHD and CVD risk were observed for African Americans, although the estimates were not statistically significant (Ford, 2013). By 2030, it is estimated that nearly 44% of the U.S. population will have some form of CVD (Go et al., 2014).

According to the Heart and Stroke Statistics 2014 Update from the American Heart Association, deaths due to CVD account for nearly one third of all deaths (Go et al., 2014). CHD was responsible for one in every six deaths in the United States in 2010. Yet declining trends in mortality due to CHD and CVD are even more dramatic than the declines in incidence. There has been a 31% decline in deaths attributable to CVD from 2000 to 2010. The rate of death due to stroke has dramatically declined from 2000 to 2010, with nearly a 36% reduction. Better control of hypertension is likely a primary reason for such great reductions in stroke mortality, along with improvements in the control of diabetes, cholesterol, and smoking cessation (Go et al., 2014).

CVD is associated with a wide range of risk factors that eventually lead to clinical manifestations. While the etiologic pathways are likely complex, the American Heart Association has estimated the attributable fractions for CVD. The 2014 Heart Disease and Stroke Statistics Update reports that over 40% of CVD mortality was attributable to high blood pressure, 13.7% to smoking, 13.2% to poor diet, 11.9% to insufficient physical activity, and 8.8% to abnormal blood glucose levels (Go et al., 2014).

Smoking continues to be a problem in the United States. One fifth of American men continue to smoke and nearly 16% of American women continue to smoke. Alarmingly, over 18% of high school students report being current smokers. Nearly 30% of adults have not recently engaged in any aerobic leisure-time activity. The outlook on dietary behaviors is even more dismal.

Less than 1% of adults met four out of five dietary goals that include recommendations for consumption of fruits and vegetables, fish, sodium, low sugar-sweetened beverages, and whole grains. Only 12.3% of the adult population met recommended goals for fruits and vegetables. Among adolescents, less than 30% met goals for low sugar-sweetened beverage intake. As further explored in the next section, nearly 70% of the population is considered overweight or obese (Go et al., 2014). Data from 2007 to 2010 National Health and Nutrition Examination Survey show that the prevalence of diabetes, hypertension, and dyslipidemia was highest among obese individuals (Saydah et al., 2014).

Inpatient cardiovascular operations have increased 28% in the past decade (Go et al., 2014). Projected shortages of health care professionals in nursing, pharmacy, and medicine are expected to be especially problematic given the high prevalence of cardiovascular conditions (Heidenreich et al., 2011). Nurses and primary care physicians are already in short supply and the significant shortage of physicians in cardiac specialty care continues to grow (Heidenreich et al., 2011).

CVD and stroke account for more in health care expenditures than any other major group of diseases in the United States (Go et al., 2014). Approximately 17% of national health expenditures are due to CVD and these costs are expected to rise substantially with our aging population (Heidenreich et al., 2011). CVD and stroke costs the United States over $300 billion in direct expenditures and indirect estimates; over $193 billion was spent on direct costs, such as cost of physicians and health professionals, hospital services, prescription medications, and home health care (Heidenreich et al., 2011). Over $122 billion was estimated to be lost in future productivity due to CVD and stroke mortality (Heidenreich et al., 2011). Costs are projected to reach over $900 billion by 2030 (Go et al., 2014).

Obesity

Experts have found that the single most important way to improve disease outcomes and reduce health care costs is to reduce obesity rates in the United States (DeVol & Bedroussian, 2007). The prevalence of obesity has risen dramatically over the past few decades. The prevalence of obesity was around 13% in the early 1960s and rose to over 36% by 2010 (May, Freedman, Sherry, & Blanck, 2013). Alarmingly, childhood obesity has more than tripled since the 1970s (May et al., 2013). Nearly 35% of U.S. adults and 17% of youth are obese, according to data collected for the National Health and Nutrition Examination Survey (2011–2012) (Ogden, Carroll, Kit, & Flegal, 2014). In total, nearly 69% of the total U.S. population is overweight or obese (Ogden et al., 2014). While the prevalence of obesity is high across the entire nation, disparities exist across gender, socioeconomic status, race/ethnicity, and age. Examining trends since 1999, age-adjusted prevalence of obesity among adults increased for both men and women, with women having higher rates of obesity than men (May et al., 2013). The prevalence of obesity for women aged 60 and older is on the rise (Ogden et al., 2014). Higher educational attainment is associated with lower rates of obesity, and this relationship is more pronounced for women than men (May et al., 2013). Country of birth and language spoken at home are also strongly correlated with obesity. For example, obesity prevalence is 13% higher for Mexican

American men born in the United States than for men born in Mexico (May et al., 2013). Mexican American boys and non-Hispanic Black girls are two groups of children and adolescents that have particularly high rates of obesity, compared with other children (May et al., 2013). The rates of childhood obesity steadily increased for many years, but according to recent data, there is some evidence suggesting that the rates of childhood obesity are leveling off or decreasing (Ogden et al., 2014). A significant decrease in obesity among 2- to 5-year-old children was observed in 2011 to 2012 (Ogden et al., 2014).

Mortality rates are significantly higher for obese individuals. Compared to normal weight individuals, obese people are 1.4 times more likely to die and extremely obese individuals are nearly 2.5 times more likely to die (Go et al., 2014).

Obesity puts individuals at high risk for many chronic conditions including hypertension, hyperlipidemia, CVD, asthma, sleep apnea, stroke, some cancers, and diabetes. Obesity and diabetes have an interesting relationship. While it is clear that obesity is a significant risk factor for diabetes incidence, the relationship appears to be more complicated in terms of mortality among diabetics. Findings from a cross-sectional study using National Health Interview Survey data (Jackson et al., 2014) showed that mortality decreased with increasing body mass index (BMI) among individuals with diabetes. However, due to limitations in study design, further prospective studies of the relationship between obesity and diabetes are needed.

Billions of dollars of annual health care spending can be attributed to obesity (Finkelstein, Trogden, Cohen, & Dietz, 2009). The amount of health care dollars spent on obesity-related conditions may significantly impact public funding options given that lifetime Medicare costs for obese individuals are estimated to be nearly $50,000 higher than normal-weight enrollees (Go et al., 2014).

Metabolic Syndrome

"Metabolic syndrome" refers to the co-occurrence of five known risk factors for a variety of disease including CVD and stroke, kidney disease, and type 2 diabetes. These five conditions (abdominal obesity, dyslipidemia, elevated blood pressure, impaired fasting glucose, and insulin resistance) are measured by (a) waist circumference greater than or equal to 102 cm for male adults or 88 cm for female adults, (b) fasting plasma glucose of 100 mg/dL or higher, (c) blood pressure greater than or equal to 130/85 mmHg, (d) triglycerides of 150 mg/dL or higher, and (e) high-density lipoprotein cholesterol (HDL) of less than 40 mg/L for male adults and less than 50 mg/dL for female adults (Beltrán-Sánchez, Harhay, Harhay, & McElligott, 2013).

The estimated prevalence of metabolic syndrome, measured as suboptimal measures for at least three of the five conditions using National Health and Nutrition Examination Survey data, has decreased over a decade from 25.5% in 1999 to 2000 to 22.9% in 2009 to 2010 (Beltrán-Sánchez et al., 2013). However, the prevalence of all five conditions did not decrease. The prevalence of hyperglycemia and waist circumference actually increased over this time period. It is likely that decreases in elevated blood pressure and better HDL trends are related to increases in antihypertensive and lipid-modifying medications

(Beltrán-Sánchez et al., 2013). The prevalence of the population with total serum cholesterol greater than or equal to 240 mg/dL is approximately 14%, and roughly one third of the population has hypertension (Go et al., 2014). Nearly 18% of people estimated to have hypertension are not aware of it (Go et al., 2014). Among those who are aware that they are hypertensive, 75% use antihypertensive medications, yet just over half have their conditions controlled at recommended levels (Go et al., 2014).

Chronic Pain

Chronic pain has significant implications for activities of daily living, work productivity, and general quality of life. According to a systematic review of studies conducted between 1999 and 2012, 20% of adults experience chronic pain, 7% experience neuropathic pain, and 7% have severe pain (Moore, Derry, Taylor, Straube, & Phillips, 2014). National data from the Medical Expenditures Panel Survey show that the prevalence of back pain has increased by 29% from 2000 to 2007 and that chronic back pain has increased by 64% (Smith, Davis, Stano, & Whedon, 2013). These estimates are only expected to increase over time due to our aging population. There is some evidence that the prevalence of chronic low back pain has significantly increased over time. One study of North Carolina residents reported a 6% increase in prevalence of chronic, impairing low back pain from 1999 to 2006 (Freburger et al., 2009). Likewise, the percentage of individuals seeking health care increased over the same time period (Freburger et al., 2009).

Chronic pain is often the cause of a multitude of complications, ranging from physical functioning limitations to mental health consequences. A national study of Medical Expenditure Panel Survey data showed that self-reports of physical limitations, mental health problems, and daily life and social limitations have worsened over time (Martin et al., 2008).

Effective treatment is crucial in management of associated symptoms such as fatigue, depression, and sleep interference (Moore et al., 2014). In a study of patients suffering from back or neck pain using National Ambulatory Medical Care Survey data and National Hospital Ambulatory Medical Care Survey data, physician referrals, number of computed tomograms or magnetic resonance images, and narcotic use are on the rise (Mafi, McCarthy, Davis, & Landon, 2013). Physical therapy referrals and the number of radiographs remained constant over a 10-year period (Mafi et al., 2013).

Many patients need spinal interventions to relieve pain. Data from the CMS show that spinal interventional techniques, including epidural steroid injections, facet joint interventions, and sacroiliac joint interventions, increased over 100% from 2000 to 2008 (Manchikanti, Pampati, Falco, & Hirsch, 2013).

Pain associated with back and neck problems is a very common encounter in clinical practice and is associated with substantial health care costs. An estimated $35 billion was spent on chronic back pain in 2007 and costs are expected to continue to rise given the increase in prevalence and an increase in the aging of the population (Smith et al., 2013). Patients with spinal problems spend nearly twice as much in medical costs than those without spinal problems and these costs are on the rise (Martin et al., 2008). It appears that a small group of patients with chronic back pain account for a disproportionate share of health care expenditures (Smith et al., 2013).

Sleep Disorders

Millions of Americans live with sleep disorders. The International Classification of Sleep Disorders recognizes over 80 different sleep-related disorders (Skaer & Sclar, 2010). Some of the most common include insomnia and obstructive sleep apnea. Sleep disorders are associated with many chronic conditions, such as diabetes, CVD, obesity, chronic pain, and depression and anxiety (Chapman et al., 2013; Liu, Croft, et al., 2013). Many chronic medical conditions also cause disordered sleep (Skaer & Sclar, 2010). According to national data from the 2010 Behavioral Risk Factor Surveillance System, nearly one third of Americans aged 45 years and older reported less than 6 hours of sleep per day on average (Liu, Wheaton, Chapman, & Croft, 2013). Just over 4% reported sleeping 10 or more hours per day on average (Liu, Wheaton, et al., 2013). Individuals reporting short or long sleep duration, compared to optimal sleepers (7–9 hours per day), had significantly higher odds of obesity, frequent mental distress, CHD, stroke, and diabetes after controlling for sociodemographic factors (Liu, Wheaton, et al., 2013). In addition to significant increased risks for chronic disease, sleep problems are also associated with drowsy driving and fatal and nonfatal motor vehicle crashes (Wheaton, Shults, Chapman, Ford, & Croft, 2014).

Insomnia is the most prevalent sleep disorder (Skaer & Sclar, 2010) and has been shown to have negative effects on functioning, memory, and work performance (Kessler et al., 2011). Stress, medical or psychiatric conditions, and medications can all be causes of insomnia or co-occur frequently with insomnia (Skaer & Sclar, 2010). Absenteeism and accidents are significantly higher for individuals with insomnia (Skaer & Sclar, 2010).

Obstructive sleep apnea, a sleep disorder causing intermittent cessation of breathing or reduced airflow, has been reported to affect about 5% of the adult population (Skaer & Sclar, 2010). It is likely that prevalence of this sleep disorder has been on the rise, given its linkage with obesity, which has also been on the rise. Gender differences in the use of health services by those with sleep disorders have also been found with women with sleep apnea more likely to utilize health services than men (Skaer & Sclar, 2010).

Disordered sleep is associated with significant economic and societal costs. Although it is difficult to find recent estimates, billions of dollars are spent directly on sleep disorders and billions more are lost in reduced work productivity (Skaer & Sclar, 2010). One recent study estimated that the equivalent of over $60 billion in lost work productivity due to insomnia alone occurs each year in the United States (Kessler, 2010). The good news with obstructive sleep apnea is that once this illness is properly treated with weight reduction or continuous positive airway pressure (CPAP), health care expenditures significantly decline (Skaer & Sclar, 2010).

Geriatric Conditions

Trends in health outcomes and health care utilization will be greatly affected by our rapidly aging population. It has been estimated that the number of adults 65 years of age or older will double between 2010 and 2050 (CDC, 2013b). Many of the diseases that affect the older population will be discussed in other chapters. In particular, cardiovascular conditions and cancer are conditions that disproportionately affect older populations (CDC, 2013b). Chronic lower respiratory diseases, stroke, Alzheimer's, diabetes, and influenza/pneumonia are also leading causes of death in older populations (CDC, 2013b). Furthermore, it is highly likely that individuals will experience more than one condition at a time (CDC, 2013b).

While leading causes of death are of concern for older adults, day-to-day living and quality of life are greatly affected by additional diseases. Depression, arthritis, osteoporosis, and asthma are also highly prevalent conditions among older populations (CDC, 2013b). Poor physical health and limitations are frequently reported by older people (CDC, 2013b). Approximately 75% of adults 80 years old or older report some kind of disability (CDC, 2013b).

Arthritis is the most common disability reported among U.S. adults because of the aging population and increases in the prevalence of risk factors such as obesity (CDC, 2013c; Hootman, Helmick, & Brady, 2012). Arthritis affects 50% of adults 65 years of age and older, and women are more likely to have arthritis than men (Hootman et al., 2012). Osteoarthritis is the most common type of arthritis, afflicting over one third of the 65 and older population (Hootman et al., 2012). Over 45% of adults aged 65 and older report activity limitations due to arthritis and approximately 25% report severe pain (Hootman et al., 2012). Although the causal relationship remains unclear, individuals with arthritis are significantly more likely to also be diagnosed with CVDs than those without arthritis (Ong, Wu, Cheung, Barter, & Rye, 2013).

Older adults are also at higher risk of injuries due to falling; one in three adults aged 65 or older fall causing moderate to severe injuries, such as hip fractures and head traumas (CDC, 2013b). Fall-related injuries and hospitalizations have been on the rise and rates for fall-related injuries may top 5.7 million per year by 2030 (Orces & Alamgir, 2014; see Figure 2.5). Vaccine-preventable diseases, such as influenza and pneumonia, are leading causes of death and hospitalization for older adults (CDC, 2013b).

Health care costs are also expected to rise significantly with the aging population and the chronic conditions they experience. In fact, approximately 95% of costs associated with older Americans are for chronic diseases, and health care costs are three to five times higher for persons aged 65 or older than younger individuals (CDC, 2013b). Much of these costs will fall upon Medicare, with projected costs increasing from $555 billion in 2011 to $903 billion in 2020 (CDC, 2013b). Over $120 billion is spent on medical care and lost earnings associated with arthritis alone (CDC, 2013c).

Cancer-Related Conditions

Although cancer remains one of the most prevalent chronic conditions, there have been positive trends over time showing reductions in overall cancer

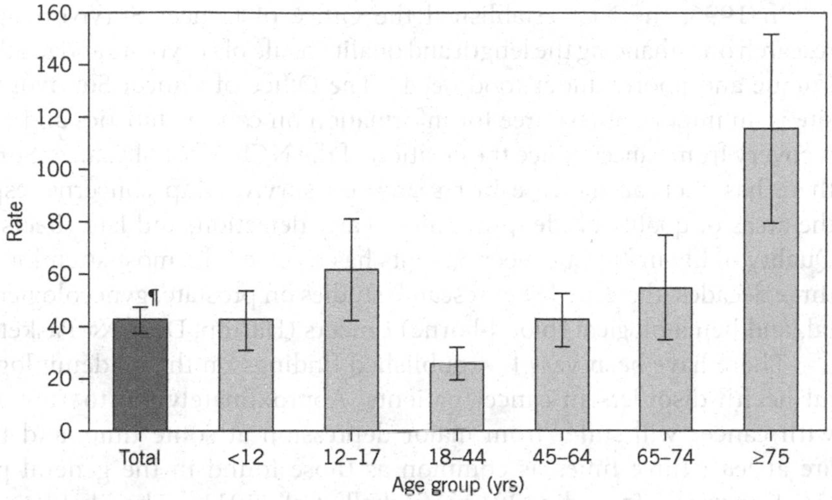

Figure 2.5 Rate* of nonfatal, medically consulted fall injury episodes,† by age group.

* Per 1,000 population.

† Annualized rates of injury episodes for which a health care professional was contacted either in person or by telephone for advice or treatment. An injury episode refers to a traumatic event in which the person experienced one or more injuries from an external cause.

¶ 95% confidence interval.

Source: www.cdc.gov/mmwr/preview/mmwrhtml/mm6104a8.htm

incidence and mortality. Delay-adjusted and age-adjusted cancer incidence rates have steadily decreased since the 1990s (Edwards et al., 2014). However, the majority of the decrease in overall cancer incidence has been for men; the incidence rates for women have remained stable. Unfortunately, not all cancer incidence rates have decreased. For men, there have been increases in melanoma, non-Hodgkin's lymphoma, leukemia, myeloma, and cancers of the pancreas, kidney, liver, and thyroid (Edwards et al., 2014). For women, incidence rates increased for melanoma, leukemia, myeloma, and cancers of the uterus, thyroid, kidney, pancreas, and liver (Edwards et al., 2014).

Overall, cancer mortality rates have also decreased over time. Over the past decade (2001–2010), death rates have declined for 11 of the 17 most common cancers in men and 15 of the 18 most common cancers in women (Edwards et al., 2014). However, pancreatic cancer and liver cancer mortality rates have increased over the past decade for men and women. Death rates for melanoma, cancer of soft tissue, increased for men, and mortality due to cancer of the uterus increased for women (Edwards et al., 2014).

Cancer survivorship is defined by the National Cancer Institute (NCI) as "anyone who has been diagnosed with cancer, from the time of diagnosis through the balance of his or her life" (www.cancer.gov/newscenter/newsfromnci/2011/survivorshipMMWR2011, accessed June 9, 2014). The numbers of survivors are now over 12 million and the numbers have increased dramatically as the baby boomers in the United States reached middle and old age. Breast cancer survivors are the largest group of cancer survivors (22%), followed by prostate cancer survivors (19%) and colorectal cancer survivors (10%). Over half of all survivors are 65 years of age and older.

In 1996, the NCI established the Office of Cancer Survivorship to focus research on enhancing the length and quality of life of survivors and to address their unique and poorly understood needs. The Office of Cancer Survivorship's website is an important resource for information on cancer statistics and research on recovery from cancer. Since the creation of the NCI Office of Cancer Survivorship, there has been an increase in research on survivorship concerns, especially in the areas of quality of life, prevention, early detection, and late effects of cancer. Quality of life in breast cancer patients has received the most attention in the last three decades; there are fewer research studies on prostate, gynecological, colorectal, and hematological (blood-borne) cancers (Harrop, Dean, & Paskett, 2011).

There have been very few published findings on the epidemiology of mental health disorders in cancer patients. Approximately 9% to 16% of patients with cancer will suffer from major depression at some time, and these rates are at least three times as common as those found in the general population (Li, Fitzgerald, & Rodin, 2012; Mitchell et al., 2011). The likelihood of major depression is highest when patients have difficult physical symptoms, when they have a history of psychiatric disorders, and when they have advanced cancer (Lo, et al., 2010). Rates of combined mood disorders in cancer patients are found to range between 30% and 40% (Mitchell et al., 2011).

The diagnosis of psychiatric disorders in cancer survivors is complicated by the effects of cancer-related fatigue, anorexia, insomnia, and cognitive impairment, which overlap with symptoms of depression (Li et al., 2012), and with the changing emotional experience of the cancer patient over the cancer continuum. Our understanding of the risk for psychiatric problems in cancer survivors is also complicated by the paucity of longitudinal studies of survivors.

Although the majority of cancer patients will not have been diagnosed with depression or another mood disorder, there is a national effort to attempt to assess all cancer patients for the risk of psychosocial distress periodically across the continuum of cancer care and survivorship (Anderson et al., 2014; Zebrack, Burg, & Vaitones, 2012). A recent population-based study of psychosocial care services received by cancer survivors found that over half of survivors report that since their diagnosis of cancer they have never received counseling, or participated in support groups, or even had a discussion with a health care provider about their psychosocial concerns, specifically how cancer may have affected their emotions or their relationships with other people (Forsythe et al., 2013). Breast cancer survivors were the most likely to say they had some discussion with health care providers while prostate cancer survivors were the least likely to have had a discussion with their provider. Overall, evidence of the rates of use of psychosocial supportive services by cancer patients is varied. One study found that half of outpatient medical oncology patients had used some sort of supportive care service, with the most common being mental health counseling (30%), nutrition services (26%), and physical therapy (15%) (Kumar et al., 2012).

Most cancer patients will continue to be followed by their treating oncologist for a period of time after their treatment is complete. However, when cancer is treated effectively, cancer survivors will be referred back to their usual source of medical care, often with little or no communication between the treating oncologist and primary care physician or the other specialists involved in the patient's care team. This "transition" in the care of the cancer survivor can be problematic. If the primary care provider has no communication with the treating oncologist, then the cancer survivor's needs for care (e.g., screening for recurrences and treatment toxicities) and cancer treatment follow-up may not be met. Primary care providers are not specifically trained in cancer follow-up care and are not necessarily confident in their ability to care for cancer survivors (Burg, Grant, & Hatch, 2005).

In 2005, in an attempt to raise awareness of the unique care needs of cancer survivors, the Institute of Medicine issued the report "From Cancer Patient to Cancer Survivor: Lost in Transition" (Hewitt, Greenfield, & Stovall, 2005). Among the recommendations in this report was that every cancer patient should be provided with a "survivorship care plan," a personalized document produced by the treating oncologist summarizing the patient's tumor characteristics, treatment received, and follow-up care needs including guidelines for screening for recurrence and secondary cancers and screening for cancer-related side effects. Although the support for the concept of care plans is widespread, few cancer centers have actually initiated the practice of providing care plans to patients. Thus, to date, most cancer survivors will have no clear documentation of their follow-up care needs. This breakdown in continuity of care is a source of concern and anxiety for the cancer survivor.

The national costs associated with cancer care are substantial. Just based on population changes alone, costs of cancer care are projected to be between $125 and $158 billion, and these costs are highest in the last year of life (Mariotto, Yabroff, Shao, Feuer, & Brown, 2011).

CONCLUSION

The BHS in the primary care setting will be primarily concerned with helping patients with the lifestyle and behavioral changes needed to control and prevent the common chronic illnesses. According to the World Health Organization (WHO), lifestyle and behavior are believed to account for 20% to 25% of disease around the world (WHO, www.who.int/trade/glossary/story050/en/). Behaviors that currently have the most impact on rates of chronic disease are smoking, alcohol consumption, excess weight and obesity, diet and nutrition, and physical activity (Ezzati & Riboli, 2013).

In order to be optimally effective in primary care practice the BHS should also be armed with the most recent evidence of how individual behavior and environment intersect to impact the course of chronic illness. Having a "long view" of epidemiologic trends in health and illness is also important in helping primary care patients understand and respond appropriately to the changing environment.

REFERENCES

Ali, M. K., Bullard, K. M., Saddine, J. B., Cowie, C. C., Imperatore, G., & Gregg E. W. (2013). Achievement of goals in U.S. diabetes care, 1999–2010. *New England Journal of Medicine*, *368*(17), 1613–1624.

American Diabetes Association. (2013). Economic costs of diabetes in the U.S. in 2012. *Diabetes Care, 36*(4), 1033–1046.

Anderson, B. L., DeRubeis, R. J., Berman, B. S., Gruman, J., Champion, V. L., Massie, M. J., . . . Rowland, J. H. (2014). Screening, assessment, and care of anxiety and depressive symptoms in adults with cancer: An American Society of Clinical Oncology guideline adaptation. *Journal of Clinical Oncology*, 32, 1605–1619.

Barrett, R., Kuzawa, C. W., McDade, T., & Armelagos, G. J. (1988). Emerging and re-emerging infectious diseases: The third epidemiologic transition. *Annual Review of Anthropology*, 27, 247–271.

Beltrán-Sánchez, H., Harhay, M. O., Harhay, M. M., & McElligott S. (2013). Prevalence and trends of metabolic syndrome in the adult U.S. population, 1999–2010. *Journal of the American College of Cardiology*, *62*(8), 697–703.

Burg, M. A., Grant, K., & Hatch, R. (2005). Caring for patients with cancer histories in community-based primary care settings: A survey of primary care physicians in the southeastern U.S. *Primary Health Care Research and Development*, 6(3), 244–250.

Centers for Disease Control and Prevention. (2013a). *Untreatable: Report by CDC details today's drug-resistant health threats*. Retrieved February 2015 from www.cdc.gov/media/releases/2013/p0916-untreatable.html

Centers for Disease Control and Prevention. (2013b). *The state of aging and health in America 2013*. Atlanta, GA: Centers for Disease Control and Prevention, U.S. Department of Health and Human Services.

Centers for Disease Control and Prevention. (2013c). Prevalence of doctor-diagnosed arthritis and arthritis-attributable activity limitation—United States, 2010–2012. *Morbidity and Mortality Weekly Report*, 62(44), 869–873. doi:mm6244a1

Centers for Disease Control and Prevention. (2014). *National diabetes statistics report: Estimates of diabetes and its burden in the United States, 2014*. Atlanta, GA: U.S. Department of Health and Human Services.

Centers for Medicare & Medicaid Services. (2013). *Chronic conditions among Medicare beneficiaries, chartbook* (2012 ed.). Baltimore, MD: Centers for Medicare & Medicaid Services.

Chapman, D. P., Presley-Cantrell, L. R., Liu, Y., Perry, G. S., Wheaton, A. G., & Croft, J. B. (2013). Frequent insufficient sleep and anxiety and depressive disorders among U.S. community dwellers in 20 states, 2010. *Psychiatric Services*, *64*(4), 385–387.

Chen, H. Y., Baumgardner D. J., & Rice J. P. (2011). Health-related quality of life among adults with multiple chronic conditions in the United States, behavioral risk factor surveillance system, 2007. *Prevalent Chronic Diseases*, *8*(1), A09.

The Council of State Governments. (2006). Costs of chronic diseases: What are states facing. Retrieved from http://hit.state.tn.us/Reports/ChronicTrendsAlert120063050306.pdf

DeSantis, C. E., Lin, C. C., Mariotto, A. B., Siegel, R. L., Stein, K. D., Kramer, J. L., . . . Jemal A. (2014). Cancer treatment and survivorship statistics, 2014. *CA: A Cancer Journal for Clinicians*, *64*(4), 252–271.

DeVol, R., & Bedroussian, A. (2007). *An unhealthy America: The economic burden of chronic disease—Charting a new course to save lives and increase productivity and economic growth*. Santa Monica, CA: Milken Institute.

Edwards, B. K., Noone, A., Mariotto, A. B., Simard, E. P., Boscoe, F. P., Henley, S. J., . . . Ward, E. M. (2014). Annual report to the nation on the status of cancer, 1975–2010, featuring prevalence of comorbidity and impact on survival among persons with lung, colorectal, breast, or prostate cancer. *Cancer*, *120*(9), 1290–1314.

Ezzati, M., & Riboli, E. (2013). Behavioral and dietary risk factors for noncommunicable diseases. *New England Journal of Medicine*, *369*, 10:954–964.

Finkelstein, E. A., Trogdon, J. G., Cohen, J. W., & Dietz, W. (2009). Annual medical spending attributable to obesity: Payer- and service-specific estimates. *Health Affairs (Millwood)*, *28*(5), 822–831.

Forsythe, L. P., Kent, E. E., Weaver, K. E., Buchanan, N., Hawkins, N. A., Rodriguez, J. L., . . . & Rowland, J. H. (2013). Receipt of psychosocial care among cancer survivors in the United States. *Journal of Clinical Oncology*. Advance online publication. doi: 10.1200/JCO.2012.46.2101.

Freburger, J. K., Holmes, G. M., Agans, R. P., Jackman, A. M., Darter, J. D., Wallace, A. S., . . . Carey, T. S. (2009). The rising prevalence of chronic low back pain. *Archives of Internal Medicine*, *169*(3), 251–258.

Freeman, E., McGuire, C. A., Thomas, J. W., & Thayer, D. A. (2014). Factors affecting costs in medicaid populations with behavioral health disorders. *Medical Care, 52*(Suppl. 3): S60–S66.

Gaziano, J. M. (2010). Fifth phase of the epidemiologic transition: The age of obesity and inactivity. *JAMA, 303*(3), 275–276.

Go, A. S., Mozaffarian, D., Roger, V. L., Benjamin, E. J., Berry, J. D., Blaha, M. J., . . . American Heart Association Statistics Committee and Stroke Statistics Subcommittee. (2014). Heart disease and stroke statistics—2014 update: A report from the American Heart Association. *Circulation, 129*(3), e28–e292.

Harrop, J. P., Dean, J. A., & Paskett, E. D. (2011). Cancer survivorship research: A review of the literature and summary of current NCI-designated cancer center projects. *Cancer Epidemiology, Biomarkers & Prevention, 20*(10), 2042–2047.

Heidenreich, P. A., Trogdon, J. G., Khavjou, O. A., Butler, J., Dracup, K., Ezekowitz, M. D., . . . Woo, Y. J. (2011). Forecasting the future of cardiovascular disease in the United States a policy statement from the American Heart Association. *Circulation, 123*(8), 933–944.

Hewitt, M. E., Greenfield, S., & Stovall, E. (2005). National Cancer Policy Board Committee on Cancer Survivorship: Improving Care and Quality of Life. *From Cancer Patient to Cancer Survivor: Lost in Transition* (p. 506). Washington, DC: National Academies Press.

Hootman, J. M., Helmick, C. G., & Brady, T. J. (2012). A public health approach to addressing arthritis in older adults: The most common cause of disability. *American Journal of Public Health, 102*(3), 426–433.

Huntley, A. L., Johnson, R., Purdy, S., Valderas, J. M., & Salisbury, C. (2012). Measures of multimorbidity and morbidity burden for use in primary care and community settings: A systematic review and guide. *Annals of Family Medicine, 10*(2), 134–141.

Jackson, C. L., Yeh, H., Szklo, M., Hu, F. B., Wang, N. Y., Dray-Spira, R., & Brancati, F. L. (2014). Body-mass index and all-cause mortality in U.S. adults with and without diabetes. *Journal of General Internal Medicine, 29*(1), 25–33.

Kessler, R. C., Berglund, P. A., Coulouvrat, C., Hajak, G., Roth, T., Shahly, V., . . . Walsh, J. K. (2011). Insomnia and the performance of US workers: Results from the America insomnia survey. *Sleep, 34*(9), 1161–1171.

Kindig, D. A., & Cheng, E. R. (2013). Even as mortality fell in most US counties, female mortality nonetheless rose in 42.8 percent of counties from 1992 to 2006. *Health Affairs, 32*(3), 451–458.

Kumar, P., Casarett, D., Corcoran, A., Desai, K., Li, Q., Chen, J., & Mao, J. J. (2012). Utilization of supportive and palliative care services among oncology outpatients at one academic cancer center: Determinants of use and barriers to access. *Journal of Palliative Medicine, 15*(8), 923–930.

Li, M., Fitzgerald, P., & Rodin, G. (2012). Evidence-based treatment of depression in patients with cancer. *Journal of Clinical Oncology, 30*(11), 1187–1196.

Liu, Y., Croft, J. B., Wheaton, A. G., Perry, G. S., Chapman, D. P., Strine, T. W., . . . Presley-Cantrell, L. (2013). Association between perceived insufficient sleep, frequent mental distress, obesity and chronic diseases among U.S. adults, 2009 behavioral risk factor surveillance system. *BMC Public Health, 13*, 84. doi:10.1186/1471-2458-13-84

Liu, Y., Wheaton, A. G., Chapman, D. P., & Croft , J. B. (2013). Sleep duration and chronic diseases among U.S. adults age 45 years and older: Evidence from the 2010 behavioral risk factor surveillance system. *Sleep, 36*(10), 1421–1427.

Lo, C., Zimmermann, C., Rydall, A., Walsh, A., Jones, J. M., Moore, M. J., . . . & Rodin, G. (2010). Longitudinal study of depressive symptoms in patients with metastatic gastrointestinal and lung cancer. *Journal of Clinical Oncology, 28*(18), 3084–3089.

Mafi, J. N., McCarthy, E. P., Davis, R. B., & Landon, B. E. (2013). Worsening trends in the management and treatment of back pain. *Journal of the American Medical Association-Internal Medicine, 173*(17), 1573–1581.

Manchikanti, L., Pampati, V., Falco, F. J., & Hirsch, J. A. (2013). Growth of spinal interventional pain management techniques: Analysis of utilization trends and Medicare expenditures 2000 to 2008. *Spine (Phila Pa 1976), 38*(2), 157–168.

Mariotto, A. B., Yabroff, K. R., Shao, Y., Feuer, E. J., & Brown, M. L. (2011). Projections of the cost of cancer care in the United States: 2010–2020. *Journal of the National Cancer Institute, 103*(2), 117–28.

Martin, B. I., Deyo, R. A., Mirza, S. K., Turner, J. A., Comstock, B. A., Hollingworth, W., & Sullivan, S. D. (2008). Expenditures and health status among adults with back and neck problems. *Journal of the American Medical Association*, *299*(6), 656–664.

May, A. L., Freedman, D., Sherry, B., & Blanck H. M. (2013). Obesity—United States, 1999–2010. *MMWR. Surveillance Summaries: Morbidity and Mortality Weekly Report. Surveillance Summaries/CDC*, *62*, 120–128.

Mitchell, A. J., Chan, M., Bhatti, H., Halton, M., Grassi, L., Johansen, C., & Meader, N. (2011). Prevalence of depression, anxiety, and adjustment disorder in oncological, hematological, and palliative-care settings: A meta-analysis of 94 interview-based studies. *The Lancet Oncology*, *12*(2), 160–174.

Moore, R., Derry, S., Taylor, R. S., Straube, S., & Phillips, C. J. (2014). The costs and consequences of adequately managed chronic non-cancer pain and chronic neuropathic pain. *Pain Practice*, *14*(1), 79–94.

Murray, C. J., Atkinson, C., Bhalla, K., Birbeck, G., Burstein, R., Chou, D., . . . U.S. Burden of Disease Collaborators. (2013). The state of U.S. health, 1990–2010: Burden of diseases, injuries, and risk factors. *JAMA*, *310*(6), 591–606.

National Center for Health Statistics (US). (2014). Health, United States, 2013: With special feature on prescription drugs. Hyattsville, MD: U.S. Department of Health and Human Services. Retrieved from http://www.cdc.gov/nchs/data/hus/hus13.pdf

Ogden, C. L., Carroll, M. D., Kit, B. K., & Flegal, K. M. (2014). Prevalence of childhood and adult obesity in the United States, 2011–2012. *Journal of the American Medical Association*, *311*(8), 806–814.

Omran, A. (2005). The epidemiologic transition: A theory of epidemiology and population change. *The Milbank Quarterly*, *83*(4), 731–757.

Ong, K. L., Wu, B. J., Cheung, B. M., Barter, P. J., & Rye, K. (2013). Arthritis: Its prevalence, risk factors, and association with cardiovascular diseases in the United States, 1999 to 2008. *Annals of Epidemiology*, *23*(2), 80–86.

Orces, C. H., & Alamgir, H. (2014). Trends in fall-related injuries among older adults treated in emergency departments in the USA. *Injury Prevention: Journal of the International Society for Child and Adolescent Injury Prevention*, *20*(6), 421–423.

Ornstein, S. M., Nietert, P. J., Jenkins, R. G., & Litvin, C. B. (2013). The prevalence of chronic diseases and multimorbidity in primary care practice: A PPRNet report. *Journal of the American Board of Family Medicine*, *26*(5), 518–524.

Saydah, S., Bullard, K. M., Cheng, Y., Ali, M. K., Gregg, E. W., Geiss, L., Imperatore, G. (2014). Trends in cardiovascular disease risk factors by obesity level in adults in the United States, NHANES 1999–2010. *Obesity*, 22(8), 1888–1895.

Selvin, E., Parrinello, C. M., Sacks, D. B., & Coresh, J. M. (2014). Trends in prevalence and control of diabetes in the United States, 1988–1994 and 1999–2010. *Annals of Internal Medicine*, *160*(8), 517–525.

Skaer, T. L. & Sclar, D. A. (2010). Economic implications of sleep disorders. *Pharmacoeconomics*, 28(11), 1015–1023.

Smith, M., Davis, M. A., Stano, M., & Whedon, J. M. (2013). Aging baby boomers and the rising cost of chronic back pain: Secular trend analysis of longitudinal medical expenditures panel survey data for years 2000 to 2007. *Journal of Manipulative and Physiological Therapeutics*, *36*(1), 2–11. doi:10.1007/s13142-012-0110-2

United Health Foundation. (2013). *America's health rankings: A call to action for individuals and their communities* (2013 ed.). Retrieved from http://cdnfiles.americashealthrankings.org/SiteFiles/Reports/AnnualReport2013-r.pdf

Wheaton, A. G., Shults, R. A., Chapman, D. P., Ford, E. S., & Croft, J. B. (2014). Drowsy driving and risk behaviors—10 states and Puerto Rico, 2011–2012. *Morbidity and Mortality Weekly Report*, *63*(26), 557–562.

Zebrack, B., Burg, M. A., & Vaitones, V. (2012). Distress screening: An opportunity for enhancing quality cancer care and promoting the oncology social work profession. *Journal of Psychosocial Oncology*, *30*(6), 615–624.

THREE

THEORIES OF HEALTH BEHAVIOR AND BRIEF BEHAVIORAL PRACTICE MODELS

KATHERINE SANCHEZ AND MARY ANN BURG

CONCEPTUALIZING HEALTH BEHAVIOR

To a large degree the training of health professionals tends to focus more on the clinical and technological aspects of health care and less on prevention and the psychology of health behavior. The increasing opportunity for living healthy lives and longer life spans over the last two centuries is less due to medical technology than the advent of sanitation, vaccinations, and prevention activities. Research is helping us understand that the human behavior side of health care in regard to prevention and health maintenance often trumps technology in the balance of factors leading to healthy outcomes. It is the role of the behavioral health specialist (BHS) to tackle the less precise yet enormously important aim of engaging humans to impact their own health.

There is a growing body of evidence on how to best engage humans in being their own stewards of good health. The best evidence for behavioral health science is built through the scientific process of developing, testing, and refining *theories of health behavior*.

> Ideally, theories summarize the state of cumulative knowledge. They specify key constructs and relationships and the underlying scientific explanations of the processes of change and link behavior change to constructs in a systematic way. They describe how, when and why change occurs. They allow investigators to understand why and how interventions succeed or fail. Rigorous testing of theoretical principles forms a basis for future interventions. (Michie & Johnston, 2012, p. 4)

Health behavior theories are only as good as the empirical evidence generated to support them, and thus it is necessary to continually test theoretical models and their hypothesized pathways in clinical trials and in longitudinal research studies across a variety of contexts and with diverse patients. The evidence from these studies then informs practitioners which interventions or parts of interventions are useful in which contexts and for which conditions.

In this chapter, we hope you will be challenged to think about how health is conceptualized—to consider how these ideas about health might influence your patients; to consider your own choices in responding to health challenges; and how the physical, social, and political context we live in shapes our health choices and behaviors. You will also be introduced to current evidence-based brief interventions that derive from the theories of health behavior.

DEFINITIONS OF HEALTH

Have you ever thought about what the word *health* means to you? Definitions of health are critical to how health behavior theory is developed; therefore, serious consideration of what "health" means is an important activity for any behavioral health professional. Here are some of the ways health has been defined.

> Health is a state of complete physical, mental and social well-being and not merely the absence of disease or infirmity. (World Health Organization, 1946)
>
> In order to qualify as a healthy person someone must have the ability, given standard or reasonable circumstances, to reach the person's set of vital goals. (Nordenfelt, 2007)
>
> Health is an adaptive state, constantly reestablishing itself through interactions between the many biological, social, emotional, and cognitive factors in a person's life. (Sturmberg, 2014)
>
> Health is a state of well-being emergent from conducive interactions between individuals' potentials, life's demands, and social and environmental determinants. Health results throughout the life course when individuals' potentials—and social and environmental determinants—suffice to respond satisfactorily to the demands of life. (Bircher & Kuruvila, 2014)
>
> Health is a result of our behaviors, our individual genetic predisposition to disease, the environment and the community in which we live, the clinical care we receive, and the policies and practices of our health care, government, and other prevention systems. (United Health Foundation, 2012)

For some individuals, the definition of health is the lack of illness, especially people who have not yet been challenged with a health problem. Often children and young adults view health—if they think much about it at all—as the lack of illness. People who view health in this way may have little concern about engaging in unhealthy activities and are less likely to be motivated to engage in lifestyle choices aimed at the prevention of health problems.

Many people will never consider the value of health until they are faced with their own health crisis. Once faced with the reality of an acute or chronic illness, individuals may redefine health as a return to normal—that is, how they felt prior to their illness and perhaps how able they are to achieve their goals. Thus, individuals may be motivated to engage in actions that are hoped to push them into recovery.

This drive to return to normal can be a special challenge when an illness leads to long-term disability or chronic disease. Because we all end up having chronic health problems and inevitably will experience the problems of aging if we live long enough, the definition of health is typically reinvented over an individual's lifetime. Health may be redefined as living as best as one can in spite of the problems of chronic illness and aging. The motivation to engage in healthy behaviors may be most easily tapped for patients who have personally experienced the challenge of chronic, long-term, and progressive disease, and whose desire to achieve the highest possible level of functioning is paramount.

It can be useful when you begin working with a new patient to ask the patient, "What does being healthy mean to you?" This question might initially be met with confusion, especially if the patient has never thought about his or her own definition of health. You may try to engage the patient with a follow-up question, such as: "When did you feel you were at your healthiest, and what made that the healthiest time for you?" Most people will be able to dwell on those times in their lives they felt healthy and consider what the conditions were that made them feel that way, including being free of illness or disease, being able to fulfill their family and social roles, and/or being able to work toward personal goals. This exercise of helping the patient derive his or her own personal definition of health can be transformed into a discussion of how the patient can work with the BHS to regain or finally achieve some of those personal health goals.

FACTORS AFFECTING INDIVIDUAL HEALTH BEHAVIORS

Health scholars have developed many opinions and conceptual models about the determinants of health for individuals and populations. The primary categories of health determinants are:

- Patient behavior (lifestyle, personal involvement in health)
- Genetics
- Environment
- Access to medical care
- Social and health policy

In a 1993 *Journal of the American Medical Association* article, McGinnis and Foege published data that showed that 50% of U.S. mortality was linked to unhealthy behaviors including tobacco use, lack of physical activity, poor dietary practices, substance abuse, and risky sexual behaviors (McGinnis and Foege, 1993). Research suggests that patient behavior has more impact on poor health outcomes than the other determinants of health and that changing health behaviors has the greatest potential for improving quality of life for persons across diverse groups in the population (Fisher et al., 2011). The BHS's focus is patient behavior, and how to work with an individual patient's current situation and the patient's strengths in order to move the patient forward into the healthy condition he or she personally defines as the goal. However, in order to be most effective, the BHS needs to be informed about how an individual patient's ability to or likelihood of engaging in newer, healthier behaviors is conditioned by the patient's genetics, environment, health care access, and the policies that affect access.

Behavior change theories are important in the conceptualization of factors involved in behavior change, for informing the research on behavioral change effectiveness, and in the development of behavioral change counseling approaches. In the next section, we review theories of health behaviors that inform the types of behavioral health interventions we utilize in the practice of behavioral health care. We will first examine two theories: the *Behavioral Model of Health Services Use* and the *Health Belief Model* that conceptualize the interpersonal and intrapersonal system of factors involved in why, when, and how patients access health care. Second, we examine two theories that conceptualize health behavior as a function of the way health care is delivered, the *Chronic Care Model* and the *Common Factors Model*. Then we turn to looking behavioral counseling modalities that are derived from theories of health behavior.

THEORIES OF HEALTH BEHAVIOR

The Behavioral Model of Health Services Use

The Behavioral Model was developed by Andersen in the late 1960s to provide a theoretical framework for health services utilization (Andersen, 1995; Andersen & Newman, 1973). Initially focusing on the family as the unit of analysis, the model was an attempt to understand why families use health services, to define and measure access to health care, and to facilitate the development of policies that promote access to health care. Later, the model shifted its focus to the individual because of difficulties in measuring the heterogeneity of families, and the relative ease of measuring effects of family characteristics on the individual.

The initial model of the 1960s described the individual's use of health care services as a function of the individual's predisposing characteristics, enabling resources, and need or illness level. It was suggested that use of health care services, like hospital admissions and emergency care, would be explained by predisposing biological needs associated with age and gender. Use of services such as dental care would be explained by predisposing social structure factors (education, ethnicity, family size), enabling resources (insurance, income) available to address those problems, and health beliefs. Health beliefs are attitudes, values, and knowledge about medical care, physicians, and disease that influence an individual's behavior toward health care services. Like the other predisposing characteristics, they are not the reason people use health services, but might explain differences in the use of services. Andersen speculated that health beliefs are essential to an improved understanding of some types of health services, but enabling resources and need are overall better predictors of differences in use of the medical care system.

During the 1970s the model evolved to include the health care delivery system and the numerous changes that had occurred during the previous decade to improve access to health care (Aday & Andersen, 1974). Health policy had established numerous programs to finance care, such as Medicaid,

Medicare, and Special Supplemental Nutrition Program for Women, Infants, and Children (WIC), and to address organizational issues, such as health maintenance organizations (HMOs) and family practice specialization, to gain equal access for various groups in the population. Consumer satisfaction was added as an outcome of health services utilization to reflect the increasing buying power and medical knowledge of the health of the health care consumer (Aday & Andersen, 1974; Andersen, 2008). These additions to the model are reflected in the "Enabling" variables under "Contextual Characteristics" and "Outcomes" in Figure 3.1.

In the 1980s (phase 3), the model expanded to include personal health practices, such as diet, exercise, and self-care, which interact with the health care delivery system to affect outcomes. Health status, as perceived by the individual and as evaluated by the professional, was added to the outcome measures; see "Outcomes" in Figure 3.1. Improved health status and consumer satisfaction were thought to be essential for health policy as indicators of effective and efficient access as they pertain to health care utilization. In the 1990s (phase 4), as outcome measurement improved, the arrows were added to the model to reflect how health outcomes can then affect subsequent predisposing, enabling, and need characteristics of the individual and his or her use of the health care delivery system (Andersen, 2008).

In the last phase of the model (phase 5), Andersen (2008) formally added the contextual determinants of health care utilization. These are organizational, provider, and community characteristics that are measured in the aggregate. Andersen divided them up as the individual characteristics had been divided, according to those that predispose, enable, and suggest. Also added to the health behaviors list was the process of medical care, which reflects the behavior of providers as they interact with patients. Measures of the process of medical care might include test ordering, prescriptions, and quality of communication.

Application of the Model

To respond to the urgent demands to better identify and treat mental health concerns among underserved minority groups studies have applied the Behavioral Model of Health Services Use. Specifically, understanding how patient characteristics such as socioeconomic status, ethnicity, health beliefs and attitudes, and accessibility to medical care influence the underutilization of services have been examined (Bazargan, Bazargan-Hejazi, & Baker, 2005; Gelberg, Andersen, & Leake, 2000; Wu, Erickson, & Kennedy, 2009).

As described by Gelberg et al. (2000), the *Behavioral Model for Vulnerable Populations* applies the original Behavioral Model of Health Services Use to underserved groups to identify challenges in obtaining needed health services in order to provide improved access and ultimately to improve their health status. The addition of the *predisposing vulnerable* domain includes social structure characteristics such as acculturation, immigration status, living conditions, and literacy. The *enabling vulnerable* domain includes characteristics that enable an individual's ability to use health care services should the need arise, such as personal resources, insurance status, affordability of medical care, income, receipt of public benefits, competing needs, and availability of information. The *need vulnerable* domain includes conditions of special relevance to vulnerable populations such as mental health or substance abuse.

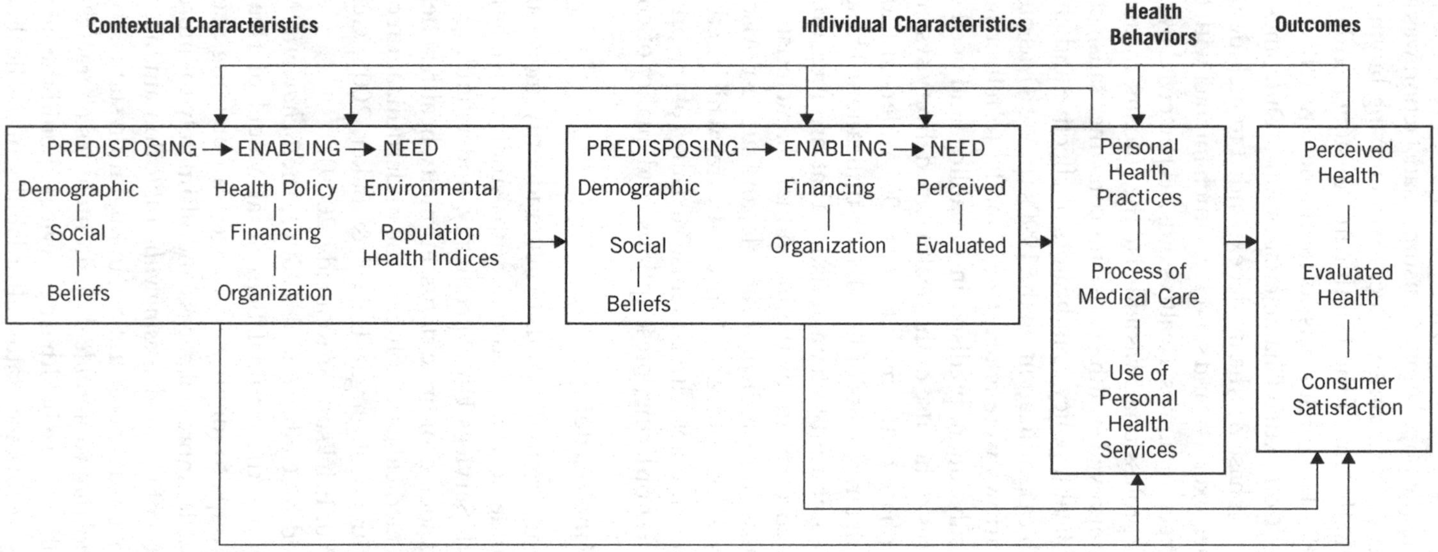

Figure 3.1 Phase 5 of the Behavioral Model of Health Services Use including contextual and individual characteristics.

Source: Andersen (2008).

To access health services, an individual must perceive some illness—either self-reported or evaluated and diagnosed by a health professional. To determine the effectiveness of the Behavioral Model with vulnerable populations, Bazargan et al. (2005) examined depression (self-report, diagnosed, and treated) among a Hispanic and African American population in public housing in Los Angeles. Their findings indicated a high incidence of depression, both by self-report and diagnosed by a physician, which was not being treated. The ability to speak English and affordability were the greatest predictors of use of antidepressant medication.

Other studies confirm that the characteristics of the Behavioral Model that accurately predicted receipt of medical treatment included perceived health status, affordability, financial strain, and continuity of medical care. Interestingly, the presence of comorbid chronic disease, though often a predictor of better identification and treatment of underlying depression, also contributes to poor medication compliance and financial strain in vulnerable populations. These findings lend support to that component of the Behavioral Model that unless the patient perceives a need, or until that need reaches a certain severity level, the depression is unlikely to get identified, after which barriers in the health care delivery system prohibit access for vulnerable populations.

The Health Belief Model

Originally conceptualized by Rosenstock (1966), the Health Belief Model (HBM) grew out of public health researchers' observation of the widespread apathy on the part of people to accept measures for the prevention, screening, and detection of diseases such as tuberculosis, cervical cancer, dental caries, rheumatic fever, polio, and influenza. Because these early prevention efforts were usually provided free or at a very low cost, and yet remained widely avoided, it became necessary to understand preventive behavior. A theory was needed to explain the behavior of people not currently suffering from disease and those oriented to the avoidance of disease. The theory needed to not overlook potential barriers to services and still consider the behavior of people being charged little or nothing for services. In 1974, a comprehensive collection of 20 years of empirical research on the HBM was published in a monograph (Becker, 1974), which broadened the application of the model from preventive health behavior to include "illness behavior" (Kirscht, 1974) and "sick role behavior" (Becker, 1974).

The basic tenets of the HBM suggest that in order for a person to take action to avoid a disease, there would need to be an individual perception of susceptibility and seriousness. The likelihood of action would also be influenced by the perceived benefits to taking action weighed against the barriers associated with it. Perceived susceptibility and seriousness are in part determined by knowledge and cognitive ability, and are the impetus for taking action. However, the direction of the preventive action is thought to depend upon the effectiveness and availability of various courses of action. For example, cancer-screening behaviors may be strongly mediated by feelings of susceptibility regarding a very serious disease, and a real conviction that there is no effective, or possibly unavailable, prevention or treatment.

Perceived susceptibility to a disease includes a subjective perception of risk among individuals, which ranges from those who deny any possibility of contracting a condition to a more moderate concern for the possibility of a disease occurring, to a genuine fear of dangerous illness. *Perceived seriousness* also varies considerably and is marked by feelings of emotional distress about a disease, complex implications of its effects on a person's job, family, and social relations, and questions about whether it will lead to death or disability. In order for preventive health behavior to occur, an individual will need to perceive that action can actually reduce the threat of disease (*perceived benefit*), and such actions are not outweighed by *perceived barriers* such as being inconvenient, expensive, unpleasant, painful, or upsetting.

According to the HBM, though an individual's perception of susceptibility and seriousness provides a force that may lead to action, and the individual might perceive an effectiveness that is believed to be available, there are still other modifying factors, which some individuals may require in order to initiate action to prevent a disease. Such modifying factors included *cues to action*, thought to trigger preventive health behavior, which might include mass public health media campaigns, reminder postcards from the dentist, or the illness of a loved one. The strength of the cues necessary to initiate action is contingent upon the perceived seriousness of and susceptibility to a disease.

The final modifying factors included in the model were an individual's demographic, sociopsychological, and structural variables. These variables affect the perceptions of seriousness, susceptibility, benefits, and barriers and contribute to the likelihood of taking preventive behavioral health action. All of the factors of the HBM are thought to operate in a risk–benefit conflict that is different for each individual, can change across time, and is influenced considerably by life circumstances. The components of the HBM are depicted in Figure 3.2.

Application of the Model

A decade after the HBM's inception, Janz and Becker (1984) conducted a comprehensive, critical review of studies published between 1974 and 1984, which applied the four fundamental HBM components to preventive health behaviors, sick-role behaviors, and illness behaviors. Analysis of preventive health behavior was examined with regard to numerous health conditions and the preventive behaviors thereof, such as influenza inoculation, screening programs for genetically inherited diseases, breast cancer, and high blood pressure. Studies that examined risk factor behaviors such as cigarette smoking, drinking and driving, and post-myocardial infarction lifestyle changes were also included in the review. Studies of sick-role behaviors included in the review examined chronic disease regimens for conditions such as hypertension, diabetes, and end-stage renal disease. Studies of illness behaviors included in the review examined beliefs about susceptibility and severity and formed a "threat of illness" index. These studies examined a range of populations such as low-income mothers in a pediatric clinic and employees of a large urban medical center covered by an HMO.

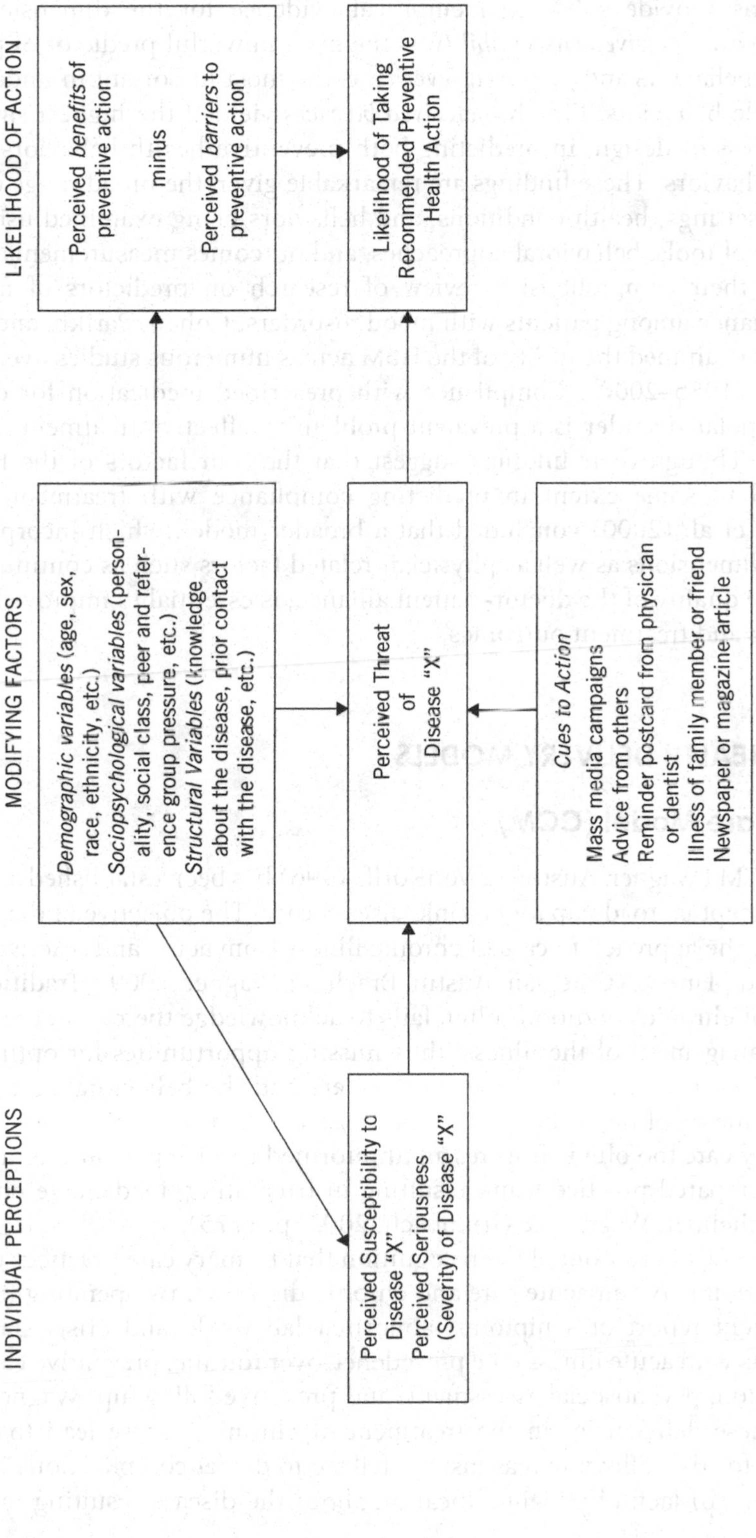

Figure 3.2 The Health Belief Model (HBM).
Source: Becker, Drachman, & Kirscht (1974).

Janz and Becker's overall evaluation of prospective and retrospective studies of the HBM found each dimension to be significantly associated with the health-related behaviors under study. They concluded that numerous investigations provide substantial empirical evidence for the dimensions of the HBM, with *perceived susceptibility* as the most powerful predictor of preventive health behaviors and *perceived severity* as the most important in understanding sick-role behaviors. Finally, *perceived barriers* yielded the highest significance, regardless of design, in predicting both preventive health behaviors and sick-role behaviors. These findings are remarkable given the broad range of populations, settings, health conditions, and behaviors being examined using a wide variety of tools, behavioral approaches, and outcomes measurements.

In their comprehensive review of research on predictors of medication compliance among patients with mood disorders, Cohen, Parikh, and Kennedy (2000) examined the utility of the HBM across numerous studies over a 15-year period (1985–2000). Compliance with prescribed medication for depression and bipolar disorder is a prevalent problem in effective treatment (Lin et al., 1995). Though their findings suggest that the four factors of the HBM were helpful to some extent in predicting compliance with treatment regimens, Cohen et al. (2000) concluded that a broader model, which incorporates the HBM dimensions as well as physician-related factors such as continuity of care and the quality of the doctor–patient alliance, is essential to improve both compliance and treatment outcomes.

BEHAVIORAL HEALTH DELIVERY MODELS

The Chronic Care Model (CCM)

The CCM (Wagner, Austin, & VonKorff, 1996) has been established as an intrinsic conceptual roadmap for chronic disease care. The objective of the CCM is to change the approach to care of chronic illness from acute and reactive to proactive and planned (Coleman, Austin, Brach, & Wagner, 2009). Traditional treatment of chronic conditions often fails to acknowledge the role of the patient in self-management of the illness, thus missing opportunities for optimal health by failing to educate the patient or understand the behavioral and psychosocial elements of his or her disease process. The treatment of chronic disease in primary care too often "features an uninformed passive patient interacting with an unprepared practice team, resulting in frustrating, inadequate encounters" (Bodenheimer, Wagner, & Grumbach, 2002, p. 1775).

The CCM grew out of the recognition that primary care practices make little distinction between acute care and chronic disease, thus operating in response to patient report of symptoms, abnormal lab work, and crisis stabilization. Patients with acute illness take precedence over routine, preventive care, disease education, psychosocial assessment, and proactive follow-up. Wagner suggests that these deficiencies in the treatment of chronic disease lead to poor outcomes for the following reasons: (a) failure to detect complications in a timely manner, (b) lack of patient education about the disease resulting in failure to self-manage and regulate the illness, (c) lower quality of care, and (d) undetected psychosocial distress.

Wagner's seminal work examined randomized controlled trials, successful chronic care programs, and disease management programs in national health systems in Western Europe and found similarities among these organized efforts. Their seminal article, "Organizing Care for Patients With Chronic Illness," is the most widely cited model on care for patients with chronic disease in the medical literature, and has been adapted to the treatment of numerous disease processes across multiple settings (Wagner et al., 1996).

An essential feature of the CCM is evidence-based, planned care, a notion that often meets resistance by practitioners who prefer the idea that each patient is unique and requires an individualized plan of care. Evidence-based planned care operates by protocol, with clinical guidelines and an organizational plan for treating diseases in a systematic way with proven effectiveness. The central features of successful programs of chronic disease management and planned care include practice redesign, patient education, expert system, and information.

Practice redesign requires the primary care practitioner to plan the way that clinical services are delivered, including the management of appointments and follow-up and the delegation of key clinical tasks to non physician members of the health team (Wagner et al., 1996). *Patient education* requires teaching competencies and offering behavioral change support to the patient and the family in order to enhance the self-management of the disease and affect lifestyle changes that are often essential to successful outcomes.

Expert system refers to the need for specialized care in the treatment of complicated disease and is most commonly achieved through referral or consultation with specialists. Such outside referrals often result in fragmented care and increased cost, and have not demonstrated increased expertise by the primary care practitioner. However, Wagner found collaborative care strategies to be most promising, wherein specialists and primary care physicians are colocated in the same setting and manage patients collaboratively, resulting in improved outcomes, integrated care, and increased expertise on the part of the primary care practitioner.

Lastly, in Wagner's CCM, *information* is required in order for a practice to improve the delivery of chronic illness care. A patient registry may be used to successfully track patient outcomes, to contact them with reminders and feedback, and to assist them in successfully adhering to a protocol of planned care. The electronic medical record (EMR) and other computer information systems have become powerful tools since the initial inception of the CCM (Coleman et al., 2009).

The CCM later evolved into "a multidimensional solution to a complex problem" (Bodenheimer et al., 2002, p. 1776), with the addition of three overlapping organizations: the entire community, the health care system, and the provider organization (Wagner et al., 2005). Thereby, the four elements of the original CCM previously described as necessary for practice redesign (self-management support, decision support, delivery system design, and clinical information systems) were now described as operating within the health care system that itself exists in the larger community. In the newer model, resources

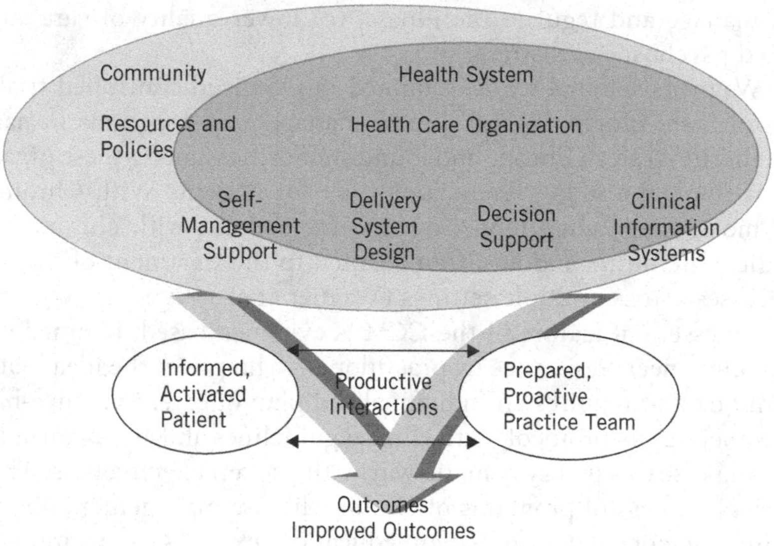

Figure 3.3 The Chronic Care Model (CCM).
Source: Wagner et al. (2005).

and policies in the community affect the delivery of medical care and many community-based resources can improve patient self-management. The health care organization, and its view of how chronic disease is managed and reimbursed, has a significant influence on the implementation of improvements and the pursuit of quality care of chronic disease. Ideally, an informed, activated patient interacts with a prepared, proactive practice team that results in improved outcomes (Figure 3.3).

Wagner's CCM applied to the treatment of mental disorders in primary care has come to be known as *integrated health care* or *collaborative care* (Thielke, Vannoy, & Unutzer, 2007; Unutzer, Schoenbaum, Druss, & Katon, 2006). It represents a comprehensive treatment model that approaches the management of mental health disorders as though they were a chronic illness and has proven to be most effective.

Numerous, randomized clinical trials have indicated the effectiveness of collaborative care over usual care (Asarnow et al., 2005; Roy-Byrne, Katon, Cowley, & Russo, 2001; Schoenbaum et al., 2002; Unutzer et al., 2002). The CCM has been widely adopted in numerous national quality improvement initiatives that have influenced more than 1,500 primary care practices in the United States and internationally (Berenson et al., 2008; Coleman et al., 2009). It also forms the foundation and informs the development of the Patient-Centered Medical Home (PCMH) model of health care delivery.

Application of the Model

In 2002, citing numerous challenges, varied interpretations to the medical home definition, and reimbursement problems for physicians, the American Academy of Pediatrics (AAP) released a new policy statement with an operational definition of the medical home (Sia et al., 2002). The statement listed ten specific services that should be provided by a medical home and a designated physician. It also detailed 37 additional services to operationalize the desirable characteristics of a medical home (Sia et al., 2002). Again, the emphasis historically has been on repairing the fragmented system of care experienced by children with special health care needs (Sia, Tonniges, Osterhus, & Taba, 2004).

In 2007, the American Academy of Family Physicians, the AAP, the American College of Physicians, and the American Osteopathic Association developed the Joint Principles of the PCMH to describe the characteristics of a PCMH (Patient-Centered Primary Care Collaborative, 2007). These principles include a personal physician, a physician-directed medical practice, a whole-person orientation, coordinated/integrated care, quality and safety, enhanced access, and payment.

The provision of all services from a single health care provider will help establish a relationship in which the patient trusts and confides. A whole-person orientation means the medical home takes responsibility for providing all of the patient's health care needs, either personally or by referring to appropriate, qualified professionals (Patient-Centered Primary Care Collaborative, 2007). Coordination of care across multiple, complex systems and the patient's community is optimally achieved through technologies such as the EMR and health registries (Patient-Centered Primary Care Collaborative, 2007). The EMR also provides consistent and timely information in an emergency and can help avoid inappropriate use of drugs or accidental overmedication. Enhanced access such as open scheduling and expanded hours can facilitate entry into care for people whose lives are continuously disrupted by poverty and other chaotic events.

A critical component of the PCMH is its continuity of care. Over time, a better understanding of each patient's unique issues evolves. Behavioral and mental health assessments are often done as a "snapshot." For example, what looks like depression may, in time, be more clearly identified as bipolar disorder. Disorders such as receptive/expressive language delays in children can be monitored to ensure patients receive necessary services at school and across grade levels. Since some disorders are genetic, other siblings, cousins, and adult relatives can be identified and offered evaluations or given referrals as appropriate. The PCMH is an integrated, total wellness model (Davis, Schoenbaum, & Audet, 2005).

Findings from several PCMH models document improved quality, reduced errors, and increased satisfaction when patients identify with a PCMH (Rosenthal, 2008). Patient autonomy and choice also contribute to satisfaction. The evidence from multiple settings suggests the ability of medical homes to advance health through organized, coordinated care (Rosenthal, 2008). Because people from ethnic minority groups and underserved populations experience episodic and fragmented care and because of the high prevalence of chronic medical, dental, mental health issues similar to those of children with special health care needs, it is important to establish a medical home that is accessible and patient-centered and provides high-quality care to vulnerable populations.

Using Medicare beneficiaries' health care as an example, virtually all spending growth in recent years is associated with patients who were treated for five or more conditions (Thorpe & Howard, 2006). Vulnerable populations are at increased risk for multiple comorbidities (Williams, Neighbors, & Jackson, 2003), which requires comprehensive care that meets or arranges all of a patient's conditions and coordinates care across systems. The PCMH model in its current evolution strives to include primary care practices as the primary source of care coordination and management of chronic diseases, especially as they occur in vulnerable populations (Berenson et al., 2008).

The Common Factors Model

In spite of numerous theoretical models and conceptual frameworks, efforts to understand successful health outcomes, especially as they relate to adherence to treatment regimens, remain elusive. In his seminal research on the role of the physician in medication compliance, Davis (1963) found that patterns of communication were strongly associated with patients' failure to comply with doctors' advice. Characteristics of physicians that correlated with poor adherence with treatment included being formal, rejecting, controlling, disagrees completely with the patient, or interviews the patient at length without subsequent feedback (Davis, 1963). These findings have been supported and replicated in the literature for 50 years (DiMatteo, 2004; Ong, Dehaes, Hoos, & Lammes, 1995).

Because clinicians bring to their practice their own theory, knowledge, and experience, it has become imperative to examine and describe the essential components of those interactions that patients deemed successful. The Common Factors theory explains and predicts behavior change in patients, based on the therapeutic alliance and belief in the treatment, as opposed to the treatment itself (Spielmans, Pasek, & McFall, 2007). "Common factors" are the elements that occur in any practitioner–patient relationship and include patients' expectations of change based solely on the fact that they are seeking help through a professional relationship, opportunities to express feelings and troubles to a warm, receptive professional, and acquiring a sense of self-efficacy and mastery. These factors are considered exclusive of specific techniques such as exposure, behavioral strategies, cognitive restructuring, or any combination thereof (Reid, Kenaley, & Colvin, 2004). In their analysis, Reid et al. suggest, "In brief, common factors are the primary engines of change in patients, dwarfing whatever effects may be contributed by specific techniques" (p. 72).

It has been well established since the 1980s that psychotherapy is effective (Wampold, 2001). And although we have considerable evidence that psychotherapies work, we have little evidence as to why they work (Sprenkle & Blow, 2004). Saul Rosenzweig (1936) is credited with originating the Common Factors Model. In his seminal article, he introduced the notion with a quote from Lewis Carroll's *Alice in Wonderland*: "At last the Dodo bird said, 'Everybody has won, and all must have prizes'" (declared at the end of a chaotic foot race in which contestants could begin to run when they felt like it) (Reisner, 2005, p. 378). Rosenzweig radically contended that positive results in treatment are the consequence of "common factors" to all therapies. Further, he suggested that all treatments are effective and this success is not proof of the underlying theoretical constructs (Rosenzweig, 1936). Research reviews and meta-analyses have failed to find differential effects, in different forms of treatments, from contrasting theoretical orientations; this effect was labeled "the Dodo Bird Verdict" (Reisner, 2005).

In one early, groundbreaking meta-analysis of intervention research, Smith & Glass (1977) concluded that the data yielded a result consistent with the Dodo Bird Verdict. "Despite volumes devoted to the theoretical differences among different schools of psychotherapy, the results demonstrate negligible differences in the effects produced by different therapy types" (p. 760). Wampold (2001) and Wampold et al. (1997) also conducted large-scale meta-analyses of the current mental health treatment literature and came to a similar conclusion: "The evidence is overwhelmingly unsupportive of the specificity of unique ingredients of any therapy" (Wampold, 2001, p. 210).

Jerome Frank (1974) was considered a pioneer of the Common Factors Model. He suggested that the role of the psychotherapist could be found in all cultures. He compares the role played by the clinician to that of the shaman. Both the shaman and the clinician have credibility within their culture: They bring about change in people, they help patients deal with their environments, and they rely on the power of science as defined by the larger culture (Frank, 1974).

An unfortunate catchphrase, "the dodo bird verdict" was then coined by the supporters of the Common Factors Model (Luborsky, Singer, & Luborsky, 1975). The phrase implies that it does not matter what one does in the therapeutic relationship. In fact, a number of common factors may bring about therapeutic change, the personality of the clinician being one significant factor examined in clinical outcomes (Reisner, 2005). Sprenkle and Blow (2004) suggest that when we refer a close friend or relative to a clinician, we are far more inclined to consider the personal qualities and virtues of that clinician over their theoretical orientation. Clinician personality characteristics associated with a strong therapeutic alliance include "being flexible, experienced, honest, respectful, trustworthy, confident, interested, alert, friendly, warm, and open" (Ackerman & Hilsenroth, 2003, p. 28).

Common factors are those characteristics that contribute to change in the patient, without regard to any specific theoretical approach or model, independent of structured techniques (Sprenkle & Blow, 2004). The practitioner–patient alliance is the most familiar of the common factors, and is truly pantheoretical (Messer & Wampold, 2002). The therapeutic alliance is "the joint product of the clinician and patient together focusing on the work of therapy" (Sprenkle & Blow, 2004, p. 122). In their meta-analysis of therapeutic alliance, Martin, Garske, and Davis (2000) identified three themes in the definition of alliance: (a) the collaborative nature of the relationship, (b) the affective bond between patient and clinician, and (c) the patient's and clinician's ability to agree on treatment goals and tasks.

In the third edition of his seminal book, *Persuasion and Healing*, Jerome Frank and his daughter Julia (1991) offer the *four shared components* of successful interventions: (a) an emotionally charged confiding relationship with a helping person; (b) a setting that is judged to be therapeutic, in which the patient believes the professional can be trusted to provide help; (c) a clinician who offers a credible rationale or plausible theoretical scheme for understanding the patient's symptoms; and (d) a clinician who offers a credible ritual or procedure for addressing the patient's symptoms (Frank & Frank, 1991). Wampold (2001) argues that these four components alone can explain the majority of outcomes in mental health treatment.

Additionally, Frank and Frank (1991) identified six elements common to the rituals or procedures of mental health treatment:

1. The clinician combats the patient's demoralization and alienation by establishing a strong relationship.
2. The clinician links hope for improvement to the process of therapy, which heightens the patient's expectation.
3. The clinician offers new learning experiences.
4. The patient's emotions are aroused and reprocessed.
5. The clinician facilitates a sense of mastery or self-efficacy.
6. The clinician offers opportunities for the patient to practice new behaviors.

Application of the Model

Support for the effectiveness of therapy is described by Hubble, Duncan, and Miller (1999) in their *Handbook for the Common Factors*, a comprehensive collection of research and literature to support the theory of common factors. In their chapter "Directing Attention to What Works," Hubble et al. describe how treatment should accommodate the patient's theory of change. Patients enter therapy with their own ideas of how their problems started and how they need to be solved. According to Messer and Wampold (2002), some of the most powerful interaction effects in mental health treatment may be produced by how the treatment interacts with the patient's belief that it will work or is consistent with the patient's culture or worldview.

There is far more evidence for other factors contributing to change than the specific approach or technique employed by the clinician (Duncan & Miller, 2006). In fact, researchers have repeatedly found that a positive therapeutic alliance is one of the best predictors of outcomes across different treatment settings. Finally, perhaps the greatest source of change comes from within the patient—strengths, resources, and motivations—as the "engine of change" (Tallman & Bohart, 1999, p. 91).

Table 3.1 lists six attributes derived from health behavior change theories and models that are cross-cutting concepts about what is required within patients to engage them in successful health behavior change (Whitlock, Orleans, Pender, & Allan, 2002). These attributes, along with the development of a strong therapeutic alliance, trust with the patient, and exploring their competencies with their own health, offer hope for treatment as a clinical process that affirms patients' strengths.

TABLE 3.1 Attributes From Health Behavior Change Theories and Models That Predispose an Individual to Successful Behavior Change

1. Strongly wants and intends to change for clear, personal reasons
2. Faces a minimum of obstacles (information processing; physical, logistical, or environmental barriers) to change
3. Has the requisite skills and self-confidence to make a change
4. Feels positively about the change and believes it will result in meaningful benefit(s)
5. Perceives the change as congruent with the individual's self-image and social group(s) norms
6. Receives reminders, encouragement, and support to change at appropriate times and places from valued persons and community sources, and is in a largely supportive community/environment for the change

Source: Whitlock, Orleans, Pender, & Allan (2002).

BRIEF BEHAVIORAL CHANGE PRACTICE MODELS, INTERVENTIONS, AND TECHNIQUES

The Context of Care and What the BHS Can Accomplish

The practice context in which the BHS works will shape the opportunities for behavioral health interventions with patients. Current behavioral change interventions are often taught as systems of therapy or "practice models" that have been derived from the conceptual roadmaps of the common health behavior theories, and that operate with distinguishable principles of change and tasks used to engage the patient in change. Common behavioral change practice models are cognitive behavioral therapy (CBT), solution-focused therapy (SFT), and motivational interviewing (MI). These behavioral change practice models are often referred to as "brief therapies" given the limited number of patient encounters they require for change. Brief therapies make sense in the current health care environment in primary care settings because of the limits of health insurance for mental health counseling and because brief patient encounters limit opportunities for longer term psychodynamic interventions.

Depending on the context of patient care, the BHS may or may not be able to fully employ the standard practice models. What the BHSs can accomplish when helping patients with behavior change is often constrained by the length of time they are scheduled to spend with patients and the number of sessions allowed for seeing patients. Different practice contexts allow for more or less focused time with patients, and the number of sessions and the amount of time allowed per session are often determined by billing practices and patients' health insurance. Furthermore, in some settings, BHS's services may be submitted to billing but not in other settings.

It is important for BHSs to learn how to adapt behavioral health interventions to the context in which they work. It is valuable to know the principles and methods of the evidence-based behavioral change *brief therapies* such as CBT, SFT, and MI. It is also essential that the BHS understands how to utilize "on-the-spot" *brief interventions* if the time they have with patients is constrained by the practice context, billing practices, or insurance plans. The brief therapies and brief interventions are similar in that the focus of the engagement is typically goal setting for behavioral change and involve a "here and now" solution focus rather than a historical or psychodynamic exploratory focus typical of the traditional psychotherapies. Both brief interventions and brief therapies also require that the BHS be active in setting the direction of the therapeutic encounter.

A third, and the most flexible, level of brief behavioral change approaches is the use of *behavioral change techniques*. These are discrete and interchangeable tools derived from behavioral health theories and the common practice models, CBT, MI, and SFT. These discrete tools can be utilized at any time and in any context in lieu of a formal therapeutic process.

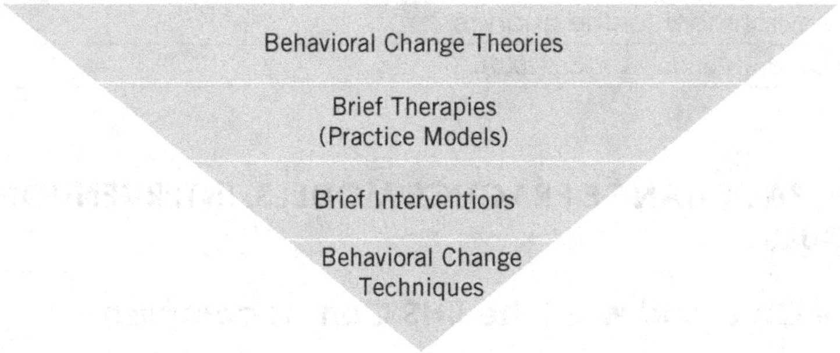

In the remainder of this chapter, we review three levels of behavioral intervention: brief therapies, brief interventions, and behavioral change techniques that allow the BHS great flexibility in working with patients in all practice contexts.

Brief Therapies

Brief therapies are systematic and planned therapeutic approaches, involving patient assessment, goal setting, focused change strategies, and measurable change assessment. Brief therapy usually requires a series of therapeutic encounters with the patient and follow-up sessions to reinforce behavioral change. Some of the most common brief therapy modalities in use today are CBT, MI, and SFT. It is not possible to review each of these modalities in detail in this book but we will review the primary practice principles for each modality and provide sources for more detailed procedures for each modality.

Cognitive Behavioral Therapy (CBT) is actually a family of evidence-based therapeutic interventions aimed at assisting patients to change identified problem thoughts and behaviors. CBT blends the concepts of behaviorism and cognitive theory into a practice modality. Behaviors are believed to be shaped by both innate motivations and learning (behavioral theory), as well as by our repetitive patterns of thought called *cognitive schemas* or *core beliefs* (cognitive theory). These cognitive schemas often include *distortions*, *misconceptions*, and *irrational thoughts* that are automatic interpretations of situations often leading to self-defeating behavior and interfering with an individual's desire to engage positive changes. For example, a patient who is referred to the BHS for sleeping disorder may, upon questioning, reveal that he wakes up and cannot return to sleep because he starts ruminating on how he is not accomplishing enough at work to get his boss to see him as a candidate for a promotion. Upon further questioning, the patient may reveal that he has always felt he is not good enough to be a leader and these feelings of inadequacy lead to his failure to speak his mind at staff meetings and therefore not having his ideas about how to improve the company heard. Thus, he is stuck in a repetitive cycle of distorted thoughts and self-defeating behaviors that essentially drive him to exhaustion and render him less effective at work and passed over for promotions. His primary care provider is also concerned about his elevated blood pressure and increased level of anxiety.

In the CBT model of practice, the BHS will, over the course of several sessions with the patient, attempt to use *disputation techniques* to help the patient see the irrationality of his automatic thoughts. Albert Ellis, one of the founders of cognitive therapy, used humor to engage the patient in seeing the irrationality of such thoughts, and would refer to habitual, self-defeating cognitive schema as "mustabation." The BHS supports the patient in identifying his automatic and often extreme or irrational cognitive schema and then tries to have the patient acknowledge how these schema support or interfere with the patient's goals, such as being viewed as a valued member of the company team. Once the patient has identified the irrational and/or self-defeating cognitions and associated behaviors, often with the use of a "cognitive diary," the patient is ready to practice replacing these automatic responses with more functional habits of thinking. There is evidence that CBT can help decrease the risk of recurrent CVD and recurrent acute myocardial infarction (Gullisson et al., 2011), decrease insomnia (Garland et al., 2014; Mitchell, Gehrman, Perlis, & Umscheid, 2012), and reduce anxiety (Cape, Whittington, Buszewicz, Wallace, & Underwood, 2010). CBT has also been demonstrated to help patients cope with chronic pain. CBT can be effectively administered face-to-face or via Internet-administered CBT and group CBT.

Motivational Interviewing (MI) was developed by William R. Miller in the early 1980s and was originally aimed at reducing maladaptive behavior, especially problem drinking; but MI has been shown to be an effective tool for promoting positive behavior change in a variety of targets including reducing alcohol and tobacco use, reducing sedentary behavior, and improving self-monitoring and confidence in change (Lundahl et al., 2013; Miller & Rose, 2009). The primary principle of MI is Prochaska's concept of readiness for change (Prochaska, DiClemente, & Norcross, 1992). The MI therapist aims to help patients resolve ambivalence about changing problematic behaviors or ambivalence about engaging in adaptive behaviors by helping patients verbalize their arguments against and for change ("change talk"). MI in practice is a very collaborative process, wherein therapists never confront or try to impose change on patients but instead work empathically with patients through stages of discovering their values and concerns about change and then supporting their desires for change by developing a change plan in the context of those values and concerns.

> In the first phase, the interviewer focuses on eliciting change talk to elicit intrinsic motivation for change. When sufficient motivation appears to be present, the interviewer transitions to a second phase of strengthening commitment to change, focusing on converting motivation into commitment to specific change goals and plans. (Miller & Rose, 2009, p. 7)

MI is useful when the patient has a specific target behavior that requires change; it is not intended for working with a patient for more substantial psychosocial therapeutic goals such as the treatment of mood disorders. MI can be used as a tool within the context of more extended psychotherapy approaches, such as CBT. It is appropriately used either in a brief encounter or in a short number of visits with the BHS. Clinical improvements, such as change in body mass index and improved cardiovascular health, are found to occur only when MI is accompanied by a sustained process of therapeutic follow-up and supportive change interventions over time (Butler et al., 2013). Additionally, there is evidence that primary care providers can be easily trained to successfully use MI techniques to engage patients during single routine medical visits in discussion of change and to help them increase their intentions to change (Butler et al., 2013). This training can be initiated by the BHS so that all providers in the primary care setting can initiate and/or help reinforce an MI intervention with patients.

Solution Focused Therapy (SFT) is a brief therapy aimed at helping patients identify their goals and resolve barriers to achieving their goals by acknowledging their personal strengths and personal history of goal achievement. An underlying theme of SFT is that change is best approached via solution building rather than problem solving and aims for small changes that can often lead to broader changes in the patient's life. SFT was developed in the 1980s by a team of therapists at the Milwaukee Brief Family Therapy Center led by two social workers, Insoo Kim Berg and her husband Steve de Shazer. SFT starts with the assumption that all patients are motivated and that the therapist's job is to discover what the patient wants to be different, the "*seeds*" of which already reside within the patient. The therapist also engages in compliments that acknowledge the patient's strengths, history of past successes, and progress in finding current solutions. The following box lists four key tasks for the typical first session of SFT and gives examples of opening questions (Iveson, 2002; p. 150).

Notice the *miracle question*, "If tonight while you were asleep a miracle happened and it resolved all the problems that bring you here, what would you be noticing different tomorrow?" This is a key component of SFT designed to

Four Key Tasks for Solution-Focused Therapy: First Session

Tasks of Therapist	Examples of Opening Questions
Find out what the person is hoping to achieve from the meeting or working together.	What are your best hopes of our work together? How will you know if this is useful?
Find out what the small, mundane, and everyday details of the person's life would be like if these hopes were realized.	If tonight while you were asleep a miracle happened and it resolved all the problems that bring you here, what would you be noticing different tomorrow?
Find out what the person is already doing or has done in the past that might contribute to these hopes being realized.	Tell me about the times the problem does not happen. When are the times that bits of the miracle already occur?
Find out what might be different if the person made one very small step toward realizing these hopes.	What would your partner/doctor/colleague notice if you moved another 5% toward the life you would like to be leading?

engage the patient in future thinking and to connect with a successful image of him- or herself as having found a solution. SFT is expected to take three to five sessions at most and may be useful in only one session with a patient.

SFT has not been subjected to clinical trials or efficacy studies; so far the evidence for the outcomes of SFT is based on the clinical observations of SFT practitioners (Franklin, 2011). Still, there is reason to expect SFT approaches to be useful in helping patients move toward positive change, for example, increasing activity for the purpose of weight management. The SFT tools of using the "miracle question," engaging patients in remembering their successes (even small ones) in creating change, and using compliments to reinforce the patient's belief in his or her own efficacy are certainly useful tools for any behavioral intervention.

Brief Interventions

A brief intervention can occur in any practice context and in short patient encounters. The Substance Abuse and Mental Health Services Administration (SAMHSA) is the federal government's agency that leads public health efforts to advance behavioral health. SAMHSA distinguishes brief therapies (practice models) from brief interventions (Colorado Clinical Guidelines Collaborative, 2008). A brief intervention is defined by SAMHSA as the brief (3–15 minutes) encounter occurring over possibly one to three sessions wherein the BHS attempts to accomplish the following: feedback about personal risk, explicit advice to change, emphasis on patient's responsibility for change, and presentation of a variety of ways to effect change. The brief intervention is enhanced when there is the establishment of a therapeutic alliance between the patient and the practitioner.

SAMHSA's SBIRT (Screening, Brief Intervention and Referral to Treatment) program is an example of an evidence-based brief intervention approach designed for early intervention with patients with substance abuse problems (SAMHSA, 2015). All health providers can be taught to use SBIRT techniques (Table 3.2).

The U.S. Preventive Task Force Five As construct is a similar brief intervention approach.

In 2002, the Counseling and Behavioral Interventions Work Group of the U.S. Preventive Services Task Force (USPSTF) was formed to assess the best evidence for behavioral health strategies to date and to synthesize all the best evidence into a unifying and user-friendly guideline to encourage the use of

TABLE 3.2 SBIRT Technique

	The health care provider
Screening	Assesses a patient for risky substance use behaviors using standardized screening tools. Screening can occur in any health care setting.
Brief Intervention	Engages a patient showing risky substance use behaviors in a short conversation, providing feedback and advice.
Referral to Treatment	Provides a referral to brief therapy or additional treatment to patients who screen in need of additional services.

SBIRT, Screening, Brief Intervention and Referral to Treatment program.
Source: SAMHSA (2015).

behavioral counseling in primary care settings. The guideline they adopted, the Five As Organization Construct for Clinical Counseling, had been previously used by the National Cancer Institute and the Canadian Preventive Task Force (Whitlock et al., 2002). The USPSTF adopted this guideline to help health care providers organize their approach to "minimal contact" behavioral counseling interventions with patients and act as a "catalyst" for health behavior change. It has relevance for any provider of behavioral health counseling and to any context in which behavioral counseling takes place. The five As are *Assess, Advise, Agree, Assist, Arrange* (Table 3.3).

Behavioral Change Techniques

There are emerging critiques of the traditional approaches to behavioral intervention research that evaluate health behavior outcomes as a result of patient exposure to packaged therapeutic modalities such as CBT, since in practice these modalities engage many specific therapeutic techniques within a therapeutic encounter with a patient, and thus research cannot specify which details of the intervention actually affect behavior change (Whitlock et al., 2002). There is a movement among health behavior researchers to move the science of evidence-based health behavior change forward by "unpacking" modalities into their component techniques and subjecting these techniques to empirical analysis.

Behavioral change techniques (BCTs) are the observable, specific, interchangeable, and replicable evidence-based tools the BHS can enlist in helping to support a patient as he or she attempts to make health behavior changes. Michie and Johnston (2012) refer to BCTs as the "active ingredients" of behavioral health work with patients. In an attempt to begin to specify the unique and observable techniques health behavior practitioners utilize in their work with patients, Michie and her research colleagues at University College, London, have developed a taxonomy of 16 groups of behavioral interventions and 93 specific BCTs. The major groups of behavioral interventions include:

i. Goals and planning
ii. Feedback and monitoring
iii. Social support
iv. Shaping knowledge
v. Natural consequences
vi. Comparison of behavior
vii. Associations
viii. Repetition and substitution
ix. Comparison of outcomes
x. Reward and threat
xi. Regulation
xii. Antecedents
xiii. Identity
xiv. Scheduled consequences
xv. Self-belief
xvi. Covert learning

TABLE 3.3 Definitions and Strategies for the Five As

The Five As	Definition	Strategies
Assess	Ask about/assess behavioral health risk(s) and factors affecting choice of behavior change goals/methods.	■ Employ focused questions ■ Use standardized assessment tools
Advise	Give clear, specific, and personalized behavior change advice, including information about personal health harms and benefits.	■ Reinforce the importance of behavior in health ■ Link behavior change to patient's context (family, social, past health) ■ Express confidence in patient's ability to change ■ Acknowledge patient's previous success in making changes ■ Provide "anticipatory advice" for avoidance of risky behaviors (e.g., drugs, tobacco, alcohol)
Agree	Collaboratively select appropriate treatment goals and methods based on the patient's interest in and willingness to change the behavior.	■ Support patient in being actively involved in his or her behavior change and gain a sense of personal control ■ Engage in realistic expectations
Assist	Using behavior change techniques (self-help and/or counseling), aid the patient in achieving agreed-upon goals by acquiring the skills, confidence, and social/environmental supports for behavior change, supplemented with adjunctive medical treatments when appropriate.	■ Teach self-management and problem-solving/coping skills ■ Explore ambivalence when the motivation to change is low ■ Provide self-help materials ■ Model and rehearse behavioral change ■ Engage patient in contingency contracting ■ Educate about stress management techniques ■ Utilize telephone counseling
Arrange	Schedule follow-up contacts (in person or by telephone) to provide ongoing assistance/support and to adjust the treatment plan as needed, including referral to more intensive or specialized treatment.	■ Refer to longer term specialized behavioral counseling to support change ■ Schedule follow-up in a short period

Source: Whitlock et al. (2002), p. 277.

The 93 BCTs in this taxonomy are too lengthy to cover in this chapter, but it may be useful for readers to review the specific BCTs for the first behavioral intervention, "Goal Setting" (Table 3.4).

TABLE 3.4 Behavioral Change Techniques for Goal Setting

No.	Label	Definition	Examples
1. Goals and planning			
1.1	*Goal setting (behavior)*	Set or agree on a goal defined in terms of the behavior to be achieved	Agree on a daily walking goal (e.g., 3 miles) with the person and reach agreement about the goal. Set the goal of eating five pieces of fruit per day as specified in public health guidelines
1.2	*Problem solving*	Analyze, or prompt the person to analyze, factors influencing the behavior and generate or select strategies that include overcoming barriers and/or increasing facilitators (includes "Relapse Prevention" and "Coping Planning")	Identify specific triggers (e.g., being in a pub, feeling anxious) that generate the urge/want/need to drink and develop strategies for avoiding environmental triggers or for managing negative emotions, such as anxiety, that motivate drinking. Prompt the patient to identify barriers preventing the patient from starting a new exercise regime, for example, lack of motivation, and discuss ways in which they could help overcome them, for example, going to the gym with a buddy
1.3	*Goal setting (outcome)*	Set or agree on a goal defined in terms of a positive outcome of wanted behavior	Set a weight loss goal (e.g., 0.5 kilogram over 1 week) as an outcome of changed eating patterns
1.4	*Action planning*	Prompt detailed planning of performance of the behavior (must include at least one of context, frequency, duration, and intensity). Context may be environmental (physical or social) or internal (physical, emotional, or cognitive) (includes "Implementation Intentions")	Encourage a plan to carry condoms when going out socially on weekends. Prompt planning the performance of a particular physical activity (e.g., running) at a particular time (e.g., before work) on certain days of the week

(continued)

TABLE 3.4 Behavioral Change Techniques for Goal Setting (*continued*)

No.	Label	Definition	Examples
1.5	*Review behavior goal(s)*	Review behavior goal(s) jointly with the person and consider modifying goal(s) or behavior change strategy in light of achievement. This may lead to resetting the same goal, a small change in that goal or setting a new goal instead of (or in addition to) the first, or no change	Examine how well a person's performance corresponds to agreed goals (e.g., whether they consumed less than one unit of alcohol per day), and consider modifying future behavioral goals accordingly (e.g., by increasing or decreasing alcohol target or changing type of alcohol consumed)
1.6	*Discrepancy between current behavior and goal*	Draw attention to discrepancies between a person's current behavior (in terms of the *form, frequency, duration, or intensity* of that behavior) and the person's previously set outcome goals, behavioral goals, or action plans (goes beyond self-monitoring of behavior)	Point out that the recorded exercise fell short of the goal set
1.7	*Review outcome goal(s)*	Review outcome goal(s) jointly with the person and consider modifying goal(s) in light of achievement. This may lead to resetting the same goal, a small change in that goal, or setting a new goal instead of, or in addition to, the first	Examine how much weight has been lost and consider modifying outcome goal(s) accordingly, for example, by increasing or decreasing subsequent weight loss targets
1.8	*Behavioral contract*	Create a written specification of the behavior to be performed, agreed on by the person, and witnessed by another	Sign a contract with the person, for example, specifying that they will not drink alcohol for 1 week
1.9	*Commitment*	Ask the person to affirm or reaffirm statements indicating commitment to change the behavior	Ask the person to use an "I will" statement to affirm or reaffirm a strong commitment (i.e., using the words "strongly," "committed," or "high priority") to start, continue, or restart the attempt to take medication as prescribed

Source: Michie et al. (2013).

Behavioral Activation

Behavioral activation was originally designed to treat depression within a brief therapeutic episode. Dimidjian, Barrera, Martell, Muñoz, and Lewinsohn (2011) defined behavioral activation as:

> a structured, brief psychotherapeutic approach that aims to (a) increase engagement in adaptive activities (which often are those associated with the experience of pleasure or mastery), (b) decrease engagement in activities that maintain depression or increase risk for depression, and (c) solve problems that limit access to reward or that maintain or increase aversive control. (Dimidjian, et al., 2011, p. 3–4)

The activated patient is defined as "understanding one's role in the care process and having the knowledge, skill, and confidence to manage one's health and health care" (Hibbard & Greene, 2013, p. 207). We highlight behavioral activation in this chapter because it is a technique that is very portable and teachable and thus has great application to the primary care setting. It has been used effectively in primary care settings for helping patients achieve lifestyle changes in chronic disease management and especially when patients have comorbid depression and chronic disease (Greene & Hibbard, 2012; Ludman et al., 2013).

Low levels of patient activation have even been found to be associated with risk of rehospitalization (Mitchell et al., 2014) and with higher costs of hospitalization (Hibbard, Greene, & Overton, 2013). Interventions designed to increase activation have demonstrated that patients can be helped to increase their levels of activation in terms of self-efficacy, self-care, and chronic disease management, adhere to treatment guidelines, engage in routine screening, and engage in regular exercise, and studies have shown improvements in clinical outcomes in chronic disease as a result of behavioral activation (Hibbard & Green, 2013).

Behavioral activation packages may include some or all of the following: activity monitoring, assessment of life goals and values, activity scheduling, skills training, relaxation training, contingency management, procedures targeting verbal behavior, and procedures targeting avoidance, but the most typical approaches used in practice are activity monitoring and scheduling (Kanter et al., 2010).

Hibbard, Stockard, Mahoney, and Tusler (2004) developed the *Patient Activation Measure (PAM)* that has been used in clinical trials of behavioral activation. The measure is short and easy to administer, including only eight items (Table 3.5). The scale is scored between 0 and 100 points and then categorizes the subject into four levels of activation. Using this brief questionnaire with a patient can not only provide a measure of their level of activation but can also serve as a stepping off point for addressing ways the patient might start increasing overt behaviors, which can lead to improvements in the patient's thoughts and moods and thereby enhance success in health maintenance. The PAM score can also be used to determine the primary care patient's need for behavioral health services and for signaling the amount of support needed from all the primary care team members to keep the patient well and reduce health care costs and emergency

TABLE 3.5 Patient Activation Measure (PAM)*

1) When all is said and done, I am the person who is responsible for taking care of my health.
2) Taking an active role in my own health care is the most important thing that affects my health.
3) I am confident that I can tell whether I need to go to the doctor or whether I can take care of a health problem on my own.
4) I am confident that I can follow through on medical treatments I may need to do at home.
5) I have been able to maintain (keep up with) lifestyle changes, such as eating right or exercising.
6) I know how to prevent problems with my health.
7) I am confident I can figure out solutions when new problems arise with my health.
8) I am confident that I can maintain lifestyle changes, such as eating right and exercising, even during times of stress.

* The PAM score was calculated based on participant responses to a scale of 0 (lowest activation) to 100 (highest activation), consistent with the procedure PAM 13. The continuous score was converted to the ordinal four-category variable, reflecting the four stages of activation. Stage 1 = PAM score of 47.0 or lower; Stage 2 = PAM score of 47.1 to 55.1; Stage 3 = PAM score of 55.2 to 67.0; Stage 4 = PAM score of 67.1 and above.

department visits (Hibbard & Greene, 2013). If the PAM score is administered to all patients with chronic diseases, then those with low activation scores can be flagged by the EMR as candidates for behavioral health services, and the primary care provider can then make the referral.

CONCLUSION

In the current health care climate, the BHS plays a critical role in working with the primary care team to improve health care outcomes for patients and reduce patients' use of costly health care services. The BHS is trained to respond to patients' needs with evidence-based brief counseling tools, which can be applied in almost any patient care context, be it individual and continuity-based counseling sessions or on-the-spot brief patient encounters. As the evidence for behavioral health interventions continues to accumulate over time, it is likely that the BHS will be seen as a necessary component of every primary care setting.

REFERENCES

Ackerman, S. J., & Hilsenroth, M. J. (2003). A review of therapist characteristics and techniques positively impacting the therapeutic alliance. *Clinical Psychology Review*, 23(1), 1–33.

Aday, L. A., & Andersen, R. (1974). A framework for the study of access to medical care. *Health Services Research*, 9(3), 208–220.

Andersen, R. M. (1995). Revisiting the behavioral model and access to medical care: Does it matter? *Journal of Health and Social Behavior, 36*(1), 1–10.

Andersen, R. M. (2008). National health surveys and the Behavioral Model of Health Services Use. *Medical Care, 46*(7), 647–653.

Andersen, R. M., & Newman, J. (1973). Societal and individual determinants of medical care utilization in the United States. *Milbank Quarterly, 51*, 95–124.

Asarnow, J. R., Jaycox, L. H., Duan, N., LaBorde, A. P., Rea, M. M., Murray, P., … Wells, K. B. (2005). Effectiveness of a quality improvement intervention for adolescent depression in primary care clinics—A randomized controlled trial. *JAMA-Journal of the American Medical Association, 293*(3), 311–319.

Bazargan, M., Bazargan-Hejazi, S., & Baker, R. S. (2005). Treatment of self-reported depression among Hispanics and African Americans. *Journal of Health Care for the Poor and Underserved, 16*(2), 328–344.

Becker, M. H. (1974). The Health Belief Model and sick role behavior. In M. H. Becker (Ed.), *The Health Belief Model and personal health behavior*. Thorofare, NJ: Charles B. Slack, Inc.

Becker, M. H. (Ed.). (1974). *The Health Belief Model and personal health behavior*. Thorofare, NJ: Charles B. Slack, Inc.

Becker, M. H., Drachman, R. H., & Kirscht, J. P. (1974). A new approach to explaining sick-role behavior in low-income populations. *American Journal of Public Health, 64*, 205–216.

Berenson, R. A., Hammons, T., Gans, D. N., Zuckerman, S., Merrell, K., Underwood, W. S., & Williams, A. F. (2008). A house is not a home: Keeping patients at the center of practice redesign. *Health Affairs, 27*(5), 1219–1230.

Bircher, J., & Kuruvilla, S. (2014). Defining health by addressing individual, social, and environmental determinants: New opportunities for health care and public health. *Journal of Public Health Policy, 35*(3), 363–386.

Bodenheimer, T., Wagner, E. H., & Grumbach, K. (2002). Improving primary care for patients with chronic illness. *JAMA-Journal of the American Medical Association, 288*(14), 1775–1779.

Butler, C. C., Simpson, S. A., Hood, K., Cohen, D., Pickles, T., Spanou, C., ... & Rollnick, S. (2013). Training practitioners to deliver opportunistic multiple behaviour change counselling in primary care: A cluster randomised trial. *BMJ: British Medical Journal, 346, f1191*.

Cape, J., Whittington, C., Buszewicz, M., Wallace, P., & Underwood, L. (2010). Brief psychological therapies for anxiety and depression in primary care: Meta-analysis and meta-regression. *BMC Medicine, 8*(1), 38.

Cohen, N. L., Parikh, S. V., & Kennedy, S. H. (2000). Medication compliance in mood disorders: Relevance of the Health Belief Model and other determinants. *Primary Care Psychiatry, 6*(3), 101–110.

Coleman, K., Austin, B. T., Brach, C., & Wagner, E. H. (2009). Evidence on the Chronic Care Model in the new millennium. *Health Affairs, 28*(1), 75–85.

Colorado Clinical Guidelines Collaborative. (2008). Guideline for alcohol and substance use screening, brief intervention, referral to treatment. Retrieved from www.integration.samhsa.gov/clinical-practice/sbirt/SBIRT_Brief_Therapy_Brief_Intervention_descriptions.pdf

Davis, K., Schoenbaum, S. C., & Audet, A. M. (2005). A 2020 vision of patient-centered primary care. *Journal of General Internal Medicine, 20*(10), 953–957.

Davis, M. S. (1963). Variations in patients' compliance with doctors' advice: An empirical analysis of patterns of communication. *American Journal of Public Health, 58*, 274–288.

DiMatteo, M. R. (2004). Variations in patients' adherence to medical recommendations—A quantitative review of 50 years of research. *Medical Care, 42*(3), 200–209.

Dimidjian, S., Barrera, M., Jr., Martell, C., Muñoz, R. F., & Lewinsohn, P. M. (2011). The origins and current status of behavioral activation treatments for depression. *Annual Review of Clinical Psychology, 7*, 1–38.

Duncan, B., & Miller, S. (2006). Treatment manuals do not improve outcomes. In J. Norcross, R. Levant, & L. Beutler (Eds.), *Evidence-based practices in mental health*. Washington, DC: American Psychological Association Press.

Fisher E. B., Fitzgibbon M. L., Glasgow R. E., Haire-Joshu D., Hayman L. L., Kaplan R. M., … Ockene J. K. (2011). Behavior matters. *American Journal of Preventive Medicine, 40*, e15–e30.

Frank, J. D. (1974). *Persuasion and healing* (Rev. ed.). New York, NY: Shocken.

Frank, J. D., & Frank, J. B. (1991). *Persuasion and healing: A comparative study of psychotherapy* (3rd ed.). Baltimore, MD: Johns Hopkins University Press.

Franklin, C. (Ed.). (2011). *Solution-focused brief therapy: A handbook of evidence-based practice*. New York, NY: Oxford University Press.

Garland, S. N., Johnson, J. A., Savard, J., Gehrman, P., Perlis, M., Carlson, L., & Campbell, T. (2014). Sleeping well with cancer: A systematic review of cognitive behavioral therapy for insomnia in cancer patients. *Neuropsychiatric Disease and Treatment*, *10*, 1113.

Gelberg, L., Andersen, R. M., & Leake, B. D. (2000). The behavioral model for vulnerable populations: Application to medical care use and outcomes for homeless people. *Health Services Research*, *34*(6), 1273–1302.

Greene, J., & Hibbard, J. H. (2012). Why does patient activation matter? An examination of the relationships between patient activation and health-related outcomes. *Journal of General Internal Medicine*, *27*(5), 520–526.

Gulliksson, M., Burell, G., Vessby, B., Lundin, L., Toss, H., & Svärdsudd, K. (2011). Randomized controlled trial of cognitive behavioral therapy vs standard treatment to prevent recurrent cardiovascular events in patients with coronary heart disease: Secondary prevention in Uppsala Primary Health Care project (SUPRIM). *Archives of Internal Medicine*, *171*(2), 134–140.

Hibbard, J. H., Stockard, J., Mahoney, E. R., & Tusler, M. (2004). Development of the Patient Activation Measure (PAM): Conceptualizing and measuring activation in patients and consumers. *Health Services Research*, *39*(4, Pt. 1), 1005–1026.

Hibbard, J. H., & Greene, J. (2013). What the evidence shows about patient activation: Better health outcomes and care experiences; fewer data on costs. *Health Affairs*, *32*(2), 207–214.

Hibbard, J. H., Greene, J., & Overton, V. (2013). Patients with lower activation associated with higher costs; delivery systems should know their patients' "scores." *Health Affairs*, *32*(2), 216–222.

Hubble, M. A., Duncan, B. L., & Miller, S. D. (1999). *The Heart and Soul of Change*. Washington, DC: American Psychological Association Press.

Iveson, C. (2002). Solution-focused brief therapy. *Advances in Psychiatric Treatment*, *8*, 149–156.

Janz, N. K., & Becker, M. H. (1984). The Health Belief Model—a decade later. *Health Education Quarterly*, *11*(1), 1–47.

Kanter, J. W., Manos, R. C., Bowe, W. M., Baruch, D. E., Busch, A. M., & Rusch, L. C. (2010). What is behavioral activation?: A review of the empirical literature. *Clinical Psychology Review*, *30*(6), 608–620.

Kirscht, J. P. (1974). The Health Belief Model and illness behavior. *Health Education Monographs*, 2, 387–408.

Lin, E. H. B., Vonkorff, M., Katon, W., Bush, T., Simon, G. E., Walker, E., & Robinson, P. (1995). The role of the primary care physician in patients adherence to antidepressant therapy. *Medical Care*, *33*(1), 67–74.

Luborsky, L., Singer, B., & Luborsky, L. (1975). Comparative studies of psychotherapies: Is it true that "everyone has won and all must have prizes"? *Archives of General Psychiatry*, *32*(8), 995–1008.

Ludman, E. J., Peterson, D., Katon, W. J., Lin, E. H., Von Korff, M., Ciechanowski, P., ... & Gensichen, J. (2013). Improving confidence for self care in patients with depression and chronic illnesses. *Behavioral Medicine*, *39*(1), 1–6.

Lundahl, B., Moleni, T., Burke, B. L., Butters, R., Tollefson, D., Butler, C., & Rollnick, S. (2013). Motivational interviewing in medical care settings: A systematic review and meta-analysis of randomized controlled trials. *Patient Education and Counseling*, *93*(2), 157–168.

Martin, D. J., Garske, J. P., & Davis, M. K. (2000). Relation of the therapeutic alliance with outcome and other variables: A meta-analytic review. *Journal of Consulting and Clinical Psychology*, *68*(3), 438–450.

McGinnis, J. M., & Foege, W. H. (1993). Actual causes of death in the United States. *JAMA*, *270*(18), 2207–2212.

Messer, S. B., & Wampold, B. E. (2002). Let's face facts: Common factors are more potent than specific therapy ingredients. *Clinical Psychology: Science and Practice*, *9*(1), 21–25.

Michie, S., & Johnston, M. (2012). Theories and techniques of behavior change: Developing a cumulative science of behavior change. *Health Psychology Review*, *6*, 1–6.

Michie, S., Richardson, M., Johnston, M., Abraham, C., Francis, J., Hardeman, W., ... Wood, C. E. (2013). The behavior change technique taxonomy (v1) of 93 hierarchically clustered techniques: Building an international consensus for the reporting of behavior change interventions. *Annals of Behavioral Medicine*, *46*(1), 81–95.

Miller, R. W., & Rose, G. S. (2009). Toward a theory of motivational interviewing. *American Psychologist*, *64*, 527–537.

Mitchell, M. D., Gehrman, P., Perlis, M., & Umscheid, C. A. (2012). Comparative effectiveness of cognitive behavioral therapy for insomnia: A systematic review. *BMC Family Practice*, *13*(1), 40.

Mitchell, S. E., Gardiner, P. M., Sadikova, E., Martin, J. M., Jack, B. W., Hibbard, J. H., & Paasche-Orlow, M. K. (2014). Patient activation and 30-day post-discharge hospital utilization. *Journal of General Internal Medicine*, *29*(2), 349–355.

Nordenfelt, L. (2007). The concepts of health and illness revisited. *Medicine, Healthcare and Philosophy*, *10*(1), 5–10.

Ong, L. M. L., Dehaes, J., Hoos, A. M., & Lammes, F. B. (1995). Doctor-patient communication—a review of the literature. *Social Science & Medicine*, *40*(7), 903–918.

Patient-Centered Primary Care Collaborative. (2007). Joint principles of the patient centered medical home. Retrieved February 10, 2009, from www.pcpcc.net/content/joint-principles-patient-centered-medical-home

Prochaska, J. O., DiClemente, C. C., & Norcross, J. C. (1992). In search of how people change: Applications to addictive behaviors. *American Psychologist*, *47*(9), 1102.

Reid, W. J., Kenaley, B. D., & Colvin, J. (2004). Do some interventions work better than others?—A review of comparative social work experiments. *Social Work Research*, *28*(2), 71–81.

Reisner, A. D. (2005). The common factors, empirically validated treatments, and recovery models of therapeutic change. *Psychological Record*, *55*(3), 377–399.

Rosenstock, I. M. (1966). Why people use health services. *Milbank Memorial Fund Quarterly*, *44*, 94–127.

Rosenthal, T. C. (2008). The medical home: Growing evidence to support a new approach to primary care. *Journal of the American Board of Family Medicine*, *21*(5), 427–440.

Rosenzweig, S. (1936). Some implicit common factors in diverse methods of psychotherapy. *American Journal of Orthopsychiatry*, *6*, 412–415.

Roy-Byrne, P. P., Katon, W., Cowley, D. S., & Russo, J. (2001). A randomized effectiveness trial of collaborative care for patients with panic disorder in primary care. *Archives of General Psychiatry*, *58*(9), 869–876.

Schoenbaum, M., Unutzer, J., McCaffrey, D., Duan, N. H., Sherbourne, C., & Wells, K. B. (2002). The effects of primary care depression treatment on patients' clinical status and employment. *Health Services Research*, *37*(5), 1145–1158.

Sia, C. J., Antonelli, R., Gupta, V. B., Buchanan, G., Hirsch, D., Nackashi, J., & Rinehart, J. (2002). The medical home. *Pediatrics*, *110*(1), 184–186.

Sia, C. J., Tonniges, T. F., Osterhus, E., & Taba, S. (2004). History of the medical home concept. *Pediatrics*, *113*(5), 1473–1478.

Smith, M. L., & Glass, G. V. (1977). Meta-analysis of psychotherapy outcome studies. *American Psychologist*, *32*(9), 752–760.

Spielmans, G. I., Pasek, L. F., & McFall, J. P. (2007). What are the active ingredients in cognitive and behavioral psychotherapy for anxious and depressed children? A meta-analytic review. *Clinical Psychology Review*, *27*(5), 642–654.

Sprenkle, D. H., & Blow, A. J. (2004). Common factors and our sacred models. *Journal of Marital and Family Therapy*, *30*(2), 113–129.

Sturmberg, J. P. (2014). Emergent properties define the subjective nature of health and disease. *Journal of Public Health Policy*, *35*, 414–419.

Substance Abuse and Mental Health Services Administration (SAMHSA). (2015). Brief interventions. Retrieved from www.integration.samhsa.gov/clinical-practice/sbirt/brief-interventions

Tallman, K., & Bohart, A. C. (1999). The client as a common factor: Clients as self-healers. In M. A. Hubble, B. L. Duncan, & S. D. Miller (Eds.), *The heart and soul of change*. Washington, DC: American Psychological Association Press.

Thielke, S., Vannoy, S., & Unutzer, J. (2007). Integrating mental health and primary care. *Primary Care*, *34*(3), 571–592.

Thorpe, K. E., & Howard, D. H. (2006). The rise in spending among Medicare beneficiaries: The role of chronic disease prevalence and changes in treatment intensity. *Health Affairs*, *25*(5), W378–W388.

United Health Foundation. (2012). *America's Health Rankings: A Call to Action for Individuals and Their Communities*. Retrieved from http://cdnfiles.americashealthrankings.org/SiteFiles/Reports/AnnualReport2012-r.pdf

Unutzer, J., Katon, W., Callahan, C. M., Williams, J. W., Hunkeler, E., Harpole, L., … Langston, C. (2002). Collaborative care management of late-life depression in the primary care setting—A randomized controlled trial. *JAMA-Journal of the American Medical Association*, *288*(22), 2836–2845.

Unutzer, J., Schoenbaum, M., Druss, B. G., & Katon, W. J. (2006). Transforming mental health care at the interface with general medicine: Report for the President's Commission. *Psychiatric Services*, *57*(1), 37–47.

Wagner, E. H., Austin, B. T., & VonKorff, M. (1996). Organizing care for patients with chronic illness. Milbank Quarterly, *74*(4), 511–544.

Wagner, E. H., Bennett, S. M., Austin, B. T., Greene, S. M., Schaefer, J. K., & Vonkorff, M. (2005). Finding common ground: Patient-centeredness and evidence-based chronic illness care. *Journal of Alternative & Complementary Medicine*, *11*(supplement 1), s-7.

Wampold, B. E. (2001). *The great psychotherapy debate: Models, methods, and findings*. Mahwah, NJ: Lawrence Erlbaum.

Wampold, B. E., Mondin, G. W., Moody, M., Stich, F., Benson, K., & Ahn, H.-n. (1997). A meta-analysis of outcome studies comparing bona fide psychotherapies: Empirically, "all must have prizes." *Psychological Bulletin*, *122*(3), 203–215.

Whitlock, E. P., Orleans, C. T., Pender, N., & Allan, J. (2002). Evaluating primary care behavioral counseling interventions: An evidence-based approach. *American Journal of Preventive Medicine*, *22*(4), 267–284

Williams, D. R., Neighbors, H. W., & Jackson, J. S. (2003). Racial/ethnic discrimination and health: Findings from community studies. *American Journal of Public Health*, *93*(2), 200–208.

World Health Organization. (1946). Preamble to the Constitution of the World Health Organization as adopted by the International Health Conference, New York, June 19–22, 1946 (signed on July 22, 1946, by the representatives of 61 States [Official Records of the World Health Organization, no. 2, p. 100] and entered into force on April 7, 1948).

Wu, C. H., Erickson, S. R., & Kennedy, J. (2009). Patient characteristics associated with the use of antidepressants among people diagnosed with *DSM-IV* mood disorders: Results from the National Comorbidity Survey Replication. *Current Medical Research and Opinion*, *25*(2), 471–482.

FOUR

DIABETES MANAGEMENT

ELISE BUTKIEWICZ, ANTONIA CARBONE, STUART GREEN, AMY MIANO, AND ELFIE WEGNER

S.O.A.P. NOTE FROM REFERRING PRIMARY CARE PROVIDER

S: The patient is a 52-year-old woman with type 2 diabetes and obesity who returns for diabetes follow-up. Her last office visit was 8 months ago. The patient screened positive for depression (PHQ9) at that time but denied thoughts of harm to self or others. She refused treatment at that time. She continues to report episodes of depressed mood and anhedonia. The patient acknowledges she has not been taking her insulin as prescribed. She rarely checks her fasting blood glucose but recently the values have been above 200 mg/dL. She continues to have both polyuria and polydipsia that have not improved or worsened since her last appointment. Her vision is worsening by self-report. Last eye exam was 2 years ago. Last A1c 8 months ago was 10.2%. She does not exercise regularly and has difficulty following healthy eating guidelines (eats "four biscuits" for breakfast sometimes and drinks sweetened drinks throughout the day). She reports difficulty motivating herself to exercise or even to keep scheduled medical appointments.

O: Vital signs: Temperature 98.7, heart rate (HR) 104, BP 140/70, weight 260, height 69.25 in. BMI 38.1, HgA1c 11.3%

General: Alert, oriented X3, well groomed, good eye contact. Appears sad, not tearful, denies suicidal thoughts or hypomania/mania. PHQ9 score of 12.

HEENT: Pupils—pupils equal, round, react to light, accommodation, throat—clear, neck—normal thyroid

Lungs: Clear

Heart: Regular rate and rhythm (RRR), no murmur

Abdomen: Obese, nontender, negative organomegaly

Extremities: 2+ deep tendon reflexes (DTRs), 5/5 motor strength, no pedal edema, no lesions, 2+ pedal pulses, decreased monofilament sensation bilaterally

A: a) DM2, uncontrolled, without complications. b) Depression. c) Obesity

P: 1) **Type 2 diabetes**: Reviewed labs and A1c goal of less than 7.0 with the patient. Encouraged glucometer glucose checks fasting and 2 hours postprandial at dinner. Instructed to increase long-acting insulin by 4 units subcutaneous daily. Continue oral diabetes medication. Repeat labs prior to next appointment in 3 months. Referral made to the certified diabetes educator (CDE), ophthalmologist, podiatrist, behavioral health specialist.

2) **Depression**: Referred to the behavioral health specialist for further assessment, treatment, and linkage to community resources.
3) **Obesity**: Referred to CDE for diabetes education and nutritional counseling. Referred to the behavioral health specialist for assistance with weight loss.

INTRODUCTION

The fundamental challenge in partnering with persons with diabetes to improve health outcomes is that while the clinical treatment and education occur in the health care provider's office, patients' health behaviors occur on an ongoing basis outside the provider's office, in the patient's home, school, community, and workplace. The key to ongoing positive outcomes is patient self-management, and the key role of the health practitioner and health system is self-management support (Haas et al., 2014; Knowler et al., 2002). How can the integrated behavioral health specialist (BHS) help the health care team meet the challenge of creating sustainable behavioral change in working with the diabetic patient?

The BHS has a variety of roles to play in the practice and on the health care team, including (of most importance):

- Facilitate collaboration between community agencies and the primary care practice. For example, the BHS can establish a collaborative relationship with agencies that offer the patients enhanced access to community programs for pre-diabetic or diabetic care (Ackermann, Finch, Brizendine, Zhou, & Marrero, 2008; Knowler et al., 2002).
- Review and suggest changes needed to strengthen the practice's methods for communicating with its patients, including patient education materials, e-mail and other electronic messaging, including practice-selected or health system apps, signage in the office, advertising or solicited media coverage of practice services and events, and presentations to the community, at screenings or other community events.
- Provide and coordinate or supervise counseling services offered to patients by the BHS, other counselors, interns, and students.
- Develop and coordinate innovative approaches to diabetes care, including group visits, patient navigation, and other peer support initiatives.
- Provide and coordinate educational programs for patients on stress management, depression, motivational methods, and other critical topics in diabetes self-care.
- Function as a consultant and educator to colleague practitioners, including physicians, nurses and other care professionals, providing input both informally, as opportunities arise, and through formal presentations on such critical diabetes-related topics as motivational interviewing, adherence, and common diabetes-related comorbidities, including depression, chronic pain (neuropathy), and substance use (including tobacco).

OVERVIEW OF DIABETES

The Physiology of Diabetes

Diabetes mellitus is a chronic disease characterized by persistent hyperglycemia, or abnormally elevated blood glucose. The two major forms of the disease are type 1 and type 2 diabetes. Each form has a different pathophysiology and demographic profile, but the end result is hyperglycemia and end-organ damage if hyperglycemia is not controlled through lifestyle modifications such as diet, exercise, and/or medications.

Type 1 diabetes, formerly called juvenile diabetes, is characterized by the destruction of islet cells in the pancreas, which produce insulin. The body's immune system attacks the islet cells destroying the body's ability to make insulin. Insulin is the hormone that allows cells to absorb glucose from the blood. Without insulin, the glucose accumulates dangerously in the blood causing the symptoms of diabetes and damaging body organs. In addition, the cells do not absorb enough glucose to provide energy and ensure proper cellular function. Fatigue and organ dysfunction can result. Type 1 diabetes occurs mostly in children, adolescents, and young adults under the age of 30, although 5% to 10% of type 1 occurs in adults over 30 (Powers, 2012). The cause is unknown but involves genetic, environmental, and immunologic factors. The treatment is strict glucose control through the use of subcutaneous insulin.

Type 2 diabetes, formerly called adult-onset diabetes, is caused by a combination of insulin resistance, impaired insulin secretion, and increased glucose production. Subtypes of type 2 diabetes include maturity-onset diabetes of the young (MODY) and gestational diabetes of pregnancy. The disease develops gradually as normal glucose tolerance progresses to impaired glucose tolerance to overt diabetes under the influence of risk factors such as obesity, inactivity, genetics, and a high carbohydrate diet (Powers, 2012).

Glucose intolerance is primarily caused by insulin resistance. The body manufactures plenty of insulin but its cells have developed a resistance to insulin, preventing the insulin from allowing glucose into the cells. Simultaneously, the liver releases excessive glucose. The result is a dangerous accumulation of glucose in the blood, causing fatigue, weakness, urinary frequency, and eventually, damage to organs as in type 1 diabetes. However, the pancreas continues to pump out more and more insulin to try to overcome the insulin resistance. After many years, the pancreas becomes depleted of insulin and type 2 patients may require subcutaneous insulin as well. This type of diabetes is initially treated with a variety of oral medications but most patients will eventually require administration of subcutaneous insulin.

Impact of Diabetes on the Patient

The early stages of diabetes may be asymptomatic; however, as hyperglycemia worsens, frequent urination, frequent thirst, fatigue, and weakness will occur. Severe, acutely elevated glucose levels can cause dehydration, electrolyte changes, and acidosis, which can be life-threatening and require intensive hospital management. Emergent manifestations of diabetes include diabetic ketoacidosis (DKA) for uncontrolled type 1 diabetes and hyperglycemic hyperosmolar state (HHS) for type 2. DKA is a life-threatening complication of type 1 diabetes caused by severe deficiency of insulin leading to high glucose and release of fatty acids and ketones, causing acid accumulation in the blood. Symptoms can develop rapidly over 24 hours and include nausea, vomiting, abdominal pain, lethargy, and shortness of breath. Electrolyte changes, dehydration, and severe acid accumulation in the blood can lead to central nervous system depression, coma, and death. HHS occurs in type 2 diabetes and is characterized by elevated glucose levels in the blood and dehydration, without acidosis. Patients develop gradual symptoms of polyuria, weakness, and weight loss, progressing to mental confusion, lethargy, and coma if untreated (Powers, 2012).

Less severe but chronically elevated glucose levels cause insidious damage to multiple organs slowly over time. Diabetes can cause cardiovascular disease including ischemic heart disease, stroke, peripheral vascular disease, sexual dysfunction, and multi-infarct dementia. Heart disease and stroke are the leading causes of death in diabetics. Other complications include neuropathy (i.e., nerve damage), kidney disease, and retinopathy.

Diabetic neuropathy correlates directly with the duration of diabetes and the degree of poor glucose control. Obesity and smoking increase the risk. The most common presentation, peripheral neuropathy, causes nerve toxicity in the nerves of the feet and hands, resulting in numbness, tingling, sharp and/or burning pains. Eventually, sensory and position-sense loss occur, increasing the risk of falls and often the development of ulcers in the lower extremities. Excessive sweating or lack of sweating can also occur. The autonomic nerves of the heart, genitourinary tract, and gastrointestinal tract can be affected as well. Cardiac effects include high resting heart rate and orthostatic hypotension (drop in blood pressure when standing suddenly). Genitourinary problems include bladder-emptying problems such as incontinence (uncontrolled urine loss), erectile dysfunction, and female sexual dysfunction. Gastrointestinal nerve damage can result in gastroparesis or lack of stomach motility. Symptoms include bloating, poor appetite, nausea, and vomiting. The small and large bowel can be affected as well, resulting in constipation or diarrhea (Powers, 2012).

Diabetic nephropathy is a form of kidney disease resulting directly from the effect of excess glucose on the renal blood vessels at the site of renal filtration, the glomerulus. The first sign is protein leakage from the kidney that worsens, finally becoming irreversible and causing a progressive decrease in renal function. This occurs in 20% to 40% of diabetics. Smoking accelerates progression of renal decline and blood pressure control delays it (Powers, 2012).

Diabetic retinopathy is the number one cause of adult blindness in the United States and affects the vision of more than half of adult diabetics. Years of uncontrolled glucose and poorly controlled blood pressure cause damage to the blood vessels of the retina, the light-sensitive tissue at the back of the eye. With yearly dilated eye exams, adequate control of blood sugar, blood pressure, and cholesterol levels, and surgery if needed, 90% of all cases of blindness from diabetes can be prevented (Leading Causes of Blindness, 2008).

Diabetics are vulnerable to all types of infections including pneumonia, urinary tract, skin and bone infections. The impact of these diabetes-related illnesses can be devastating. Diabetes is the leading cause of end-stage renal disease (ESRD) resulting in dialysis, nontraumatic lower extremity amputations, and adult blindness. Smoking can accelerate many chronic diabetes complications, especially cardiovascular and renal disease.

Screening for Diabetes

The American Diabetes Association (ADA) recommends screening everyone over the age of 45 years every 3 years for diabetes, and earlier if they are overweight (BMI greater than 25 kg/m^2) and have one additional risk factor for diabetes (habitually inactive, family history, member of a high-risk ethnic population, history of diabetes during pregnancy, high blood pressure, abnormal blood fats, have polycystic ovary syndrome, previous diagnosis of prediabetes, other clinical symptoms associated with insulin resistance, or have a history of vascular disease; American Diabetes Association, 2014). Diabetes is diagnosed by a fasting glucose greater than 126 mg/dL, a glucose greater than 200 mg/dL 2 hours after an oral glucose challenge, or a hemoglobin A1c greater than or equal to 6.5%. A random plasma glucose concentration greater than 200 mg/dL accompanied by classic symptoms of diabetes (polyuria, polydipsia, weight loss) is also sufficient to diagnose diabetes (Powers, 2012). Patients who are at very high risk for progression to diabetes (age less than 60 years, BMI greater than or equal to 35 kg/m^2, family history of diabetes in a first-degree relative, elevated triglycerides, reduced HDL, hypertension, or A1c greater than 6.0%) and those with prediabetes, glucose intolerance, or an A1c of 5.7% to 6.4% should be monitored annually to determine if diagnostic criteria for diabetes are present. Risk assessment questionnaires have also been evaluated to identify patients at high risk of developing diabetes in an effort to prevent or delay progression of diabetes. The questionnaires showed that as risk classification increased, the mean A1c increased. Factors used to classify a patient's risk included the number of high-risk parents, physical activity, BMI, and previous diagnosis of high blood sugar (Rowan et al., 2014).

Early Intervention With Diabetes

Patients with glucose intolerance, or prediabetes, should be monitored regularly. Significant ongoing behavioral change in diet and activity level has the potential to reduce or even reverse glucose intolerance. If diabetic patients are able to initiate behavioral change, they can delay or avoid the onset of full-blown diabetes. The Diabetes Prevention Program study (Translating the Diabetes Prevention Program into the Community: The DEPLOY Pilot Study) showed that weight loss of 5% to 7%, dietary changes, 30 minutes of exercise five times per week, and metformin therapy are all means to delay the onset of diabetes (Ackermann et al., 2008; Powers, 2012). Behavioral changes, however, were more effective than medication (58% vs. 31% reduction in development of diabetes).

Prevention of acute and chronic complications of diabetes requires changes in diet, exercise habits, weight loss, frequent medical visits, and adherence to medication regimens, which may include oral medications or injectables such as insulin. Glucose should be maintained in a normal range of fasting between 80 mg/dL and 120 mg/dL and 2 hours after meals less than 180 mg/dL. Frequent blood sugar monitoring is important especially for insulin-requiring diabetics who may have five insulin shots daily. Some insulin-dependent diabetics use insulin pumps, where insulin is continuously infused via a needle embedded in the skin, which reduce insulin injections but require maintenance and frequent blood glucose monitoring.

Visits to the primary care medical home and/or endocrinologist are recommended every 3 months to monitor blood pressure, perform foot exams, and laboratory tests such as the hemoglobin A1c test (identifies degree of glucose control over the prior 3 months), cholesterol, renal function, and urine protein levels. Yearly dilated eye exams are necessary.

An important component of diabetes care is diabetes education and diabetes self-management. When available, an excellent resource is a certified diabetes educator (CDE), usually available at Diabetes Centers of Excellence, in endocrinology offices, or in some cases in primary care settings (Grigg, Ning, & Santana, 2014). Patients with complications of diabetes may also require regular visits to specialists such as the podiatrist, nephrologist, cardiologist, neurologist, wound care specialist, chronic pain specialist, physical or occupational therapist, psychologist, or psychiatrist.

Medical nutrition therapy is very important in diabetes management. Recommendations include reductions in carbohydrates, choosing carbohydrates with a low glycemic index and that are high in fiber. Reductions in animal fats are important as is a high intake of vegetables and fruits (five to seven servings per day). Patients with renal disease must watch their salt and protein intake. Weight reduction is an important factor with a 5% to 7% weight loss being as effective as metformin for reducing fasting blood glucose levels and more effective than metformin for reducing post-load glucose levels (Knowler et al., 2002). Evaluation of obese patients for bariatric surgery and weight loss medications may be beneficial.

Exercise has many benefits, which include lowered body fat, increased muscle mass, weight loss, decreased risk of heart disease, and lower blood pressure. Exercise also lowers blood glucose (during and following exercise) and increases insulin sensitivity. The ADA recommends 150 min/wk of moderate aerobic physical activity over the course of at least 3 days with additional resistance training (Colberg et al., 2010). Diabetics, especially type 1 diabetics, should be aware that their glucose may drop during exercise and be prepared by increasing snacks before and during exercise and increasing the frequency of glucose testing before, during, and after exercise.

Medications and Diabetes

Patients with diabetes often require several medications to obtain adequate glucose control. Initial treatment usually consists of oral metformin. Metformin is considered an optimal first-line treatment due to its efficacy, low cost, and lack of propensity to cause hypoglycemia and weight gain. Additional agents may be prescribed with metformin or another first-line agent if the patient presents with diabetes that has progressed (A1c greater than or equal to 7.5%) or if the patient does not obtain adequate glucose control with metformin alone. Additional agents are selected by taking into account patient-specific factors, as there are advantages and disadvantages for each medication. Some agents commonly used include, but are not limited to, incretin mimetics (exenatide [Byetta], liraglutide [Victoza], exenatide XR [Bydureon]), DPP-4 inhibitors (sitagliptin [Januvia], saxagliptin [Onglyza], linagliptin [Tradjenta], alogliptin [Nesina]), and sulfonylureas (glipizide, glyburide, and glimepiride). Insulin is selected as initial therapy in patients presenting with severe diabetes such as those with an A1c greater than 9% or patients who are unable to maintain adequate glucose control with other medications (Tamez-Perez, Proskauer-Pena, Hernrndez-Coria, & Garber, 2013).

Medications used for the treatment of diabetes are available in various dosage forms. Some medications used for the treatment of diabetes may be taken orally, which include, but are not limited to, metformin, glipizide, and sitagliptin. Other medications are available only in injectable formulations such as exenatide and liraglutide.

Medication delivery systems for insulin include insulin pen devices, insulin pumps, and inhaled insulin. Insulin pen devices are often preferred over a vial and syringe because pen devices eliminate the need for patients to draw up insulin from a vial and are more compact and discreet. Therefore, pen devices may limit or eliminate the cognitive and emotional burden of diabetes management (Fry, 2012). Patients using pen devices may be better controlled than those who use a vial and syringe (Seggelke et al., 2014). In order to use a pen device, the patient must select the dose using a dial and the dose is released by pushing a button. Continuous subcutaneous insulin infusion pumps allow for administration of insulin via a programmable pump (Health Quality Ontario, 2009). Pumps were developed in an effort to provide patients with tight glucose control to prevent complications such as eye, kidney, and nerve problems that may occur in patients with diabetes. Improved technology has resulted in more sophisticated pump capabilities including patient alerts, records of device use, and remote access to data. Some patients may be more comfortable than others utilizing devices offering more advanced technological features. Comfort with technology, dexterity, and a patient's vision should be considered when helping patients select an insulin delivery device. Traditionally insulin was available only as an injectable formulation, but in 2014, an inhaled formulation of insulin (Afrezza) was approved by the FDA (Klonoff, 2014). Afrezza is rapid-acting insulin that is to be inhaled prior to each meal.

There are many factors that may make it difficult for patients to adhere to their medication regimens. Medication adherence may be affected by medication side effects or the required frequency of dosing. Table 4.1 describes various medication-related side effects that may occur in patients who are being treated for diabetes. Some strategies that may be used to improve adherence include hypoglycemia awareness, the use of insulin pen devices, reducing the financial burden of insulin to the patient, and providing additional support from nurses, pharmacists, and psychiatrists and other mental health professionals (Davies et al., 2013). Multidisciplinary intervention is an effective strategy for managing

TABLE 4.1 Medication-Related Factors That May Impact Patients With Diabetes

Medication-Related Factors	Specific Causes and/or Medications
Hypoglycemia (low blood sugar)	Hypoglycemia may occur with certain medications used to treat diabetes, especially in elderly patients. Symptoms of hypoglycemia may include sweating, hunger, confusion, and fatigue. When severe and prolonged, hypoglycemia may cause altered levels of consciousness, seizure, and even death (Cryer and Davis, 2003). Examples of medications used for the treatment of diabetes that may cause hypoglycemia are sulfonylureas, which include glyburide (DiaBeta, Micronase), glipizide (Glucotrol, Glucotrol XL), and glimepiride (Amaryl). Insulin may also cause hypoglycemia. Repaglinide (Prandin) and nateglinide (Starlix) can cause hypoglycemia, although the incidence is less than with sulfonylureas, and is worse if the medication is taken without a meal. Pramlintide (Symlin) may cause hypoglycemia with insulin. Medications used for the treatment of diabetes that do not cause hypoglycemia include metformin, miglitol, acarbose, sitagliptin, saxagliptin, linagliptin, alogliptin, and canagliflozin. Rosiglitazone and pioglitazone do not cause hypoglycemia but have several more serious potential adverse effects, which may preclude their use.
Weight gain	Weight gain may occur in patients taking sulfonylureas such as glyburide (DiaBeta, Micronase), glipizide (Glucotrol, Glucotrol XL), and glimepiride (Amaryl). Weight gain may also occur in those taking repaglinide (Prandin), or nateglinide (Starlix) or those taking insulin. Pioglitazone (Actos) and rosiglitazone (Avandia) may also cause weight gain. Medications used for the treatment of diabetes that do not cause weight gain include metformin, miglitol, acarbose, sitagliptin, saxagliptin, linagliptin, alogliptin, canagliflozin, pramlintide, exenatide (Byetta), liraglutide (Victoza), and exenatide XR (Bydureon).
Diarrhea, flatulence, abdominal discomfort	Diarrhea is a common side effect of metformin and may occur in up to 50% of patients. Some methods to diminish the gastrointestinal side effects of metformin include using an extended-release formulation of the medication and starting the medication at a low dose and increasing the dose in 500 mg increments on a weekly basis until target dose is reached. Diarrhea, flatulence, and abdominal discomfort may occur in a large percentage of patients taking acarbose (Precose) or miglitol (Glyset), but these side effects usually lessen after 4–8 weeks of treatment. Doses of miglitol and acarbose should be titrated to reduce potential gastrointestinal side effects. Sulfonylureas such as glyburide (DiaBeta, Micronase), glipizide (Glucotrol, Glucotrol XL), and glimepiride (Amaryl) may cause indigestion although it is a less common side effect of sulfonylureas. Exenatide (Byetta), liraglutide (Victoza), and exenatide XR (Bydureon) may cause diarrhea. The incidence of diarrhea is highest with exenatide (Byetta).

(continued)

TABLE 4.1 Medication-Related Factors That May Impact Patients With Diabetes (*continued*)

Medication-Related Factors	Specific Causes and/or Medications
Nausea	Sulfonylureas such as glyburide (DiaBeta, Micronase), glipizide (Glucotrol, Glucotrol XL), and glimepiride (Amaryl) may cause nausea. Metformin can cause nausea, especially upon initiation of treatment. Pramlintide (Symlin) may cause nausea and vomiting. Exenatide (Byetta), liraglutide (Victoza), and exenatide XR (Bydureon) may cause nausea and vomiting.
Headache	Sulfonylureas such as glyburide (DiaBeta, Micronase), glipizide (Glucotrol, Glucotrol XL), and glimepiride (Amaryl) may cause headache. Exenatide (Byetta), liraglutide (Victoza), and exenatide XR (Bydureon) may cause headache.
Frequent dosing	Repaglinide (Prandin) and nateglinide (Starlix) are dosed three times daily. Acarbose (Precose) and miglitol (Glyset) are dosed three times daily. Pramlintide (Symlin) requires three additional injections each day because it cannot be mixed with insulin.

patients with diabetes and may improve patient outcomes (Jiao et al., 2014). When pharmacists are integrated into diabetes care teams to provide diabetes education, significant decreases in A1c may be seen (Bluml, Watson, Skelton, Manolakis, & Brock, 2014).

Patients with diabetes may have other conditions requiring the use of medications, which may impact their glucose control. For example, patients taking "atypical" antipsychotics for the treatment of schizophrenia, bipolar disorder, or depression in combination with other antidepressants may experience increases in blood sugar. Some atypical antipsychotics—olanzapine, quetiapine, aripiprazole, risperidone—have the potential to increase blood glucose (Pramyothin & Khaodhiar, 2010). In addition, antidepressant medication such as fluoxetine can cause hypoglycemia while taking the medication or hyperglycemia upon discontinuation of the medication (Prozac [fluoxetine; prescribing information] Indianapolis, IN: Eli Lilly and Company; July 2014.)

PSYCHOSOCIAL ASSESSMENT

Completing routine psychosocial assessment of patients with diabetes will help the BHS identify emotional and other factors that may impact diabetes self-care and health outcomes. Performing a comprehensive assessment early in treatment and addressing any concerns that come to light may prevent or ameliorate problems with self-care. Further, comprehensive assessment introduces the patient to the resources and support available through a BHS within the primary care practice. Table 4.2 lists diabetes-related psychosocial assessment factors along with diabetes-specific points to consider.

TABLE 4.2 Psychosocial-Related Factors That May Impact Patients With Diabetes

Psychosocial-Related Factors	Specific Considerations
History/stage of diabetes	■ Emotional response to diabetes and coping mechanisms. Consider using Problem Areas in Diabetes (PAID) questionnaire for assessment. ■ Experience with multigenerational family diabetes.
Concurrent medical conditions	■ Nondiabetic experiences with loss, medical expenses, and physical limitations can lower the patient's threshold for diabetes-related stresses. ■ Diabetes-related conditions such as renal failure, visual impairment, obesity, pain, and neuropathy further complicate capacity for self-care.

Physical limitations	■ Effects of neuropathy:
	  ■ Reduced manual dexterity (difficulty with insulin injections)
	  ■ Ambulation difficulties
	  ■ Visual impairment (difficulty with glucose testing and injections)
	  ■ Shortness of breath
	  ■ Amputations

Use of durable medical equipment	■ Assess need and availability. May benefit from physical therapy/occupational therapy evaluation.

Medications	■ Is the person with diabetes able to describe:
	  ■ Medications and purpose?
	  ■ Medication regimen accurately?
	  ■ A plausible method for adherence to prescribed regimen?
	■ Is there evidence of medication nonadherence?
	■ Is the patient experiencing side effects of the medication?
	■ Are there competing medication costs?
	■ Assess complexity of medication routine. Who sets up, reminds, administers, renews, and picks up diabetes supplies and medications if the patient is not independent in medication routine?

Financial status	■ Does the individual have health insurance? ■ Can the individual afford medications and supplies? (Glucose test strips range in cost from $.50 to $1.50 or more per strip. Free glucometers that may be distributed to physician offices by manufacturers' representatives frequently require use of the more costly test strips.)
Cognitive status	■ Forgetfulness, confusion, impaired decision making, and other factors can diminish ability to manage diabetes routine without support. Consider using the VA-SLUMS (Veterans Administration-St. Louis University Mental Status) cognitive screening tool available online (http://familymed.uthscsa.edu/geriatrics/tools/SLUMS.pdf).
Education/literacy level	■ Does the patient need help understanding self-care techniques, routines, nutrition, etc.? ■ Avoid medical jargon. ■ Explore options for adapting instructions and routines as needed, including creating visual prompts if necessary. ■ Use language translation services whenever necessary.

(continued)

TABLE 4.2 Psychosocial-Related Factors That May Impact Patients With Diabetes (*continued*)

Psychosocial-Related Factors	Specific Considerations
Behavioral health concerns, past and current	■ Depression, anxiety, eating disorders, trauma, loss history, personality disorders, other major psychiatric disorders, and substance use may all impact the patient's ability to self-manage diabetes care.
Use/misuse of alcohol and other substances, past and current	■ Both alcohol use and smoking raise blood sugar levels and increase the likelihood of medical complications in persons with diabetes (www.cdc.gov). ■ How does use of alcohol and other substances interrelate with the patient's family/friend network?
Diabetes-specific emotional distress	■ See discussion of Problem Areas in Diabetes (PAID) questionnaire.
Change history and readiness to change	■ Explore prior experience with making changes in daily behaviors (quitting smoking, exercising, losing weight, changing diet, etc.). ■ Assess stage of change, decisional balance regarding improving diabetes self-care behaviors.
Current self-care behaviors/barriers to self-care	■ Quality of the patient's current diabetes self-care, facilitators, barriers. See discussion of Self-Care Inventory (SCI-R).
Family responsibilities/ stresses	■ Does the patient need assistance coping with caregiving for other family members (i.e., child care, elder care, care of disabled family member). ■ Are there adequate, stable finances or competing financial demands that interfere with purchasing supplies or needed equipment?
Work responsibilities/ stresses	■ Does the patient have the ability (time, privacy, hygienic conditions) during the work day for blood glucose testing, medications, and other needs? ■ Is the patient experiencing any diabetes-related discrimination? ■ What are the patient's coping techniques? ■ Assess organizational and time management skills.

Tools for Diabetes-Specific Psychosocial Assessment

There is an abundance of diabetes-specific screening and assessment tools, including the Hypoglycemia Fear Survey, the Teen Adjustment to Diabetes Scale (TADS), the Diabetes Eating Problem Survey, the Diabetes Distress Scale (DDS), the Diabetes Coping Measure, the ATT39, and the Confidence in Diabetes Scale, among many others (Dunn, Smartt, Beeney, & Turtle, 1986; Polonsky et al., 2005; Shepard, Vajda, Nyer, Clarke, & Gonder-Frederick, 2014; Van der Ven et al., 2003; Wisting, Froisland, Skrivarhaug, Dahl-Jorgensen, & Ro, 2013; Wysocki, 1993). Familiarity with existing screening and assessment tools will provide the BHS with a foundation for dialogue specific to patients with diabetes.

The following is an overview of two diabetes-specific tools that are simple to use and relevant to most patients with diabetes. These tools may be used in combination with general assessment of self-efficacy and readiness to change, as well as with routine assessment of depression and anxiety.

The *Problem Areas in Diabetes (PAID) questionnaire* (Exhibit 4.1) assesses emotional distress and comprises 20 diabetes-specific items that ask the respondent to rate, from "not a problem" to "serious problem," the degree to which various feelings are a problem for him or her. A product of the Diabetes Attitudes, Wishes, and Needs (DAWN) study, the PAID questionnaire and its scoring instructions are readily accessible on the Internet at www.DAWNstudy.com. The PAID questionnaire can be used to assess and monitor emotional adjustment to diabetes over time and to identify specific areas of distress that may require more in-depth attention (Welch, Jacobson, & Polonsky, 1997).

The *Diabetes Self-Care Inventory-Revised Version (SCI-R)* (Exhibit 4.2) can be used to better understand a patient's self-care activities and to assess how behavioral health interventions are affecting self-care activities over time. SCI-R scores are associated with other variables known to impact self-care, such as self-efficacy, self-esteem, depression, and anxiety (Weinger, Butler, Welch, & La Greca, 2005).

BEHAVIORAL FACTORS IN DIABETES

The two major behavioral factors in diabetes care are the numerous tasks required to manage the condition and the psychosocial factors that impact each patient's ability to perform these tasks (Meichenbaum & Turk, 1987).

Diabetes self-management involves a complicated, demanding, and relentless treatment routine that impacts virtually all aspects of a patient's life (work, school, family, and friends). A typical day in the life of a person living with diabetes will vary according to the type of diabetes (1 or 2), disease status, comorbidities, and treatment regimen. Especially significant is whether the treatment plan includes oral medication, a combination of oral and injectable medication, or insulin alone. Examples of ideal daily self-care tasks include checking glucose at least two times daily, reading food labels, keeping a food diary, keeping a glucose level log, meal planning, counting carbohydrates/portion sizes, eating timely meals, exercising daily and self-treatment of potential hypoglycemia, taking medications as prescribed and as variably necessary based on continuous assessments of glucose levels, and arranging and keeping multiple medical appointments.

In an essay that illustrates not only the demanding nature of diabetes but also the disease's emotional impact, one particularly diligent man with insulin-dependent diabetes described his days as follows:

> Every morning the first thing I do is search my apartment for my blue case. In it is my ... glucometer, lancet, syringes, and other blood glucose testing paraphernalia ... I test my blood at least four times a day: in the morning, before lunch, before dinner, and before bedtime. On days when I exercise, I may test two times before vigorous activity to ensure my blood sugar is high enough and one time after I exercise to ensure

Exhibit 4.1 Problem Areas in Diabetes Questionnaire (PAID)

Problem Areas in Diabetes Questionnaire (PAID)

DAWN
Diabetes Attitudes Wishes & Needs

INSTRUCTIONS: Which of the following diabetes issues are currently a problem for you?
Circle the number that gives the best answer for you. Please provide an answer for each question. Please bring the completed form with you to your next consultation where it will form the basis for a dialogue about how you are coping with your diabetes.

Patient name: Completion date: Interview date:

	Not a problem	Minor problem	Moderate problem	Somewhat serious problem	Serious problem
1. Not having clear and concrete goals for your diabetes care?	0	1	2	3	4
2. Feeling discouraged with your diabetes treatment plan?	0	1	2	3	4
3. Feeling scared when you think about living with diabetes?	0	1	2	3	4
4. Uncomfortable social situations related to your diabetes care (e.g., people telling you what to eat)?	0	1	2	3	4
5. Feelings of deprivation regarding food and meals?	0	1	2	3	4
6. Feeling depressed when you think about living with diabetes?	0	1	2	3	4
7. Not knowing if your mood or feelings are related to your diabetes?	0	1	2	3	4
8. Feeling overwhelmed by your diabetes?	0	1	2	3	4
9. Worrying about low blood sugar reactions?	0	1	2	3	4
10. Feeling angry when you think about living with diabetes?	0	1	2	3	4
11. Feeling constantly concerned about food and eating?	0	1	2	3	4
12. Worrying about the future and the possibility of serious complications?	0	1	2	3	4
13. Feelings of guilt or anxiety when you get off track with your diabetes management?	0	1	2	3	4
14. Not "accepting" your diabetes?	0	1	2	3	4
15. Feeling unsatisfied with your diabetes physician?	0	1	2	3	4
16. Feeling that diabetes is taking up too much of your mental and physical energy every day?	0	1	2	3	4
17. Feeling alone with your diabetes?	0	1	2	3	4
18. Feeling that your friends and family are not supportive of your diabetes management efforts?	0	1	2	3	4
19. Coping with complications of diabetes?	0	1	2	3	4
20. Feeling "burned out" by the constant effort needed to manage diabetes?	0	1	2	3	4

changing how we care for diabetes

www.dawnstudy.com

novo nordisk®

(*continued*)

Exhibit 4.1 Problem Areas in Diabetes Questionnaire (PAID) *(continued)*

Problem Areas in Diabetes Questionnaire (PAID)

Ways to identify patient emotional distress

Diabetes can be demanding and cause emotional distress. It is vital that clinicians are able to identify diabetes-related emotional distress in their patients. Validated practical strategies are available to promote an open dialogue and help to flag when serious emotional distress exists.

One tool that has proven very helpful to healthcare professionals is the Problem Areas in Diabetes (PAID) scale, a simple, one-page questionnaire.

Why the PAID scale?

PAID has high acceptability and scientific validity as evidenced by more than 60 scientific papers and scientific research abstracts.

The PAID measure of diabetes related emotional distress correlates with measures of related concepts such as depression, social support, health beliefs, and coping style, as well as predicts future blood glucose control of the patient.
The questionnaire has proven to be sensitive to detect changes over time following educational and therapeutic interventions.

What is the PAID scale?

The PAID is a self-report pencil and paper questionnaire that contains 20 items that describe negative emotions related to diabetes (e.g. fear, anger, frustration) commonly experienced by patients with diabetes. Completion takes approximately five minutes.

Scoring of the questionnaire

Each question has five possible answers with a value from 0 to 4, with 0 representing "no problem" and 4 "a serious problem". The scores are added up and multiplied by 1.25, generating a total score between 0 – 100. Patients scoring 40 or higher may be at the level of "emotional burnout" and warrant special attention. PAID scores in these patients may drop 10-15 points in response to educational and medical interventions.
An extremely low score (0-10) combined with poor glycaemic control may be indicative for denial.

How to use the PAID scale?

In a clinical setting, the PAID can be administered routinely (e.g. annual review) and/or ad hoc as a diagnostic tool.
The patient can be asked to complete the questionnaire before consultation (waiting room) or at the beginning of the consultation.
Together with the patient, the clinician can calculate the total score and invite the patient to elaborate on problem areas that stand out (high scores) and explore options for overcoming the identified issues. This may include referral to a mental health specialist.

Novo Nordisk 2006. Adapted from DAWN Interactive 2. Text by Frank Snoek and Garry Welch.

that I have not gone too low. If I feel strange sometime during the day, I will test again … I write the data in my log book, in which I keep a tally of my glucose levels ... I project where I want [my glucose level] to be throughout the remainder of the day, whether I can eat, how much I can eat, how much insulin I should inject, and whether I can exercise or must wait to get my sugars higher.

Usually [for the first reading of the day], I come in at ___ the [glucose level] goal I have set for myself. If I meet this goal, give or take ten points, I feel a sense of accomplishment, a willingness to meet the day. If the read-out is much above ___ my mood changes abruptly. "A poor beginning," I say to myself, "What did I do? What on earth did I eat yesterday?" The next few minutes are spent reconstructing my last night's meals and insulin injections, adjusting my dose for the day, and thinking about what I can eat for breakfast.

Exhibit 4.2 Self Care Inventory-Revised Version (SCI-R)

This survey measures what you *actually do*, not what you are advised to do. How have you followed your diabetes treatment plan in the past 1-2 months?

	Never	Rarely	Sometimes	Usually	Always	
1. Check blood glucose with monitor	1	2	3	4	5	
2. Record blood glucose results	1	2	3	4	5	
3. If type1:Check ketones when glucose level is high	1	2	3	4	5	Have type 2 diabetes
4. Take the correct dose of diabetes pills or insulin	1	2	3	4	5	Not taking diabetes pills or insulin
5. Take diabetes pills or insulin at the right time	1	2	3	4	5	Not taking diabetes pills or insulin
6. Eat the correct food portions	1	2	3	4	5	
7. Eat meals/snacks on time	1	2	3	4	5	
8. Keep food records	1	2	3	4	5	
9. Read food labels	1	2	3	4	5	
10. Treat low blood glucose with just the recommended amount of carbohydrate	1	2	3	4	5	Never had low blood glucose
11. Carry quick-acting sugar to treat low blood glucose	1	2	3	4	5	
12. Come in for clinic appointments	1	2	3	4	5	
13. Wear a Medic Alert ID	1	2	3	4	5	
14. Exercise	1	2	3	4	5	
15. If on insulin: Adjust insulin dosage based on glucose values, food, and exercise	1	2	3	4	5	Not on insulin

> I do not expect to be perfect, and I know there are times when things get out of control either because I ate too much or injected too little ... There have been many times when I have thought I was low—when I even felt low—and my meter has told me the opposite and vice versa ... Many times I can think of no good reason for the discrepancy. When my mental image of my physical self conflicts with my meter, I have a problem. Do I doubt myself, or do I doubt my meter? ... The discrepancy between the reading and my expectation makes me redouble my efforts to remember what I could have forgotten, what I might have done wrong. Only when I remember do I feel in control once again. (Cevetello, 2011)

Emotional distress (most commonly depression, anxiety, and the psychological impact of stressors) will negatively impact the ability of patients to engage in optimal self-care (Anderson, Freedland, Clouse, & Lustman, 2001; Jacobson, de Groot, & Samson, 1994; Rubin & Peyrot, 1992). Psychological factors other than depression and anxiety will also directly impact self-care. These factors include cognitive capacity, self-efficacy, and readiness to change, among others. The clarity and organization of the patient's thinking, and such key factors as the patient's intelligence, attention skill, working memory, and social acuity will inevitably determine the patient's ability to understand and implement self-management strategies. These qualities will also impact motivation by enhancing or limiting the patient's understanding of the consequences of poor self-management. Patients with limited cognitive skills, limited literacy, or impaired auditory processing will also struggle to use helpful informational resources and supports. Similarly, social skills deficits will tend to limit the social support on which chronic disease self-management critically relies. Self-efficacy is fundamental to a patient's motivation and ability to self-manage chronic disease and lifestyle changes. Both of these factors, as well as others, will determine whether the patient moves along the change continuum from precontemplation to action (Prochaska & DiClemente, 1983). Motivation to change is the crux on which all of the desired behavioral changes depend. Given the proper motivation, a patient will use tools and supports already at hand to produce desired change, or can easily be helped to acquire additional tools and support as and if needed (Prochaska, Norcross, DiClemente, 2007).

Children and Adolescents With Diabetes

It is often acknowledged that diabetes is the entire family's disease, as the care needs of the patient with diabetes touch and overlap virtually all aspects of the family's routine. At no time is this more evident than when the patient is a child or teen. For BHSs in primary care settings the focus of support can be the parent as much as the child or teen. Stress related to caring for a child with diabetes affects both the child and the parent in (a) increased risk for poor mental health outcomes for parents, (b) potential impairment of parents' ability to manage the child's illness, (c) increased stress experienced by the child, and (d) negative influence on the child's diabetes self-management (Streisand, Swift, Wickmark, Chen, & Holmes, 2005). Furthermore, diabetes-related parenting stress is associated with parents' level of confidence in their ability to manage the child's diabetes, owning much of the responsibility for the child's diabetes management, and high levels of worry about a possible episode of severe low blood glucose level (Streisand et al., 2005). All of these are areas of potential intervention and support. Finding the balance between age-appropriate independence and safety in managing the child or teen's diabetes is a complex and constantly shifting process in which the BHS can be of assistance.

As a child with diabetes grows, care and parenting challenges shift. In the infant and toddler years, key challenges involve keeping up with the complex and rapidly changing insulin demands of the growing child. This complexity can make finding reliable and safe childcare difficult and can have negative consequences on the family's income. School-age children are faced with stigma and "feeling different" from peers and adults along with increasing responsibility for their own diabetes care (Ayala & Murphy, 2011).

In children with diabetes, the major family challenge is to maintain normal developmental expectations for the child's behavior and relations with others. The temptation to overfocus on the child's illness and to lessen expectations for the child's functioning is significant. A common pathological family dynamic is for the child's diabetic episodes to arise as a mechanism for shifting attention away from other problematic family relationships, especially those in the parents (Minuchin et al., 1975; Minuchin & Fishman, 1979).

The shift in responsibility for self-care continues through adolescence. Parents may prematurely hand over responsibility to adolescents out of weariness of conflicts and intense management demands, but many teens do not have the problem-solving skills and maturity to manage their diabetes independently. Shared responsibility for diabetes management tasks has been associated with less depression, less anger, higher diabetes self-efficacy, and better metabolic control (Helgeson, Reynolds, Siminerio, Escobar, & Becker, 2008). By ages 10 to 12 many children may be able to self-manage some aspects of their diabetes care. Parents may undermine the expected shift to self-care by encouraging dependency, reflecting parental fears and anxiety. BHSs can support parents and teens by facilitating trust and positive communication that is supportive and nonblaming (Ivey, Wright, & Dashiff, 2009).

Six months of exposure to behavioral family systems therapy developed specifically for families with diabetes has been shown to decrease family conflict, reduce nonadherence, and increase glycemic control (Wysocki et al., 2006). The method is a series of meetings with families, especially parents and adolescents, conducted by therapists, typically a dozen sessions over a 6-month period, which "targets family communication and problem solving, extreme beliefs of parents and adolescents (11–16 years old) that impede communication, and systemic barriers to problem solving" (Wysocki et al., 2006, p. 928). The intervention has four key components: problem-solving training, communication training, cognitive restructuring, and functional-structural family therapy. Steps within these components include for problem solving, problem definition, generation of solutions, group decision making, planning, implementation and monitoring of the selection solution, and renegotiation or refinement of ineffective solutions; for communication skills training, instructions, feedback, modeling, and rehearsal; for cognitive restructuring, addressing family members' irrational beliefs, attitudes, and attributions about one another's behavior; and for functional–structural family therapy, addressing, for example, weak parental coalitions and cross-generation coalitions. Of these methods, those that are emphasized depend on problems and patterns identified during initial assessment. All sessions also include providing didactic information about diabetes and "teaching the family to acquire and apply the targeted skills at home (Wysocki et al., 2006, p. 931). Both assessment and intervention are made diabetes specific by identifying diabetes-related problems that are "barriers to diabetes management or control" (Wysocki et al., 2006, p. 931), providing training in behavioral contracting targeting adolescent adherence to the diabetes regimen, having therapists co-conduct some sessions with a CDE who provides education and training in use of clinical algorithms, having parents simulate living with diabetes for 1 week, and extending the treatment focus to the youth's peers, siblings, teachers, or others in the youth's social network (Wysocki, Greco, Harris, Bubb, & White, 2001).

While many adolescents face the decisions and risks related to driving, choosing whether to smoke or use alcohol, and whether to be sexually active, diabetic teens face greater health risks associated with these activities than do nondiabetic teens. BHSs can offer supportive conversation and education to assist teens in thoughtful decision making, and can assist in developing problem-solving skills. Additionally, meeting privately at some point during office visits with the teen patient provides the opportunity for routine preconception counseling to occur to help teens understand the diabetes-specific risks of an unplanned pregnancy (Ayala & Murphy, 2011).

From the child or teen's perspective diabetes requires the integration of a complicated routine requiring heightened awareness while also working through the usual developmental tasks of forming social relationships, becoming autonomous, and separating from family. BHSs must therefore be alert to signs of stress and childhood depression. The rate of depression among youth with diabetes is almost twice that of the highest estimate of depression in youth in general. Symptoms include increased irritability, moodiness, loss of interest and pleasure, change in sleep pattern and appetite, drop in school performance, poor diabetes control, and a sense of being overwhelmed. Childhood depression has been associated with poor metabolic control and episodes of DKA (Ayala & Murphy, 2011; Delamater, 2009).

Disordered Eating and Diabetes

Eating disorders and diabetes share common ground. The near-constant attention to diabetes-specific self-care behaviors such as detailed meal planning, precision in food portions, and careful monitoring of exercise and blood glucose parallel the rigid thinking about food and body image found in nondiabetic women with eating disorders (Goebel-Fabbri, Fikkan, Connell, Vangsness, & Anderson, 2002). Although the prevalence of eating disorders among youth and adults with diabetes is reportedly inconclusive, estimates are that adolescents with diabetes may have between two and three times greater risk of developing an eating disorder than their peers without diabetes (Pereira & Alvarenga, 2007). Approximately 28% of girls and 9% of boys with type 1 diabetes scored above the cutoff for disturbed eating behavior (DEB) and one third reported skipping their insulin dose entirely at least occasionally after overeating. Estimates of the prevalence of DEB among individuals with type 1 diabetes range from 10% to 49% (Wisting et al., 2013). The prevalence of DEB has been shown to increase dramatically with age, from about 33% for females between ages 14 and 16 to nearly 50% for females between ages 17 and 19, as well as with weight (highest rates with obese patients; Wisting et al., 2013). DEBs place patients with diabetes at risk for serious complications such as visual impairment, kidney failure, and cardiovascular disease (Pereira & Alvarenga, 2007).

For the assessment of eating behavior, Pereira and Alvarenga (2007) suggest that the clinician use the following questions, and avoid naming specific disordered eating behaviors:

How do you feel when you eat beyond what was planned for your meal?
What do you do (or what do you believe you need to do) after you feel that you ate more than you planned?
How do you feel your weight will change when you have an episode of overeating?
As a person with diabetes, how do you think that having diabetes affects your eating and your weight?
What techniques do you believe to be most effective to balance your weight and manage your diabetes?

BHSs who are attuned to DEBs can help identify concerns about weight, body image, and self-esteem by incorporating these topics into their routine discussions with patients with diabetes. Routine and annual screenings for disturbed eating and increased psychosocial focus are recommended for young patients with type 1 diabetes especially among females, older adolescents, and individuals with higher BMI (Wisting et al., 2013).

Stress, Anxiety, and Diabetes

Stressors are believed to impact diabetes, either causing or impacting care and outcomes. While stress can directly impact blood glucose levels, stress most directly impacts diabetes when stressful events weaken the resources and supports essential for diabetes self-management and care. Lack of health insurance, for example, will limit access to medical care and health system supports. Unemployment will increase food insecurity and nutritional deficits. Interpersonal losses, such as death or illness in the family, or divorce, will decrease social support (Walker, Gebregziabher, Martin-Harris, & Egede, 2014). The stress associated with poor social conditions (e.g., job strain) can impact development of diabetes (Baumert et al., 2014). The stressors that trigger posttraumatic stress disorder (PTSD) have also been associated with development of diabetes (Roberts et al., 2015). Those with prediabetes, at high risk for development of diabetes, may be especially impacted by stress, with increased weight as a mediating factor (Virtanen et al., 2014). Diabetes appears more prevalent in patients with anxiety (as well as depression) at baseline (Engum, 2007). Additionally, there may be a higher rate of anxiety disorders in those with diabetes (Huang, Chiu, Lee, & Wang, 2011). The essential presumed relationship between diabetes and anxiety is the heightened state of vigilance—the core feature of anxiety—that attention to the condition, and especially active self-care, of diabetes requires. There are specific aspects of diabetes self-management that are anxiety inducing, such as fear of hypoglycemic episodes and fear of injections (see discussion following). But there are mixed reports about an independent relationship between anxiety disorders and diabetes, other than etiologically (Grigsby, Anderson, Freedland, Clouse, & Lustman, 2002; Scott, 2014).

Fear of Hypoglycemia

Managing the risk of developing hypoglycemia is part of the daily routine of a person with diabetes. Persons with type 1 diabetes average 43 symptomatic episodes of hypoglycemia a year while persons with type 2 diabetes who are treated with insulin experience an average of 16 symptomatic episodes a year (Perlmuter, Flanagan, Shah, & Singh, 2008). Patients with type 1 diabetes also typically experience up to two severe hypoglycemic episodes a year while those with type 2 diabetes experience about one severe episode every 5 years. The risk of severe hypoglycemic episodes increases with the number of years of insulin treatment. While the symptoms of hypoglycemia can warn of an impending hypoglycemic episode, they can also create anxiety and fear of future episodes. Severe hypoglycemic episodes often occur during sleep, leaving individuals unable to recognize symptoms and take action to counter them. Nocturnal hypoglycemia is estimated to affect 50% of adults with diabetes and 78% of children, and is suspected to contribute to the 6% mortality rate of persons with type 1 diabetes below the age of 40 (Perlmuter et al., 2008).

It is no wonder that fear of hypoglycemia is a well-known emotional occurrence. The fear can motivate some individuals to purposely keep their blood glucose levels above recommended levels as a precaution against a hypoglycemic episode, even knowing the longer-term consequences of high blood sugar levels. Further complicating matters, individuals with anxiety can confuse symptoms of anxiety (sweating, dizziness) with warning signs of a hypoglycemic episode, leading to unnecessary overeating (Sabourin & Pursley, 2013).

BHSs should work closely with diabetic patients to reduce fears of hypoglycemia. Approaches to reduce fear and anxiety can include teaching individuals to better assess early warning signs, reinforcing strategies offered by health care providers to reduce ambiguity (testing blood glucose levels), and using cognitive strategies (decatastrophizing of certain consequences, reframing) and relaxation techniques.

Needle Phobia in Persons With Diabetes

The repeated exposure to needlesticks, especially for those who begin as children, as in type 1 diabetes, can exacerbate anxiety even to pathologic levels (Cemeroglu et al., 2014). Anxiety will fluctuate as coping skills and social supports are acquired, strengthened, or degrade. But a phobia, once established, is less likely to moderate and should be identified and treated. The recommended psychosocial assessment process should include assessment of needle-related anxiety including whether a phobic response has been established. If a needle phobia is present, treatment would consist of an evidence-based phobia treatment protocol: teaching and reinforcing new and existing relaxation skills, eliciting the patient's particular phobic response pattern, and structured exposure experiences initially in the therapist's office and then as "homework" outside the office leading to desensitization of the phobic response. Effective treatment of phobias—needle phobias or otherwise—is a well-established therapeutic intervention of short duration (typically ten sessions or less) and can even be done effectively on a self-help, bibliotherapy-guided basis. Where such treatment services are integrated and available in the primary care setting they are more likely to be accessed and used. The presence of a BHS in medical settings is therefore critical. This is especially needed in primary care settings, since more than 90% of patients with diabetes receive most of their care in primary care practices (Hiss, 1996; Rothman & Wagner, 2003).

Depression and Diabetes

The prevalence of depression among people with diabetes is approximately twice as high as for those without diabetes, affecting more than 40% of all persons with diabetes (Anderson et al., 2001; Gonzalez, Peyrot, et al., 2008; Peyrot & Rubin, 1997). The relationship between diabetes and depression is symbiotic: diabetes invites depression, and depression seems to worsen the severity of diabetes and its complications. Depression has been found to be associated with a wide variety of diabetes complications, including neuropathy, retinopathy, and sexual dysfunction (Lin et al., 2006, 2010; Naranjo, Fisher, Arean, Hessler, & Mullan, 2011). Compared to individuals with diabetes alone, those with both depression and diabetes have more symptoms, increased work disability, and increased use of medical services. Diabetes-specific emotional distress such as depression, anxiety, and stress are negatively correlated with self-care in type 1 and 2 diabetics (Weinger et al., 2005).

The relationship between depression and diabetes involves both biological and behavioral factors. The physiological aspects of depression seem to contribute to poor glycemic control, thereby increasing diabetes complications; the behavioral effects of depression seem to negatively impact self-care behaviors (adherence to diet, checking blood glucose, taking medications as prescribed, exercising).

Once depression exists in the person with diabetes, characteristic features of depression may negatively impact diabetes self-care. Depression-related withdrawal from social interaction may lessen social support. Negative thinking about the self may lessen self-efficacy and motivation. Depression-related fatigue, low energy, and poorer quality sleep are threats to the energy and activity levels required to manage diabetes. Cognitive changes associated with depression, including difficulties in concentration, may also make self-care more difficult. Neuropathic pain may exacerbate depression. The anxiety already associated with diabetes (fears of hypoglycemia, anxiety about needles) is likely to intensify.

Routine psychosocial screening and assessment of depression are recommended by the U.S. Preventive Services Task Force but is especially indicated in patients with chronic conditions including diabetes (U.S. Preventive Services Task Force, 2009). Strategies such as reminder prompts for behavioral health providers to screen for diabetes in patients with depression have been shown to be useful (Gote & Bruce, 2014). When depression is diagnosed, treatment should be provided. The current standard of care is the combination of antidepressant medication and counseling (ADA, 2013).

While treatment of depression alone has not been shown to improve self-care behaviors, comprehensive interventions that address both depression and self-care can have positive effects on both emotional status and self-care behaviors (Gonzalez, Peyrot, et al., 2008; Gonzalez, Safren, et al., 2008). The BHS is uniquely positioned to provide or arrange for counseling and facilitate increased support.

Substance Use and Diabetes

Problematic substance use is associated with poor self-care and lack of attention to health (Minugh, Rice, & Young, 1998; Zhu et al., 2015). While problematic for all those with substance use problems, such inattention to health can be disastrous for those with diabetes. The BHS should routinely screen diabetic patients for substance use problems, and encourage strong, ongoing collaborative communication between primary care and specialized substance use treatment settings (Walter & Petry, 2014).

Family Dynamics and Social Support

For most adults, including adults with diabetes, the family represents the most important source of social support. The BHS should therefore be actively interested in the patient's family relations, assessing the availability of supportive family, identifying family problems from the patient's perspective, and offering active assistance to improve the patient's relationship with family, whether through counseling directly, or taking steps to help the patient engage family members in aspects of the patient's care.

However, there are many patients who have no significant social support in their lives. This is especially problematic for people with a complex, chronic condition such as diabetes (Reeves et al., 2014). People with more social support do better with self-care behaviors (Gleeson-Kreig, Bernal, & Woolley, 2002; Lloyd, Wing, Orchard, & Becker, 1993; Wen, Shepherd, & Parchman, 2004). Friends and community organizations may also be important sources of support. People with diabetes may be much more likely to initiate and maintain exercise routines if the routines are done with supportive others. Peer illness support groups or organizations can offer strong support. In most states, the ADA offers peer support groups. These are often hospital based and can be identified through local or online self-help clearinghouses. The BHSs should create or use an existing database of support organizations for their patients and create mechanisms for getting such information to patients and encouraging them to use them. The practice could also offer group visits for patients with diabetes, which can also provide significant peer support. The BHS could organize or advise the group visit process.

Cognitive and Functional Capacity

Strong cognitive capacities and skills are required for the ideal self-management of diabetes. As described earlier, diabetes self-care is complex. Cognitive limitations or impairments from concomitant depression, other psychiatric conditions, developmental condition, or age- or disease-related changes can negatively impact the management of diabetes. Additionally, those patients in midlife with diabetes may have a greater incidence of cognitive decline than those who do not have diabetes (Rawlings et al., 2014). To address cognitive limits the BHS and team must identify the underlying condition(s) and institute appropriate treatments. Identifying and mobilizing social and structural supports for the cognitively impaired patient will be the critical intervention. This might include family support and support from daycare or residential programs.

Variability in patients' physical status will impact diabetes care and self-care. A patient who is not ambulatory will need home-based and remote services and may not be able to visit the office easily or at all. A variety of physical limitations may need accommodation. Sensory impairments will require hearing and vision adaptations. Administering medication, especially insulin injections, can be dangerous for unsupervised patients with visual impairment. Alternative means for diabetic patients to access good nutrition and exercise may need to be arranged. Screening should identify such conditions and proactively offer or arrange whatever adjustment and services are needed. The physical environment is another variable. Ideal environments for diabetes care would offer easy access to exercise- friendly areas, including safe, readily available roadways and sidewalks for bicycling and walking. Similarly, an ideal diabetes care environment would have supermarkets and other venues that make nutritious food choices easily available. Many patients do not live in such areas. The BHS should be an advocate for community improvements to address such patient needs.

Finances

The affordability of diabetes medication and supplies (e.g., glucometer, needles, test strips) is a care barrier for many patients. The BHS can help patients apply for medicines through drug company patient assistance programs (see the section "Resources for Persons with Diabetes"). The BHS should be well-versed in available resources, including insurance and benefit options, and relevant community services. Whenever possible, lower-cost generic medicines should be prescribed. Other financial issues that impact persons with diabetes include food insecurity, funds for transportation to medical appointments, costs for gym and exercise equipment access, housing instability, and even affordability of copayments for medical care. The BHS should be a lead advocate in resolving financial barriers that may impact patients' health and care.

BRIEF COUNSELING METHODS

Stress management and *brief action planning* are brief counseling methods that can improve diabetes self-care (Gutnick et al., 2014; Surwit et al., 2002).

Stress management is a term commonly used (and understood by patients) for how people deal with life's challenges and the problematic human responses that commonly arise. In terms of clinical outcomes, studies suggest a relationship between stress and blood glucose levels and diabetes-related problems. A study by Faulenbach et al. showed that postprandial glucose levels were higher during acute psychological stress. There are a variety of stress management approaches (Sobol-Pacyniak, Szymczak, Kwarta, Loba, & Pietras, 2014). Relaxation techniques (e.g., progressive muscle relaxation, diaphragmatic breathing, meditation, yoga, tai chi, chi gong) are often taught as stress management skills. Such techniques are ideally used preventively to lower baseline levels of arousal from routine, daily stressors, and as preparation for responding to stress exacerbations. Simply learning to pay more attention to bodily tension, such as that commonly experienced in the shoulders, face, or belly, and then employing such simple measures as regularizing and deepening breathing, sighing, stretching, or repeating a self-soothing statement (silent or verbalized) can be effective in reducing dysfunctional arousal in stressful situations (Koloverou, Tentolouris, Bakoula, Darviri, & Chrousos, 2014).

Other brief counseling approaches that exist are also evidence based and have been shown to be capable of producing positive change. Such approaches include use of the 5 As model (assess or ask, advise, agree, assist, arrange) (Whitlock, Orleans, Pender, & Allan, 2002), health coaching, motivational interviewing (Lundahl et al., 2013), the 5 Rs model (relevance, risks, rewards, roadblocks, repetition) (Christie & Channon, 2014), and goal setting (Sabourin & Pursley, 2013).

Peyrot and Rubin (2007) suggest using the following solution-focused questioning in behavioral/psychosocial interventions with patients with diabetes:

1. Start with the patient's problem: *What's the hardest thing about managing your diabetes?*
2. Specify the problem: *Can you give me an example?*
3. Negotiate an appropriate goal: *Is there any reason why you should change your self-care behaviors? What is it? What is your goal for changing your self-care behavior? Is that a realistic goal?*
4. Identify barriers to goal attainment: *What could keep you from reaching your goal?*
5. Formulate strategies to achieve the goal: *How can you overcome that barrier to reaching your goal? How have you successfully dealt with that barrier before?*
6. Contract for change (or define what success would look like in measureable/observable terms): *What are your criteria for defining success? How will you reward yourself for success?*
7. Track outcomes: *How will you keep track of your outcomes?*
8. Provide ongoing support: *What will you do if you slip in your efforts? What can I do to help?*

The solution-focused questioning approach can be used by the BHS in individual and group sessions with patients, and can be incorporated as part of the BHS's role as self-management facilitator or supporter.

The key to all counseling approaches is patient motivation. The first "A" of the 5 As model is assessment of the patient's readiness to change. But when motivation is low (e.g., precontemplation), strategies to increase motivation can be implemented.

Based on extensive studies of human change, Prochaska has identified the methods most effective for moving people from precontemplation to contemplation, and they are highly related: consciousness raising and environmental change (Prochaska et al., 2007). Consciousness raising means increasing the patient's awareness of the problems and consequences associated with not changing, and the benefits of change. This is most powerfully accomplished through changes in the patient's social and physical environment. For a patient with diabetes, an example of a consciousness-raising change in the social environment would be having loved ones (such as the patient's children or other family or close supportive relations) express concern about the patient's nutritional or fitness status, or other diabetes self-management behaviors. Exposure to other people (directly or through media portrayals) experiencing diabetes-related problems or (alternatively) successful managing diabetes care or self-care would be another example. Changes in the physical environment could include signage or advertising, which highlights diabetes-related issues, or increasing the appeal and availability of positive diabetes-relevant resources, such as good nutrition or exercise. The BHS and the other health care providers in the practice should assume precontemplation as the most common status for patients, and design and promote interventions that impact the environment and raise patient consciousness.

BEHAVIORAL HEALTH ASSESSMENT AND TREATMENT SUMMARY TO REFERRING PRIMARY CARE PROVIDER

Date: October 9, 2014
To: Referring Physician
From: Behavioral Health Specialist
Regarding: Patient Jane Doe

Referral Information

Ms. Doe is a 52-year-old single woman with a 15-year history of type 2 diabetes as well as hypertension, hyperlipidemia, and morbid obesity (BMI 38.1). The patient's physician reported that Ms. Doe is having difficulty adhering to medical and nutritional recommendations related to her diagnoses. The patient was referred to the behavioral health specialist for assessment and intervention related to psychosocial factors that may be interfering with successful diabetes self-care behaviors, maintaining her depression, and making it difficult for her to address her obesity. The patient expressed to her physician a willingness to meet with the behavioral health specialist to discuss possible steps to improve self-care. The initial assessment interview took place on Wednesday, October 8, 2014.

Behavioral Observations

The patient arrived 30 minutes late for her appointment, reportedly due to transportation problems. She was alert and oriented. Her posture, body movements, and speech patterns were within normal limits. She was casually and appropriately dressed. Grooming and hygiene were within normal limits. Eye contact was within normal limits. Affect was appropriate to the situation. She denied visual or auditory hallucinations. She was capable of maintaining attention throughout the meeting, and denied problems with memory or distractibility. She scored 28 points on the Beck Depression Inventory (BDI-II), indicating moderate depression bordering on severe depression. This score was consistent with the patient's informal self-assessment. The patient denied thoughts of harm to self or others. She was cooperative throughout the interview, and appeared to have no cognitive or intellectual deficits. Literacy level appeared average. However, patient reported having difficulty clearly seeing the smaller letters on the questionnaire, and so required a large-print version of the BDI-II questionnaire. The patient completed the Problem Areas in Diabetes (PAID), scoring in the problem range for "feeling alone with your diabetes" and "feeling overwhelmed by your diabetes." She also completed the Self-Care Inventory (SCI-R) questionnaire, indicating that for most self-care tasks she "rarely" or "sometimes" incorporated most self-care tasks into her daily routine over the past 1 to 2 months.

Psychosocial Factors

Social supports: The patient is divorced and lives alone in a rented studio apartment. Two older sisters live in the state but have infrequent contact with the patient, and reportedly have health concerns that limit their mobility. Two adult children live nearby with their spouses and young children. The patient said she does not ask her children for help because "they have their own problems." The patient has a boyfriend who she has known for 7 years, and who lives nearby. They routinely eat supper together, and the patient said that it is difficult for her to "watch my diet" when she is with her boyfriend because he "eats everything I'm not supposed to eat."

Financial status: Income is solely from support payments from her ex-husband. The patient currently has no health insurance, and pays for medical appointments on a sliding fee scale. She reported difficulty affording prescribed medications and diabetic supplies. The patient reported she has a car, but said that her car is unreliable and is not always in working condition. The patient last worked about 2 years ago, at which time she worked about 30 hours a week as a cleaning person for an office-maintenance company.

Emotional/behavioral health: The patient reported low mood, with onset roughly 10 years ago when she became divorced. She said that for the past few months, almost every day, she feels sad and empty for much of the day. About a year ago, she stopped attending social activities at her church, which she used to enjoy, "because I just can't seem to make myself go." In addition, she reported an increase in appetite, including frequent snacking, drinking soda and sweetened iced tea throughout the day, and eating desserts. The patient reported feeling fatigued much of the day, with difficulty feeling motivated to start activities. The patient said she has never been treated for depression, neither with medication nor with counseling, and has never been hospitalized for psychiatric reasons. She screened negative for alcohol or drug dependence.

Health literacy: The patient was able to describe her medications and their purpose, but was not able to accurately describe her medication regimen (frequency of glucose checks, timing, amount of insulin). The patient was not able to describe a nutritionally balanced diabetic diet, nor healthy portion sizes.

Activities of daily living: The patient reported that she is independent in all activities of daily living, but that "pain in my feet" limits the distance and time she feels comfortable walking and standing. She does not currently use any durable medical equipment. The patient said that for 2 years she has not been able to work as a housekeeper due to her mobility limitations. The patient reported that since she is not working, she has adequate time during the day for diabetes-related self-care tasks. However, she reported she has difficulty seeing the glucometer display, adjusting the dosage of her insulin for injection, and generally "keeping track of what I am supposed to do, and when."

Transportation: The patient reported difficulty leaving the home for medical appointments and socialization because she relies on her boyfriend to transport her.

Cultural/spiritual factors: The patient said that she considers her religious beliefs to be a helpful resource, but she has not felt motivated to attend church services, Bible study, or social activities in over a year. She said she prays daily and finds it helpful. The patient reported that eating high-carbohydrate "comfort foods" from her family's ethnic heritage is a daily temptation.

Change history/readiness to change: The patient successfully quit smoking 20 years ago "on my own, cold turkey," after having smoked for about 10 years. Although she said that she believes it is important to make changes in a variety of her current health behaviors, she expressed a low confidence that she would actually be able to make the desired changes. She also expressed some ambivalence about making health-related changes, including saying that "I'm not sure what the benefit would really be."

Assessment

1. Moderate depression is currently untreated. The patient said she is receptive to discussing medical treatment options with the physician and beginning counseling with the behavioral health specialist.

2. Low income and lack of health insurance are causing difficulty in obtaining medications and medical supplies.
3. Eating habits are negatively impacted by emotional and health-literacy factors.
4. Chronic pain is limiting social and vocational function, and exacerbating mood disorder.
5. Visual impairment is negatively impacting on ability to perform diabetes self-care tasks.
6. Difficulty accessing transportation is limiting the patient's ability to adhere to medical recommendations, as well as limiting ability to connect with social supports.
7. Primary social support (boyfriend) appears to be hindering positive dietary change behaviors.
8. Spiritual resources could be harnessed to support positive change in mood and self-care habits.
9. The patient has a successful change history related to quitting smoking.

Treatment Plan

1. Begin weekly individual counseling services with the behavioral health specialist using cognitive behavioral therapy to address low mood and self-care behaviors. Incorporate motivational interviewing techniques to explore diabetes-related change behaviors, readiness to change, and confidence level. Elicit patient input on change priorities. Based on patient input, develop specific and measurable objectives for behavioral activation and new self-care behaviors (SMART goals). Possible areas of focus include:
   a. Encourage increased use of spiritual resources. Discuss specific strategies and develop measurable objectives.
   b. Discuss successful change strategies used by the patient in previous changes, such as quitting smoking.
   c. Discuss decisional balance (pros and cons) of changing eating behaviors.
   d. Explore ways of expanding circle of social supports, such as diabetes self-help support group and diabetes group physician visits. Encourage the patient to include boyfriend in diabetes education and support processes. Explore possibility of increasing contact with family members.
   e. Explore the patient's responses to the PAID and SCI-R questionnaires.
   f. Increase "manageability" of the patient's daily self-care routine, in collaboration with the physician. Simplify where possible. Use vision-impairment strategies or devices as needed for reminders (large-print schedule, cell phone app, etc.). Monitor successful changes.
2. Explore financial and health insurance options.
   a. Discuss possible application for long-term disability status, which would increase patient income and result in eventual eligibility for Medicare and/or Medicaid.
   b. Explore the patient's current eligibility for Medicaid under Medicaid expansion provisions of the Affordable Care Act.

   c. Assist patient with application for discounted or free medications and supplies using Rx Outreach and pharmaceutical company patient assistance programs.
3. Increase knowledge of nutritional guidelines. Provide nutritional consultation through a certified diabetes educator. Encourage the patient to invite her boyfriend to nutritional consultation sessions for support and mutual nutritional learning.
4. Explore pain management options with the primary care physician, including possible orthotics for foot pain, and possible referral to pain management service.
5. Obtain vision-assistance devices and consultation services from state agency for persons with visual impairment. Encourage the patient to meet with the primary care physician for possible change from insulin syringe to premeasured insulin pen for easier visual management.
6. Explore alternative transportation options, including paratransit options for persons with disabilities.

Initial Objectives

As a result of first conversation with the behavior health specialist, the patient developed the following beginning objectives, which she plans to initiate within the next week:

1. Schedule follow-up appointment with the primary care physician for consideration of medication to treat low mood. Schedule appointment with the behavioral health specialist to begin counseling.
2. Expand circle of social supports: The patient will call her son and her daughter once a week for a short conversation.
3. Explore health insurance options: The patient will complete online application for state Medicaid benefits.
4. Improve eating habits:
   a. Create a list of pros and cons of changing eating habits.
   b. Reduce portion of size of breads and pasta by half each time she eats.
   c. Reduce soda consumption by half and substituting water flavored with a slice of lemon.
   d. Keep a 3-day food diary to bring to nutritional consultation appointment.

Additional objectives to be developed with the patient over the course of work with the behavioral health specialist.

REFERENCES

Ackermann, R. T., Finch, E. A., Brizendine, E., Zhou, H., & Marrero, D. G. (2008). Translating the Diabetes Prevention Program into the community. The DEPLOY Pilot Study. *American Journal of Preventive Medicine*, *35*(4), 357–363. doi:10.1016/j.amepre.2008.06.035

American Diabetes Association. (2013). Standards of medical care in diabetes—2013. *Diabetes Care*, *36*(Suppl. 1), S11–S66. doi:10.2337/dc13-S011

American Diabetes Association. (2014). Standards of medical care in diabetes—2014. *Diabetes Care, 37*(Suppl. 1), S14–S80. doi:10.2337/dc14-S014

Anderson, R. J., Freedland, K. E., Clouse, R. E., & Lustman, P. J. (2001). The prevalence of comorbid depression in adults with diabetes: A meta-analysis. *Diabetes Care, 24*(6), 1069–1078.

Ayala, J. M., & Murphy, K. (2011). Managing psychosocial issues in a family with diabetes. *MCN. The American Journal of Maternal Child Nursing, 36*(1), 49–55. doi:10.1097/NMC.0b013e3181fc5e94

Baumert, J., Meisinger, C., Lukaschek, K., Emeny, R. T., Rückert, I. M., Kruse, J., & Ladwig, K. H. (2014). A pattern of unspecific somatic symptoms as long-term premonitory signs of type 2 diabetes: Findings from the population-based MONICA/KORA cohort study, 1984-2009. *BMC Endocrine Disorders, 14*(1), 87. doi:10.1186/1472-6823-14-87

Bluml, B. M., Watson, L. L., Skelton, J. B., Manolakis, P. G., & Brock, K. A. (2014). Improving outcomes for diverse populations disproportionately affected by diabetes: Final results of Project IMPACT: Diabetes. *Journal of the American Pharmacists Association: JAPhA, 54*(5), 477–485. doi:10.1331/JAPhA.2014.13240

Cemeroglu, A. P., Can, A., Davis, A. T., Cemeroglu, O., Kleis, L., Daniel, M. S., . . . Koehler, T. J. (2014). Fear of needles in children with type 1 diabetes mellitus on multiple daily injections (MDI) and continuous subcutaneous insulin infusion (CSII). *Endocrine Practice, 21*, 46–53. doi:10.4158/ep14252.OR

Cevetello, J. (2011). Evocative objects: Things we think with. Cambridge, MA: The MIT Press.

Christie, D., & Channon, S. (2014). The potential for motivational interviewing to improve outcomes in the management of diabetes and obesity in paediatric and adult populations: A clinical review. *Diabetes, Obesity & Metabolism, 16*(5), 381–387. doi:10.1111/dom.12195

Colberg, S. R., Sigal, R. J., Fernhall, B., Regensteiner, J. G., Blissmer, B. J., Rubin, R. R., . . . Braun, B. (2010). Exercise and type 2 diabetes: The American College of Sports Medicine and the American Diabetes Association: Joint position statement. *Diabetes Care, 33*(12), e147–e167. doi:10.2337/dc10-9990

Cryer, P. E., Davis, S. N., & Shamoon, H. (2003). Hypoglycemia in diabetes. *Diabetes Care, 26*(6), 1902–1912.

Davies, M. J., Gagliardino, J. J., Gray, L. J., Khunti, K., Mohan, V., & Hughes, R. (2013). Real-world factors affecting adherence to insulin therapy in patients with type 1 or type 2 diabetes mellitus: A systematic review. *Diabetic Medicine: A Journal of the British Diabetic Association, 30*(5), 512–524. doi:10.1111/dme.12128

Delamater, A. M. (2009). Psychological care of children and adolescents with diabetes. *Pediatric Diabetes, 10*(Suppl. 12), 175–184. doi:10.1111/j.1399-5448.2009.00580.x

Dunn, S. M., Smartt, H. H., Beeney, L. J., & Turtle, J. R. (1986). Measurement of emotional adjustment in diabetic patients: Validity and reliability of ATT39. *Diabetes Care, 9*(5), 480–489.

Engum, A. (2007). The role of depression and anxiety in onset of diabetes in a large population-based study. *Journal of Psychosomatic Research, 62*(1), 31–38. doi:10.1016/j.jpsychores.2006.07.009

Faulenbach, M., Uthoff, H., Schwegler, K., Spinas, G. A., Schmid, C., & Wiesli, P. (2012). Effect of psychological stress on glucose control in patients with type 2 diabetes. *Diabetic Medicine: A Journal of the British Diabetic Association, 29*(1), 128–131. doi:10.1111/j.1464-5491.2011.03431.x

Fry, A. (2012). Insulin delivery device technology 2012: Where are we after 90 years? *Journal of Diabetes Science and Technology, 6*(4), 947–953.

Gleeson-Kreig, J., Bernal, H., & Woolley, S. (2002). The role of social support in the self-management of diabetes mellitus among a Hispanic population. *Public Health Nursing, 19*(3), 215–222.

Goebel-Fabbri, A. E., Fikkan, J., Connell, A., Vangsness, L., & Anderson, B. J. (2002). Identification and treatment of eating disorders in women with type 1 diabetes mellitus. *Treatments in Endocrinology, 1*(3), 155–162.

Gonzalez, J. S., Peyrot, M., McCarl, L. A., Collins, E. M., Serpa, L., Mimiaga, M. J., & Safren, S. A. (2008). Depression and diabetes treatment nonadherence: A meta-analysis. *Diabetes Care, 31*(12), 2398–2403. doi:10.2337/dc08-1341

Gonzalez, J. S., Safren, S. A., Delahanty, L. M., Cagliero, E., Wexler, D. J., Meigs, J. B., & Grant, R. W. (2008). Symptoms of depression prospectively predict poorer self-care in patients with type 2 diabetes. *Diabetic Medicine: A Journal of the British Diabetic Association, 25*(9), 1102–1107. doi:10.1111/j.1464-5491.2008.02535.x

Gote, C., & Bruce, R. D. (2014). Effectiveness of a reminder prompt to screen for diabetes in individuals with depression. *Journal for Nurse Practitioners, 10*(7), 456–464. doi:10.1016/j.nurpra.2014.04.021

Grigg, J., Ning, Y., & Santana, C. (2014). The impact of certified diabetes educators on diabetes performance and variation among primary care sites within an integrated health system. *Journal of Primary Care & Community Health, 5*(2), 80–84. doi:10.1177/2150131913520552

Grigsby, A. B., Anderson, R. J., Freedland, K. E., Clouse, R. E., & Lustman, P. J. (2002). Prevalence of anxiety in adults with diabetes: A systematic review. *Journal of Psychosomatic Research, 53*(6), 1053–1060.

Gutnick, D., Reims, K., Davis, C., Gainforth, H., Jay, M., & Cole, S. (2014). Brief action planning to facilitate behavior change and support patient self-management. *Journal of Clinical Outcomes Management, 21*(1), 17–29.

Haas, L., Maryniuk, M., Beck, J., Cox, C. E., Duker, P., Edwards, L., . . . Youssef, G. (2014). National standards for diabetes self-management education and support. *Diabetes Care, 37*(Suppl. 1), S144–S153. doi:10.2337/dc14-S144

Health Quality Ontario. (2009). Continuous subcutaneous insulin infusion (CSII) pumps for type 1 and type 2 adult diabetic populations: An evidence-based analysis. *Ontario Health Technology Assessment Series, 9*(20), 1–58.

Helgeson, V. S., Reynolds, K. A., Siminerio, L., Escobar, O., & Becker, D. (2008). Parent and adolescent distribution of responsibility for diabetes self-care: Links to health outcomes. *Journal of Pediatric Psychology, 33*(5), 497–508. doi:10.1093/jpepsy/jsm081

Hiss, R. G. (1996). Barriers to care in non-insulin-dependent diabetes mellitus. The Michigan experience. *Annals of Internal Medicine, 124*(1 Pt. 2), 146–148.

Huang, C. J., Chiu, H. C., Lee, M. H., & Wang, S. Y. (2011). Prevalence and incidence of anxiety disorders in diabetic patients: A national population-based cohort study. *General Hospital Psychiatry, 33*(1), 8–15. doi:10.1016/j.genhosppsych.2010.10.008

Ivey, J. B., Wright, A., & Dashiff, C. J. (2009). Finding the balance: Adolescents with type 1 diabetes and their parents. *Journal of Pediatric Health Care: Official Publication of National Association of Pediatric Nurse Associates & Practitioners, 23*(1), 10–18. doi:10.1016/j.pedhc.2007.12.008

Jacobson, A. M., de Groot, M., & Samson, J. A. (1994). The evaluation of two measures of quality of life in patients with type I and type II diabetes. *Diabetes Care, 17*(4), 267–274.

Jiao, F. F., Fung, C. S., Wong, C. K., Wan, Y. F., Dai, D., Kwok, R., & Lam, C. L. (2014). Effects of the Multidisciplinary Risk Assessment and Management Program for Patients with Diabetes Mellitus (RAMP-DM) on biomedical outcomes, observed cardiovascular events and cardiovascular risks in primary care: A longitudinal comparative study. *Cardiovascular Diabetology, 13*(1), 127. doi:10.1186/s12933-014-0127-6

Klonoff, D. C. (2014). Afrezza inhaled insulin: The fastest-acting FDA-approved insulin on the market has favorable properties. *Journal of Diabetes Science and Technology, 8*(6), 1071–1073. doi:10.1177/1932296814555820

Knowler, W. C., Barrett-Connor, E., Fowler, S. E., Hamman, R. F., Lachin, J. M., Walker, E. A., & Nathan, D. M. (2002). Reduction in the incidence of type 2 diabetes with lifestyle intervention or metformin. *The New England Journal of Medicine 346*(6), 393–403. doi:10.1056/NEJMoa012512

Koloverou, E., Tentolouris, N., Bakoula, C., Darviri, C., & Chrousos, G. (2014). Implementation of a stress management program in outpatients with type 2 diabetes mellitus: A randomized controlled trial. *Hormones (Athens)*. doi:10.14310/horm.2002.1492

Leading Causes of Blindness. (2008). *NIH Medline Plus*. 3(3), 14–15.

Lin, E. H., Katon, W., Rutter, C., Simon, G. E., Ludman, E. J., Von Korff, M., . . . Walker, E. (2006). Effects of enhanced depression treatment on diabetes self-care. *Annals of Family Medicine, 4*(1), 46–53. doi:10.1370/afm.423

Lin, E. H., Rutter, C. M., Katon, W., Heckbert, S. R., Ciechanowski, P., Oliver, M. M., . . . Von Korff, M. (2010). Depression and advanced complications of diabetes: A prospective cohort study. *Diabetes Care, 33*(2), 264–269. doi:10.2337/dc09-1068

Lloyd, C. E., Wing, R. R., Orchard, T. J., & Becker, D. J. (1993). Psychosocial correlates of glycemic control: The Pittsburgh Epidemiology of Diabetes Complications (EDC) Study. *Diabetes Research and Clinical Practice*, *21*(2–3), 187–195.

Lundahl, B., Moleni, T., Burke, B. L., Butters, R., Tollefson, D., Butler, C., & Rollnick, S. (2013). Motivational interviewing in medical care settings: A systematic review and meta-analysis of randomized controlled trials. *Patient Education and Counseling*, *93*(2), 157–168. doi:10.1016/j.pec.2013.07.012

Medical Advisory Secretariat. (2009). Continuous Subcutaneous Insulin Infusion (CSII) pumps for type 1 and type 2 adult diabetic populations: An evidence-based analysis. *Ontario Health Technology Assessment Series*, *9*(20), 1–58.

Meichenbaum, D., & Turk, D. C. (1987). *Facilitating Treatment Adherence: A Practitioner's Guidebook*. New York, NY: Plenum Press.

Minuchin, S., Baker, L., Rosman, B. L., Liebman, R., Milman, L., & Todd, T. C. (1975). A conceptual model of psychosomatic illness in children. Family organization and family therapy. *Archives of General Psychiatry*, *32*(8), 1031–1038.

Minuchin, S., & Fishman, H. C. (1979). The psychosomatic family in child psychiatry. *Journal of the American Academy of Child Psychiatry*, *18*(1), 76–90.

Minugh, P. A., Rice, C., & Young, L. (1998). Gender, health beliefs, health behaviors, and alcohol consumption. *The American Journal of Drug and Alcohol Abuse*, *24*(3), 483–497.

Naranjo, D. M., Fisher, L., Arean, P. A., Hessler, D., & Mullan, J. (2011). Patients with type 2 diabetes at risk for major depressive disorder over time. *Annals of Family Medicine*, *9*(2), 115–120. doi:10.1370/afm.1212

Pereira, R. F., & Alvarenga, M. (2007). Disordered eating: Identifying, treating, preventing, and differentiating it from eating disorders. *Diabetes Spectrum*, *20*(3), 141–148. doi:10.2337/diaspect.20.3.141

Perlmuter, L. C., Flanagan, B. P., Shah, P. H., & Singh, S. P. (2008). Glycemic control and hypoglycemia: Is the loser the winner? *Diabetes Care*, *31*(10), 2072–2076. doi:10.2337/dc08-1441

Peyrot, M., & Rubin, R. R. (1997). Levels and risks of depression and anxiety symptomatology among diabetic adults. *Diabetes Care*, *20*(4), 585–590.

Peyrot, M., & Rubin, R. R. (2007). Behavioral and psychosocial interventions in diabetes: A conceptual review. *Diabetes Care*, *30*(10), 2433–2440.

Polonsky, W. H., Fisher, L., Earles, J., Dudl, R. J., Lees, J., Mullan, J., & Jackson, R. A. (2005). Assessing psychosocial distress in diabetes development of the diabetes distress scale. *Diabetes Care*, *28*(3), 626–631.

Powers, A. C. (2012). Diabetes mellitus. In D. L. Longo, A. S. Fauci, D. L. Kasper, S. L. Hauser, J. L. Jameson, & J. Loscalzo (Eds.), *Harrison's principles of internal medicine* (18 ed.; chap. 344). New York, NY: The McGraw-Hill Companies.

Pramyothin, P., & Khaodhiar, L. (2010). Metabolic syndrome with the atypical antipsychotics. *Current Opinion in Endocrinology, Diabetes, and Obesity*, *17*(5), 460–466. doi:10.1097/MED.0b013e32833de61c

Prochaska, J. O., & DiClemente, C. C. (1983). Stages and processes of self-change of smoking: Toward an integrative model of change. *Journal of Consulting and Clinical Psychology*, *51*(3), 390–395.

Prochaska, J. O., Norcross J. C., DiClemente C. C. (2007). *Changing for good: A revolutionary six-stage program for overcoming bad habits and moving your life positively forward*. New York, NY: Harper Collins.

Rawlings, A. M., Sharrett, A. Richey, S., Andrea L. C., Coresh, J., Albert, M., Couper, D., . . . Selvin, E. (2014). Diabetes in midlife and cognitive change over 20 years: A cohort study. *Annals of Internal Medicine*, *161*(11), 785–793. doi:10.7326/M14-0737

Reeves, D., Blickem, C., Vassilev, I., Brooks, H., Kennedy, A., Richardson, G., & Rogers, A. (2014). The contribution of social networks to the health and self-management of patients with long-term conditions: A longitudinal study. *PLoS One*, *9*(6), e98340. doi:10.1371/journal.pone.0098340

Roberts, A. L., Agnew-Blais, J. C., Spiegelman, D., Kubzansky, L. D., Mason, S. M., Galea, S., . . . Koenen, K. C. (2015). Posttraumatic stress disorder and incidence of type 2 diabetes mellitus in a sample of women: A 22-year longitudinal study. *Journal of the American Medical Association Psychiatry*. doi:10.1001/jamapsychiatry.2014.2632

Rothman, A. A., & Wagner, E. H. (2003). Chronic illness management: What is the role of primary care? *Annals of Internal Medicine*, *138*(3), 256–261. doi:10.7326/0003-4819-138-3-200302040-00034

Rowan, C. P., Miadovnik, L. A., Riddell, M. C., Rotondi, M. A., Gledhill, N., & Jamnik, V. K. (2014). Identifying persons at risk for developing type 2 diabetes in a concentrated population of high risk ethnicities in Canada using a risk assessment questionnaire and point-of-care capillary blood HbA1c measurement. *BMC Public Health*, *14*, 929. doi:10.1186/1471-2458-14-929

Rubin, R. R., & Peyrot, M. (1992). Psychosocial problems and interventions in diabetes. A review of the literature. *Diabetes Care*, *15*(11), 1640–1657.

Sabourin, B. C., & Pursley, S. (2013). Psychosocial issues in diabetes self-management: Strategies for healthcare providers. *Canadian Journal of Diabetes*, *37*(1), 36–40. doi:10.1016/j.jcjd.2013.01.002

Scott, K. M. (2014). Depression, anxiety and incident cardiometabolic diseases. *Current Opinion in Psychiatry*, *27*(4), 289–293. doi:10.1097/yco.0000000000000067

Seggelke, S. A., Hawkins, R. M., Gibbs, J., Rasouli, N., Wang, C. C., & Draznin, B. (2014). Effect of glargine insulin delivery method (pen device versus vial/syringe) on glycemic control and patient preferences in patients with type 1 and type 2 diabetes. *Endocrine Practice: Official Journal of the American College of Endocrinology and the American Association of Clinical Endocrinologists*, *20*(6), 536–539. doi:10.4158/ep13404.or

Shepard, J. A., Vajda, K., Nyer, M., Clarke, W., & Gonder-Frederick, L. (2014). Understanding the construct of fear of hypoglycemia in pediatric type 1 diabetes. *Journal of Pediatric Psychology*, *39*(10), 1115–1125. doi:10.1093/jpepsy/jsu068

Sobol-Pacyniak, A. B., Szymczak, W., Kwarta, P., Loba, J., & Pietras, T. (2014). Selected factors determining a way of coping with stress in type 2 diabetic patients. *BioMed Research International*, 2014, 587823. doi:10.1155/2014/587823

Streisand, R., Swift, E., Wickmark, T., Chen, R., & Holmes, C. S. (2005). Pediatric parenting stress among parents of children with type 1 diabetes: The role of self-efficacy, responsibility, and fear. *Journal of Pediatric Psychology*, *30*(6), 513–521. doi:10.1093/jpepsy/jsi076

Surwit, R. S., van Tilburg, M. A., Zucker, N., McCaskill, C. C., Parekh, P., Feinglos, M. N., . . . Lane, J. D. (2002). Stress management improves long-term glycemic control in type 2 diabetes. *Diabetes Care*, *25*(1), 30–34.

Tamez-Perez, H. E., Proskauer-Pena, S. L., Hernrndez-Coria, M. I., & Garber, A. J. (2013). AACE comprehensive diabetes management algorithm 2013. *Endocrine Practice: Official Journal of the American College of Endocrinology and the American Association of Clinical Endocrinologists*, *19*(4), 736–737. doi:10.4158/ep13210.lt

U.S. Preventive Services Task Force, Agency for Healthcare Research and Quality. (2009). Screening for depression in adults: U.S. Preventive Services Task Force recommendation statement. *Annals of Internal Medicine*, *151*(11), 784–792. doi:10.7326/0003-4819-151-11-200912010-00006

Van der Ven, N. C., Weinger, K., Yi, J., Pouwer, F., Adèr, H., Van Der Ploeg, H. M., & Snoek, F. J. (2003). The confidence in diabetes self-care scale psychometric properties of a new measure of diabetes-specific self-efficacy in Dutch and U.S. patients with type 1 diabetes. *Diabetes Care*, *26*(3), 713–718.

Virtanen, M., Ferrie, J. E., Tabak, A. G., Akbaraly, T. N., Vahtera, J., Singh-Manoux, A., & Kivimaki, M. (2014). Psychological distress and incidence of type 2 diabetes in high-risk and low-risk populations: The Whitehall II Cohort Study. *Diabetes Care*, *37*(8), 2091–2097. doi:10.2337/dc13-2725

Walker, R. J., Gebregziabher, M., Martin-Harris, B., & Egede, L. E. (2014). Relationship between social determinants of health and processes and outcomes in adults with type 2 diabetes: Validation of a conceptual framework. *BMC Endocrine Disorders*, *14*(1), 82. doi:10.1186/1472-6823-14-82

Walter, K. N., & Petry, N. M. (2014). Patients with diabetes respond well to contingency management treatment targeting alcohol and substance use. *Psychology, Health & Medicine*, *19*(6) 1–11. doi:10.1080/13548506.2014.991334

Weinger, K., Butler, H. A., Welch, G. W., & La Greca, A. M. (2005). Measuring diabetes self-care: A psychometric analysis of the self-care inventory-revised with adults. *Diabetes Care*, *28*(6), 1346–1352.

Welch, G. W., Jacobson, A. M., & Polonsky, W. H. (1997). The problem areas in diabetes scale. An evaluation of its clinical utility. *Diabetes Care*, *20*(5), 760–766.

Wen, L. K., Shepherd, M. D., & Parchman, M. L. (2004). Family support, diet, and exercise among older Mexican Americans with type 2 diabetes. *The Diabetes Educator*, *30*(6), 980–993.

Whitlock, E. P., Orleans, C. T., Pender, N., & Allan, J. (2002). Evaluating primary care behavioral counseling interventions: An evidence-based approach 1. *American Journal of Preventive Medicine*, 22(4), 267–284. doi:http://dx.doi.org/10.1016/S0749-3797(02)00415-4

Wisting, L., Froisland, D. H., Skrivarhaug, T., Dahl-Jorgensen, K., & Ro, O. (2013). Disturbed eating behavior and omission of insulin in adolescents receiving intensified insulin treatment: A nationwide population-based study. *Diabetes Care*, *36*(11), 3382–3387. doi:10.2337/dc13-0431

Wysocki, T., Greco, P., Harris, M. A., Bubb, J., & White, N. H. (2001). Behavior therapy for families of adolescents with diabetes: Maintenance of treatment effects. *Diabetes Care*, *24*(3), 441–446.

Wysocki, T., Harris, M. A., Buckloh, L. M., Mertlich, D., Lochrie, A. S., Taylor, A., . . . White, N. H. (2006). Effects of behavioral family systems therapy for diabetes on adolescents' family relationships, treatment adherence, and metabolic control. *Journal of Pediatric Psychology*, *31*(9), 928–938. doi:10.1093/jpepsy/jsj098

Wysocki, T. (1993). Associations among teen-parent relationships, metabolic control, and adjustment to diabetes in adolescents. *Journal of Pediatric Psychology*, *18*(4), 441–452. doi:10.1093/jpepsy/18.4.441

Zhu, Q., Lou, C., Gao, E., Cheng, Y., Zabin, L. S., & Emerson, M. R. (2015). Drunkenness and its association with health risk behaviors among adolescents and young adults in three Asian cities: Hanoi, Shanghai, Taipei. *Drug and Alcohol Dependence*, *147*, 251–256. doi:10.1016/j.drugalcdep.2014.10.029

RESOURCES FOR PERSONS WITH DIABETES

American Diabetes Association (ADA): www.diabetes.org Online resource in English and Spanish, with educational information, links to local association offices, professional resources, community chat rooms, and DiabetesPro SmartBrief e-mail newsletter.

TuDiabetes.org: www.tudiabetes.org (in English) and www.estudiabetes.org (in Spanish) offer video chats, blogs, groups, and forums.

BenefitsCheckup: www.benefitscheckup.org Online service developed by the National Council on Aging allows individuals to enter their income information to determine whether they are eligible for a variety of government benefits, including nutritional assistance (food stamps), government prescription assistance programs, and utility assistance.

Pharmaceutical assistance programs: Income-eligible patients without prescription medication coverage receive many medications free or at low cost. For example, insulins such as Apidra, Humalog, NovoLog, Levemir, and Lantus are available through company patient assistance programs. A comprehensive listing of available company programs can be found at www.NeedyMeds.org or by calling NeedyMeds at 800-503-6897. Similar online directories are available through Rx Assist (www.rxassist.org), Partnership for Prescription Assistance (www.pparx.org), and Goodrx.com. Online discount pharmacies such as RxOutreach (www.RxOutreach.org) may be able to provide reduced-cost medications and supplies.

Visual impairment services: State offices serving persons who are blind or visually impaired may offer assessment, in-home consultations, information/referral, vocational rehabilitation, assistive technology, social casework support, and training/equipment to support independent living.

Skilled medical home health care: Under Medicare, short-term in-home services are available for homebound persons. Services must be ordered by a physician and can include physical therapy, occupational therapy, speech-language pathology services, and "intermittent" skilled nursing, including education regarding diabetes self-care protocols.

Adult day centers: Depending on whether they are classified as social or medical, day programs may provide social activities, transportation, meals, personal care, therapeutic activities, and/or medication administration. The cost of attending may be covered by Medicaid, community Medicaid-waiver programs, or other government funding sources if paying privately is not possible.

YMCA's Diabetes Prevention Program: Healthy lifestyle education, coaching, and support. The programs provide group classes in 16 weekly sessions and eight follow-up monthly sessions. The cost is $430 but subsidies and scholarships are available for low-income populations, and some insurers cover the program. A national listing of participating YMCAs can be found at www.ymca.net/diabetes-prevention/participating-ys.html.

Nutrition supports:

- **Congregate meal centers for seniors:** Contact your local office on aging for meal center locations. A geographic search function that will provide local Office on Aging phone numbers is available at www.eldercare.gov.
- **Supplemental Nutrition Assistance Program (formerly Food Stamps)**: Contact your local/county board of social services or welfare office for instructions on how to apply. To check eligibility, patients can use BenefitsCheckup, described previously.
- **Meals on Wheels**: Home-delivered meals can be arranged for homebound older adults. Consult with your local Office on Aging for contact information.
- The BHS should develop a database of local supplementary food sources such as food banks.

Transportation: Low cost or free transportation for medical appointments is generally available for adults who are over age 60 or who receive long-term disability benefits. Contact your local/county Office on Aging for local information. For adults not over age 60 or disabled, especially those with low income or social support, the lack of transportation can pose a significant barrier to office visits. As practices and health systems become more accountable for clinical outcomes of care, including populations not covered by Medicare, the transportation issue will need to be addressed. Collaborations between large primary care practices or health systems and community agencies providing transport services may be able to develop systems that meet these needs.

Diabetes-specific assistance programs: A listing of national and state programs that assist persons with diabetes can be found on the NeedyMeds.org website by clicking Patient Savings and entering "diabetes" under the Diagnosis-Based Assistance tab (other medical conditions can also be searched). Programs listed provide a variety of supports, including assistive technology, durable medical assistance, and medical supplies.

FIVE

CARDIAC DISEASE AND BEHAVIORAL HEALTH

PAUL W. GOETZ, DEBORAH EDBERG, SANTINA WHEAT, AND CANDACE COLEMAN

S.O.A.P NOTE FROM REFERRING PRIMARY CARE PROVIDER (EMERGENCY DEPARTMENT)

S: RW is a 44-year-old male with a past medical history significant for Gastroesophageal reflux disease (GERD), chronic back pain, hyperlipidemia, and obesity. He came to the Emergency Department (ED) with a several hour history of severe abdominal/chest pain while he was sleeping at home. He took Pepcid without relief. Pain began to radiate into left arm. Drove himself to ED. Denies nausea/vomiting, diaphoresis. + Mild shortness of breath.

Past medical history: GERD × 6 years, lower back pain s/p work injury 5 years prior, HTN, Hyperlipidemia (HLD), obesity
Medications: Crestor, Lotensin, Ibuprofen, Norco prn back pain
Surgical history: L5-S1 Fusion 2013
Family history:
Grandfather—Myocardial infarction (MI) at 49 years old
Father: MI at 45 years old; s/p CABG × 2; hypertension; HLD; obesity; osteoarthritis (s/p b/l hip replacements, knee replacement); Barrett's esophagus s/p esophagectomy with Grade 3 dysplasia, smoker
Mother: COPD; chronic bronchitis (second-hand smoker)
Sister: Sjögren's
Brother: Hyperlipidemia (HLD)
Social history:
Previous smoker—10 pack-year, quit 5 years ago
Occasional marijuana, no IV drug use
Daily alcohol—two to three glasses wine, occasional scotch/beer
Lives alone, unemployed for 5 years—had been in sales, currently working at school as teacher's aide
Close family support—both parents live in town
Relatively sedentary due to back pain

O: Temp: 97.9
Pulse: 105

Respirations: 20, 96% oxygenation on room air
Blood pressure: 135/80
Gen: slightly pale, diaphoretic, visible discomfort, awake, alert & oriented x3, overweight
HEENT: atraumatic/normocephalic, moist mucous membranes, no goiter
Chest: clear to auscultation bilaterally
CV: mildly elevated rate, normal rhythm, no murmur
Abd: soft, nontender, nondistended, no hepatosplenomegaly/masses; + scar lumbar spine
Ext: no edema
Neuro: grossly normal
Labs:
CMP normal
LDL: 84; total Chol: 200; HDL 32
CBC normal
Trop: 2.3
EKG: ST segment elevation myocardial infarction (STEMI) in lateral leads
Angio: left circumflex 100%; LAD 70%
Echo: moderate hypokinetic defect with EF 50%

A: 44 yo male with PMH of GERD, HLD, and obesity. He lives alone and does have excessive alcohol intake. He presented to the ED and left circumflex was stented.

P:
1. Medically manage CAD poststent- Beta Blocker and Aspirin; plan to stent LAD in 1-2 weeks.
2. Follow patient on Beta Blocker and may need to decrease ACE but will try to optimize therapy.
3. HLD well controlled with current medication regimen.
4. Referral to behavioral health specialist for evaluation and treatment recommendations.

INTRODUCTION

Heart disease is the leading cause of death in the United States (e.g., Mathers & Loncar, 2006; Rosamond et al., 2007) and the majority of the risk factors for heart disease, which are discussed in more detail in the following, are modifiable. Therefore, understanding and addressing heart disease from a psychological and behavioral perspective are imperative. In addition to psychological and behavioral risk factors, there are a number of common psychological sequelae that are associated with receiving a cardiac diagnosis, cardiac surgery, medical management of the disease, and morbidity and mortality. The focus of the behavioral health specialist with the cardiac patient is to address not only the risk factors associated with heart disease, but to also address the psychological distress and maladaptive behaviors that can be associated with increased morbidity and mortality. This chapter reviews common psychological factors associated with cardiovascular disease (CVD) and methods of assessment in cardiac patients, and provides examples of intervention strategies to improve mental health and health behavior risk factors in CVD.

While it is important and interesting that links between the mind and heart have been established, it is equally important to understand the mechanisms involved in this relationship. One mechanism is neurobiological in nature. The vagus nerve establishes a bidirectional pathway between the brain and heart. This variability in vagal activity, in turn, creates heart rate variability (HRV; e.g., Porges, 2007). There is empirical evidence linking depression and anxiety with low respiratory sinus arrhythmia (RSA) (e.g., Thayer & Lane, 2002, 2009) and low RSA is associated with CVD (e.g., Masi, Hawkley, Rickett, & Cacioppo, 2007; Thayer & Lane, 2007). Other neurobiological mechanisms involve the dysregulation of the hypothalamic–pituitary–adrenal (HPA) axis (Stetler & Miller, 2011) and metabolic imbalances (Pan et al., 2012). In addition to the aforementioned mechanisms, health behaviors (e.g., medical adherence, smoking, diet, exercise) can largely be affected by factors such as depression and anxiety (e.g., Alcántra et al., 2014; Kessing, Pelle, Kupper, Szabo, & Denollet, 2014). Additionally, an individual's cognitive functioning (e.g., capacity to attend to and remember health information) as well as perceptions and beliefs about his or her cardiac condition also affect outcomes (e.g., Juergens, Seekatz, Moosdorf, Petrie, & Rief, 2010; Tully, Baune, & Baker, 2013).

The traditional risk factors for coronary heart disease (CHD) involve non modifiable and modifiable factors (Figure 5.1). Non modifiable factors are variables we have no control over, such as family history, gender, and age. Modifiable risk factors account for the majority of the variance in developing CHD. Specifically, the INTER-HEART study found that the following risk factors accounted for 90% and 94% of the population attributable risk in males

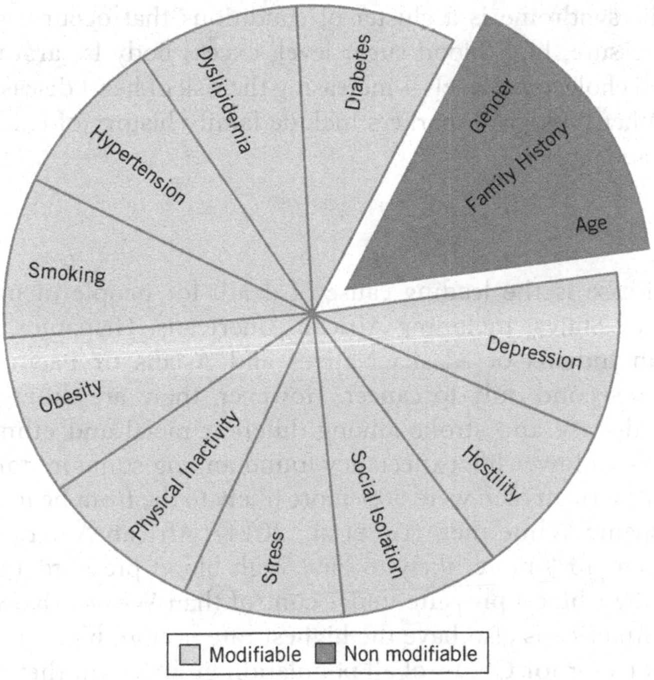

Figure 5.1 Risk factors for coronary heart disease (CHD). Adapted from Allan and Fisher (2012), p. 6. Copyright American Psychological Association.

and females, respectively: smoking, hypertension, cholesterol, diabetes, obesity, diet, sedentary lifestyle, and psychological factors such as social isolation and depression (Yusuf et al., 2004). These risk factors involve behavioral components and, therefore, opportunities for behavioral intervention.

EPIDEMIOLOGY OF CARDIAC DISEASE

CVD is common in the general population, affecting the majority of adults over 60 years old. CVD includes major physical conditions such as CHD, heart attacks (myocardial infarction [MI]), strokes, and peripheral artery disease. There are approximately 700,000 people who die of heart disease in the United States every year, one in every three deaths, making heart disease the leading cause of death for both men and women. Every year over 900,000 Americans have a heart attack. Of these, 620,000 are a first heart attack and 295,000 happen in people who have already had a heart attack (Go et al., 2014). CHD costs the United States $314.5 billion each year—including cost of health care services, medications, and lost productivity. Even though CVD mortality has declined by 31% over the past 40 years (Go et al., 2014), it is costly to treat and remains the leading cause of death in the United States and other Western countries. Consequently, addressing the factors that prevent CVD and minimizing risk factors after a cardiac event are important for prevention, quality of life, and containing health care costs.

Physiological Factors

Metabolic syndrome is a cluster of conditions that occur together—increased blood pressure, high blood sugar level, excess body fat around the waist, and abnormal cholesterol levels—increasing the risk of heart disease, stroke, and diabetes. Other biological markers include family history of cardiac disease, heart attacks, and stroke.

Ethnicity

Heart disease is the leading cause of death for people of most ethnicities in the United States, including African Americans, Hispanics, and Whites. For American Indians or Alaska Natives and Asians or Pacific Islanders, heart disease is second only to cancer. However, there are differences in the rates of heart disease and stroke among different racial and ethnic groups, which contribute to lower life expectancy found among some minorities. As of 2007, African American men were 50% more likely to die from heart disease than were non-Hispanic White men (Go et al., 2014). African American adults of both genders are 40% more likely to have high blood pressure and 27% less likely to have their blood pressure under control than Whites (Howard et al., 2006). African Americans also have the highest rate of high blood pressure—a significant risk factor for CVD—of all population groups, and they tend to develop it earlier in life than other ethnic groups (Go et al., 2014).

Men and Heart Disease

Men are at the greatest risk for cardiac disease. About 8.2% of all White men, 6.8% of Black men, and 6.7% of Mexican American men have CHD (Centers for Disease Control and Prevention National Health and Nutrition Exam Survey [CDC NHANES], 2007–2010). Between 70% and 89% of sudden cardiac events occur in men (Go et al., 2014). Heart disease may have no obvious physical signs, making it a dangerous disease and a silent killer. In fact, half of the men who die suddenly of CHD have had no previous symptoms.

Women and Heart Disease

Heart disease is the leading cause of death for women in the United States, killing nearly 422,000 each year, nearly one in every four female deaths. Following a heart attack, approximately one in four women will die within the first year, compared to one in five men (CDC National Center for Health Statistics, 1999–2010). Although heart disease is sometimes thought of as a "man's disease," around the same number of women and men die each year of heart disease in the United States. About 4.6% of all White women, 7.1% of Black women, and 5.3% of Mexican American women have CHD (CDC NHANES, 2007–2010). Despite increases in awareness over the past decade, only 56% of women recognize that heart disease is their number one killer. Like men, two thirds (64%) of women who die suddenly of CHD have no previous physical symptoms (Go et al., 2014). Heart disease is the leading cause of death for African American and White women in the United States. For Hispanic women, risk of dying from heart disease and cancer is equal, while for American Indian or Alaska Native and Asian or Pacific Islander women, heart disease is the second cause of death after cancer.

Heart Disease and Age

Many people mistakenly think of heart disease and stroke as conditions that only affect older adults. However, a large number of younger people suffer heart attacks and strokes. About 150,000 people who died from CVD in 2010 were younger than age 65 (CDC National Center for Health Statistics, 1999–2010).

PSYCHOLOGICAL FACTORS IN DISEASE MANAGEMENT AND ADHERENCE

It is well established that an individual's psychological makeup has a great impact not only on risk factors for developing CVD, but also on managing the disease and adhering to treatments and medical recommendations (e.g., Seldenrijk et al., 2015; Tully & Baune, 2014). When examining psychological factors associated with CVD, it is important to keep in mind that these factors interact with one another and are bi-directional (e.g., depressive symptoms impact exercise; exercise impacts depressive symptoms). The following is a review of common psychological and behavioral factors associated with the management of CVD and adherence to treatment. This is not an exclusive review, but rather a look at the more common sequelae likely to be seen in a primary care setting.

Mental Health and Personality Factors

Depression

Depression is characterized by sadness, sleep disturbance, anhedonia, loss of energy, feelings of worthlessness, notable change in weight, and diminished cognitive abilities such as concentration. Of note, somatic symptoms of depression are the same as certain symptoms in cardiac diseases such as coronary artery disease (CAD), including sleep disturbance and fatigue, which is important to keep in mind during assessment and treatment of depression in the cardiac population. The non-somatic symptoms of depression (depressed mood, anhedonia, feelings of worthlessness or guilt, suicidal thinking) may carry greater weight when assessing cardiac patients for depression. It is important to consult with the primary care provider to obtain relevant medical data to understand the severity of the patient's cardiac condition, which will help give a better understanding of how much of the patient's somatic symptoms may be related to the cardiac diagnosis, versus depression. However, knowing that these factors can be difficult to tease apart, especially initially, it is still important to address these symptoms, such as sleep disturbance, from a psychological perspective.

There is a plethora of research examining the relationship between cardiac health and mood, especially depression (e.g., Tully & Baune, 2014; Tully, Cosh, & Baumeister, 2014). Depression has been shown to be an independent predictor for increased mortality following MI (e.g., Frasure-Smith, Lesperance, & Talajic,1995) and individuals with current depression have a two- to threefold increased risk of CVD over a period of years (Seldenrijk et al., 2015). Moreover, research demonstrates an exposure-response relationship between depression and cardiac risk (e.g., Seldenrijk et al., 2015). The greater level or degree of depressive disorder leads to a greater risk of CVD.

Depression is also associated with poorer self-care behaviors and a generally more unhealthy lifestyle, for example, smoking and little physical activity (Bonnet et al., 2005), and poorer compliance with medications (Grenard et al., 2011). Additionally, as indicated previously, there are neurobiological influences involved in the depression–CVD relationship (e.g., Thayer & Lane 2009). More recently, researchers have begun to look at specific components of depression that may contribute to CVD and mortality. For example, Barefoot et al. (2000) found hopelessness and depressive affect to be better predictors, relative to other depressive symptoms, for reduced survival in individuals with CAD.

Like many other medical conditions, depression is more likely to be present in individuals with CVD (e.g., Lesperance & Frasure-Smith, 2000). Prevalence of depression in individuals with cardiac diagnoses is greater than in the general population (Celano & Huffman, 2011). For example, Rutledge, Reis, Linke, Greenberg, and Mills (2006) conducted a meta-analysis in which they found 21.6% of patients with heart failure experience clinical depression. Celano and Huffman (2011) indicate that 31% to 45% of patients with CAD also suffer from clinical symptoms of depression.

In addition to depression being associated with cardiac diseases themselves, patients are also at risk for developing depression following cardiac surgery (for a review, see Ravven, Bader, Azar, & Rudolph, 2013), which is associated with higher postsurgical morbidity and mortality (Blumenthal et al., 2003). After controlling for other factors, Blumenthal et al. (2003) found that patients with clinically significant depression had a two- to threefold increase in likelihood of mortality following coronary artery bypass graft (CABG). Likewise, Ho et al. (2005) found that preoperative depression was independently predictive of higher mortality at 6 months following valve surgery. This highlights the importance of depressive symptoms in preoperative screening as well as postoperative follow-up.

Anxiety

The role of anxiety in cardiac disease is less well understood. A recent systematic review found the prevalence of any anxiety disorders (excluding posttraumatic stress disorder [PTSD]) to be 15.52% in CHD patients. Prevalence of anxiety in patients with implantable-cardioverter defibrillators (ICDs) is between 11% and 28% (Magyar-Russell et al., 2011). An ICD is a device that delivers an electrical shock to mitigate arrhythmias that may be life-threatening. Depending on the characteristics of the arrhythmia, the ICD may not ever discharge for some patients, and for others, it may discharge often, which can lead to anxiety (see Sears, Matchett, Vazquez, & Conti, 2012, for a review). Like depression, anxiety is also associated with poorer cardiac outcomes. Specifically, anxiety and worry are associated with greater risk of CHD and worse outcomes (Kubzansky et al. 1997; Kubzansky, Kawachi, Weiss, & Sparrow, 1998).

Like depression, the physical symptoms of anxiety are often similar or the same as many cardiac symptoms. The physical symptoms of panic disorder are a good example (e.g., change in heart rate and respiration, light-headedness, dizziness). Therefore, it is not uncommon for patients to worry that their anxiety symptoms are due to their cardiac illness. For example, when patients are experiencing panic symptoms, they may have thoughts such as "I'm having a (another) heart attack," "I'm going to die," or "My ICD is going to go off."

The research on anxiety and CVD has largely examined anxiety as a general, singular construct, rather than looking at specific anxiety disorders or symptoms (e.g., Seldenrijk et al., 2015; Tully et al., 2011). However, recent literature in this area does suggest some common factors in the anxiety–CVD relationship. Researchers have begun looking at subgroups and specific diagnoses within anxiety. Generalized anxiety disorder (GAD) is associated with higher morbidity following cardiac surgery (Tully et al., 2011) and panic disorder specifically was associated with increased risk of CVD (Seldenrijk et al., 2015).

The mechanisms through which anxiety is linked to CVD are similar to those of depression—neurobiological (e.g., decreased vagal activity) and behavioral (e.g., physical inactivity, medication nonadherence, poor diet). Anxiety can often lead to avoidant behavior, which may result in behaviors such as not engaging in medical follow-up because of the potential of "bad news," not taking medications due to anxiety about side effects, or not exercising due to the fear of possibly having another heart attack.

Anger and Hostility

Anger is another psychological factor commonly associated with CVD. Anger and hostility are often lumped together when discussing phenomenon associated with these terms. However, it is important to distinguish anger from hostility. Hostility is described as "negative attitude toward others, consisting of enmity, denigration, and ill will" (Smith, 1994, p. 26), whereas anger is "an unpleasant emotion ranging in intensity from irritation or annoyance to fury or rage" (Smith, 1994, p. 26). Aggression is the overt behavior that results from these emotional and affective states.

Research has shown that anger and hostility are associated with increased CHD events in initially healthy individuals, as well as poorer prognosis and recurrent cardiac events in patients already diagnosed with CHD (Chida & Steptoe, 2009). There is also research to suggest that hostility may be the key risk factor related to CVD (e.g., Guerrero & Palmero, 2010; Miller, Smith, Turner, Guijarro, & Hallet, 1996; Stewart, Fitzgerald, & Kamarck, 2010). Guerreo and Palmero (2010) found that defensive hostility, specifically, was associated with greater cardiac reactivity compared to hostility in general. Stewart et al. (2010) suggest that hostility increases and may promote depressive symptoms, acting as the mechanism to which hostility increases risk for CAD.

Personality Factors

The association between certain character traits and CVD risk has been complicated. Initially, researchers were focused on Type-A behavior, which is associated with time urgency and hostility (e.g., Friedman & Rosenman, 1974). However, more recent research has raised doubts about a Type-A personality being a reliable risk factor (e.g., Razzini et al., 2008). A Type-D (distressed) personality is characterized by two primary traits: negative affectivity and social inhibition (Denollet & Pedersen, 2012). This means individuals with a Type-D personality style experience themselves, others, and the world in a generally negative light, and they tend to inhibit expressing these emotions in social contexts and keeping people at a distance (Denollet & Pedersen, 2012). This combination of traits is related to increased morbidity and mortality in patients with CAD (Razzini et al., 2008). Moreover, while a Type-D personality consists of negative affectivity, there is evidence to suggest that a Type-D personality is associated with CAD, independent of depression (e.g., Vukovic et al., 2014).

BEHAVIORAL HEALTH ASSESSMENT OF CARDIAC PATIENTS

As reviewed previously, cardiac symptoms often have overlap with somatic symptoms of depression and anxiety. Therefore, it is important to have a basic understanding of the cardiac diagnosis with which the patient is presenting. This will be important to know not only from an assessment perspective but also from a treatment standpoint. For example, a patient who presents with anxiety associated with being shocked five times by an ICD will be treated differently than a patient who has anxiety about heart failure symptoms. Familiarity with the basic symptoms of the patient's cardiac diagnosis and keeping these symptoms in mind when conducting a psychological assessment are recommended.

Clinical Interview

A thorough clinical interview will help identify cognitions, emotions, and behaviors associated with a patient's cardiac diagnosis (see Table 5.1 for specific assessment topics and questions). Obtain the patient's understanding of his or her cardiac condition. This will provide an idea of any education that may be needed for the patient, possible cognitive deficits that may interfere with self-care, or acceptance of the cardiac illness. Along the same lines, it is important to get the patient's understanding of the current medical treatment (e.g., does the patient know the names of his or her medications, what are the medications for, and the dosages?).

Gathering information about the patient's social history will provide information about current and potential social support. Support is important for cardiac patients not only from an emotional standpoint, but also from a practical perspective (e.g., help with medications, getting rides to appointments, having another set of ears to hear medical information). Depending on the type of surgery

TABLE 5.1 Cardiac Behavioral Medicine Interview Questions

Domain	Example Question Topics
Social History	– With whom does the patient reside – Employment or disability – Life stressors – Transportation method to medical appointments
Health Behaviors	– Exercise – Diet (e.g., sodium and fat intake) – Amount of fluids consumed, especially if diagnosis of congestive heart failure – Medical follow-up – Alcohol, tobacco, Illicit drug use (frequency, amount, duration of use) – Motivation and self-efficacy to change behaviors
Compliance	– Symptom reporting – Medication compliance; reminder system for medications (e.g., pillbox) – Patient's knowledge about medications
Psychiatric	– Level of alertness and orientation – Speech rhythm, rate, volume – Notable cognitive deficits (e.g., difficulties with concentration or memory) – History or depression, anxiety, or other psychiatric issues – Current depressive or anxiety symptoms (follow diagnostic criteria) – History of or current suicidal ideation – Family psychiatric history – Recent changes in weight – Change in sleep – Panic symptoms – Current psychotropic medications – Current understanding of their cardiovascular disease status

(e.g., minimally invasive versus open heart sternotomy), a patient will need postsurgical assistance with daily activities. While it is ideal for a postsurgical patient to resume daily life activities as soon as possible, there may be restrictions, such as no driving, no lifting of objects heavier than 5 to 10 pounds, and upper body mobility restrictions. Physical recovery may take 6 to 8 weeks, during which time support will be critical. The postsurgical patient may qualify for home health nursing or aides to help with medications and other home care needs.

As reviewed, health behaviors are critical to cardiac health. Obtain specific information (quantity, frequency, and duration of use) about smoking, alcohol, and illicit drug use. Also, given the association between diet and physical activity and CVD (e.g., Ahmed, Blaha, Nasir, Rivera, & Blumenthal, 2012; Bhupathiraju & Tucker, 2011), assess the patient's diet and regular exercise routine. Relatedly, inquire about adherence to medications, medical follow-up, and reporting new or exacerbation of current symptoms.

Assessment of the patient's psychiatric functioning should involve history of depression and anxiety, as well as other psychiatric issues that are uncovered during the interview. It is important to obtain, if possible, specific thoughts and emotions about the patient's cardiac illness, which would be potential targets for intervention. For example, the patient who presents with a diagnosis of CAD, has an ICD, and exhibits symptoms of depression and anxiety may have thoughts that he or she cannot engage in any enjoyable life activities for fear the ICD will discharge, and that he or she is destined to a life of sedentariness. In addition to psychiatric symptoms, it is also important to know if the patient is taking any psychotropic medications, as certain medications may be contraindicated for certain cardiac diagnoses (see Table 5.2 for common examples). In addition to a clinical interview, it is also helpful to obtain more objective data in the form of assessment instruments.

Assessment Instruments

There are a number of instruments that have been utilized to assess psychological functioning in cardiac patients. For example, the Beck Depression Inventory (BDI-II), State-Trait Anxiety Inventory (STAI), and the Patient Health Questionnaire (PHQ-9) are several common anxiety and depression assessment tools. They are brief, which would be conducive to primary care settings. Refer to Table 5.3 for a summary of brief paper/pencil instruments that may be utilized. Following is a review of a few examples.

The BDI-II is a 21-item self-report measure assessing cognitive, affective, and somatic symptoms of depression. Patients select one of several items to best describe how they have been feeling in the previous 2 weeks, where each option is associated with a score ranging from 0 to 3. A summary score is calculated, with possible scores ranging from 0 to 63. Higher scores indicate higher levels of depressive symptoms (Beck, Steer, & Brown, 1996). The inventory has been shown to be a reliable and valid measure of depression (Osman et al., 1997).

The STAI (Spielberger, Gorsuch, & Lushene, 1970) comprises 20 statements related to anxiety such as "I feel nervous and restless." Each statement is rated on a scale ranging from 1 (seldom/never) to 4 (very often). Total scores range from 20 to 80 and a higher score indicates greater levels of state anxiety. Factor

TABLE 5.2 Common Psychotropic Medication Contraindications in Cardiac Disease

Medication	Concern
Anxiolytics	Acute withdrawal from benzodiazepines (especially short acting) may be life-threatening in unstable cardiac patients. Beta-blockers should not be used as anti-anxiety agents in patients with congestive heart failure because they decrease cardiac contractility and may worsen failure.
Tricyclic antidepressants	Can have arrhythmogenic side effects and are not recommended for most coronary heart disease patients
Monoamine oxidase inhibitors (MAOIs)—antidepressants	Can induce orthostatic hypotension
Neuroleptics	Caution for patients with preexisting conduction (rhythm) issues (e.g., long QT syndrome)
Carbamazepine (mood stabilizer)	Can lead to atrioventricular conduction disturbances

Note: This table is not an all-inclusive list of possible psychotropic contraindications in cardiovascular disease (for reviews, see Kop & Plumhoff, 2012; Murray, 2000; Robinson & Levenson, 2000).

TABLE 5.3 Brief Assessment Instruments

Measure	Description
Patient Health Questionnaire (PHQ-9)	A nine-item assessment of depressive symptoms
Beck Depression Inventory (BDI-II)	A 21-item self-report measure assessing cognitive, affective, and somatic symptoms of depression
State-Trait Anxiety Inventory (STAI)	An anxiety assessment comprised of 20 statements related to anxiety such as "I feel nervous and restless"
Beck Anxiety Inventory (BAI)	A 21-item self-report instrument for measuring the severity of anxiety
Montreal Cognitive Assessment (MoCA)	Designed as a rapid screening instrument for mild cognitive dysfunction in eight domains
The Short Form-12 Health Survey (SF-12)	A measure of health-related quality of life that assesses general health constructs such as physical functioning, energy/fatigue, and pain
Perceived Stress Scale (PSS)	A 14-item assessment measuring the degree to which one perceives life events as stressful
Interpersonal Support Evaluation List (ISEL)	A 12-item measure assessing perceived social support and resources

Note: PHQ-9 (Kroenke et al., 2001), BDI-II (Beck, Steer, & Brown, 1996), STAI (Spielberger, Gorsuch, & Lushene, 1970), BAI (Beck, Epstein, Brown, & Steer, 1988), MoCA (Nasreddine et al., 2005), SF-12 (Ware, Kosinski, & Keller, 1996), PSS (Cohen, Kamarck, & Mermelstein, 1983), ISEL (Cohen, Mermelstein, Kamarck, & Hoberman, 1985).

analysis of the STAI indicates the presence of two subscales: anxiety-present and anxiety-absent (Spielberger et al., 1970). Anxiety-absent items are reversed-scored, meaning that lower scores reflect less anxiety, and a total anxiety score is obtained by adding the total scores from both subscales. The STAI has been shown to be psychometrically sound (Spielberger, Gorsuch, Lushene, Vagg, & Jacobs, 1983).

The PHQ-9 is a nine-item depression assessment tool. Major depression is present if five or more of the nine criteria have been present at least "more than half the days" in the past 2 weeks, and one of the symptoms is depressed mood or anhedonia. Other depression is present if two, three, or four criteria have been present at least "more than half the days" in the past 2 weeks, and one of the symptoms is depressed mood or anhedonia. One of the nine criteria ("thoughts that you would be better off dead or hurting yourself in some way") counts if present at all, regardless of duration. Each item is scored from 0 (not at all) to 3 (nearly every day) and total scores range from 0 to 27. A question about daily functioning was added to the questionnaire "How difficult have these problems made it for you to do your work, take care of things at home, or get along with other people?" The PHQ-9 has good reliability and validity in a clinical setting (e.g., Kroenke, Spitzer, & Williams, 2001).

BRIEF COUNSELING METHODS

In this section we address the brief counseling interventions that may be implemented for patients presenting with cardiac diagnoses in a primary care setting. A behavioral health specialist may see a cardiac patient for health maintenance (i.e., changing and maintaining health behaviors), addressing depression or anxiety related to a new cardiac diagnosis, or following an emergency department visit for a cardiac event. A cardiac patient may also be referred for coping with recovery following a cardiac surgery (e.g., depressive symptoms, lifestyle changes, or being confronted with the patient's own mortality). To date, there is no consistent evidence to suggest that psychological interventions alone reduce morbidity or mortality in patients with CVD (e.g., Whalley, Thompson, & Taylor, 2012). Earlier studies showed some positive outcomes. For example, Blumenthal et al. (1997) found that a stress management program reduced recurrence of cardiac events in patients with CHD. Ornish et al.'s (1998) intense lifestyle change program, including stress management and group support, significantly reduced coronary atherosclerosis and subjects in the program had fewer cardiac events compared to a control group. Many recent studies have been unable to find such results, as revealed in systematic reviews (e.g., Whalley et al., 2012). For example, the large multicenter ENRICHD trial (ENRICHD Investigators, 2003) involved 2,481 post-MI patients who had depression or low perceived social support. Patients were either assigned to cognitive behavioral therapy (CBT) sessions to target depressive symptoms or to a "usual care" group. At 6-month follow-up, the CBT group fared better in terms of depressive symptoms. However, there were no significant differences in terms of cardiac outcomes.

Cognitive Behavioral Therapy

CBT involves addressing maladaptive thoughts and behaviors that contribute to psychological distress such as depression and anxiety (Clark & Beck, 2010). The goal of CBT is to change thought patterns that are associated with depression or anxiety. A patient with CHD, for example, may have the thought "I am useless because I can no longer contribute to my family the way I used to." The cognitive aspect of CBT would help the patient develop a more adaptive and realistic perspective (e.g., "I cannot do some of the activities I used to, but I am still able to contribute to my family in meaningful ways"). The behavioral aspect involves interventions such as activity scheduling to increase activity and structure, utilizing social support, and developing or reengaging in activities that are positively reinforcing. If cardiac patients are functionally limited due to symptoms, coming up with more passive activities may be necessary, with the goal being to minimize time for rumination and enhance positively reinforcing behaviors.

Relaxation and Diaphragmatic Breathing

Introducing cardiac patients to relaxation and diaphragmatic breathing strategies has shown some promise in terms of psychological and physiological outcomes (Collins & Rice, 1997; Dixhoorn, 1998). Relaxation typically involves progressive muscle relaxation (PMR), which involves instructing the patient to focus on individual muscle groups and to flex the muscle group for several seconds, and then to release the tension and experience the relaxation of the muscle, with the relaxation phase being longer in duration relative to the flexing phase. The goal with PMR is to help the patient become more aware of muscle tension and to implement the practice of relaxing the muscles when tension is identified. Of note, it is recommended to ask the patient if he or she experiences pain any place in the body, and to avoid focus in that particular area. Autogenic muscle relaxation (AMR) involves focusing on a muscle group and utilizing imagery and relaxing trigger words (e.g., relax, loose, peaceful, warm) to describe the state in which the muscles are relaxed. The patient should be instructed to be mindful of how the muscles and body feel when relaxed. Again, avoid areas of the body in which the patient may be experiencing pain. Relaxation strategies should be practiced several times per day to gain the most benefit. Like most learned behaviors, the more often these strategies are practiced, the more automatic they will become. The behavioral health specialist would provide a brief introduction to these strategies and instruct the patient to extend the time on each muscle group when the patient is practicing alone. There are a variety of websites, phone apps, or audio instruction dedicated to relaxation that may be helpful for patients, especially when first learning these strategies.

Diaphragmatic breathing involves the practice of breathing from the diaphragm rather than from the chest. Breathing from the diaphragm, the primary muscle involved in respiration, decreases respiration rate and heart rate, and is associated with a relaxed state. Often when we are in a stressed state, we breathe from the chest, which can lead to hyperventilation or other irregular respiration patterns and contribute to a cycle of somatic anxiety symptoms. The exact mechanisms are not well understood but it is thought that diaphragmatic breathing changes oxygen and carbon dioxide levels, resulting in greater parasympathetic nervous system activity and physiological relaxation (for a review, see Gevirtz & Schwartz, 2003). It is often helpful for patients to learn this technique by placing one hand on the chest and another on the stomach to be able to determine how much they are utilizing their diaphragm. The goal is to have the bottom hand move more than the hand on their chest. Patients can use imagery such as picturing their stomach like a balloon and imagine it inflating as they breathe in, and deflating as they breathe out. The patient should practice diaphragmatic breathing in combination with relaxation strategies.

Health Behavior Intervention

Given the often-limited treatment time in the primary care setting, brief interventions for health behavior risk factors (e.g., smoking, poor diet, physical inactivity) may provide opportunity for more immediate change. As reviewed already, psychological interventions are often coupled with lifestyle changes for cardiac patients (e.g., Ornish et al., 1998). Enhancing self-efficacy and motivation, and encouraging behavior change should be a focus of intervention with health behaviors. Utilizing the clinical interview, it is important to assess the cognitive, environmental, and resource barriers to making these changes. Educating patients on the deleterious effects of negative health behaviors on their cardiac health is a good place to start. As well, having patients monitor their health behaviors with written journals or logs will provide the behavioral health specialist and the patient more insight into the behavior and, therefore, data to use to help change the behavior.

Complementary Interventions

Yoga

Yoga means, "joining or yoking together" and encompasses the physical, mental, and spiritual practices used to transform the body and mind. The physical practices (i.e., asana) are most well known to the West, but the breathing (i.e., pranayama) and meditation techniques are also integrated into many classes. There are many forms of yoga that emphasize different aspects of breathing, physical movement, and meditation. Hatha yoga is the form most known and commonly practiced in the West, and works through physical movement and breathing to positively impact the mind and cultivate awareness. It can be practiced in many styles, such as Ashtanga, Integral, Kripalu, Iyengar, and Bikram. It is important to determine from patients which form of yoga they are practicing, and to discuss individual physical restrictions and precautions. A Bikram class, for example, uses a set series of postures in a heated room, or extended inversion positions or vigorous breathing and would likely not be appropriate for a patient with CVD.

Yoga as a physical exercise and mindfulness practice has gained much attention recently in its treatment applications, especially since the U.S. Department of Defense funded several large studies on yoga in PTSD (Engel et al., 2015). A 2012 systematic review evaluated ten randomized controlled trials (RCTs) comparing yoga with wait-list controls, relaxation, therapy, anxiety education, or exercise. Of these ten RCTs, seven moderate- to high-quality studies found statistically significant reductions in anxiety and stress in yoga groups as compared with controls (Li & Goldsmith, 2012). Across three systematic reviews of yoga for depression, anxiety, and stress, yoga produced overall reductions of symptoms between 12% and 76%, with an average of 39% net reduction (Skowronek, Mounsey, & Handler, 2014).

In addition to improving mood symptoms that can exacerbate CVD, yoga has been used effectively in the management and reversal of CVD itself. For example, reviews of RCTs have found that yoga has favorable effects on blood pressure and cholesterol (Hartley et al., 2014; Yogendra et al., 2004). Dietary change plus yoga has been found to be associated with fewer angina episodes per week, improved exercise capacity, decreased body weight, lower serum total cholesterol levels, and less frequent revascularization procedures (Manchanda et al., 2000). In another study, yoga reduced oxidative stress and improved antioxidant defense in elderly hypertensive individuals (Patil, Dhanakshirur, Aithala, Naregal, & Das, 2014).

There are a number of purported healing mechanisms of yoga; one mechanism proposed is the measured increase in vagus nerve activity. The rubbing together of limbs and pressure from the floor stimulates mechanoreceptors in the dermis that are innervated by vagal afferent fibers (O'Keane, Dinan, Scott, & Corcoran, 2005). The increased vagal response or induction of the parasympathetic nervous system contributes to a reduction in cortisol, which lowers blood pressure and blood glucose levels. The induction of the parasympathetic nervous system also enhances immune function by decreasing inflammatory markers and increasing T cells. The behavioral health specialist may want to be familiar with local and/or Internet sources that can provide the patient with a gentle introduction to yoga practice.

BASIC NEEDS, SOCIAL SERVICES, AND COMMUNITY REFERRALS

Beyond having good primary care established, a patient with a cardiac diagnosis should have a team of providers to ensure the best care in several domains. Ideally, this team of providers would include the patient's primary care doctor, a cardiologist, a nurse, a nutritional therapist, and a behavioral health specialist. In addition to the medical treatment the patient obtains, providing education, psychological intervention and support, and community resources will help ensure the patient has the tools to engage in adaptive self-care. In addition to what has been covered in this chapter with regard to psychological intervention, cardiac patients may need practical resources such as transportation to appointments, assistance with filling a pillbox if they have limited capacity and support to do it on their own, and financial assistance to afford medications. It is also helpful to be aware of cardiac rehabilitation programs in your area. While a patient may be encouraged to exercise, he or she may need special physical assistance or cardiac monitoring to ensure safety. A team approach and these additional resources are critical to ensuring the cardiac patient is successful at engaging in adaptive self-care.

BEHAVIORAL HEALTH ASSESSMENT AND TREATMENT SUMMARY TO REFERRING PRIMARY CARE PROVIDER

Cardiac Behavioral Medicine Health and Behavior Evaluation

Subjective

Mr. W is a 44-year-old, Caucasian, single cardiac patient referred for a health and behavior evaluation. The patient recently drove himself to the emergency department with severe abdominal and chest pain, with the pain starting to radiate to his left arm. He also complained of mild shortness of breath. It was determined he had an MI, at which time he was taken to the cath lab and stented. He was discharged with medical management and a plan for a left anterior descending (LAD) stent in 1 to 2 weeks. A consultation was requested to assess the patient's psychosocial and behavioral risk factors for heart disease and to identify any psychosocial or behavioral barriers to heart health and recovery.

Objective

Mr. W has a bachelor's degree in business and worked in a sales department for 15 years. Most recently he had been on disability after a work injury 5 years ago and recently started working part time as a teacher's aide at a local high school. He stated that he did well in school ("As and Bs") and denied having difficulty with reading or writing.

Social History

Mr. W was married for 10 years and divorced 3 years ago. He is not in contact with his ex-wife. He currently lives alone and does not have a significant other or children. Both of his parents live in the city (within a few miles of him). He has a good relationship with his parents, who are both retired, and they have been supportive financially and emotionally. He does not have any siblings but does have a number of "very close" friends. When he is not working, he usually spends time at his parents' house or with friends.

The patient reports the following life stressors: current medical situation and financial hardship.

Mr. W reports having minimal coping strategies. Specifically, he stated that when he feels stressed, anxious, or down, he typically "retreats," isolating himself from others and he tends to ruminate on whatever is bothering him. He has good social support, primarily consisting of his parents and several close friends. However, it seems he does not utilize this support when needed.

Health Behaviors

Mr. W reported that he smoked tobacco cigarettes "on occasion" (about 10 packs a year) and quit 5 years ago without lapses or relapses. He denied current cravings or urges. He stated that he quit using "the patch." He smokes marijuana cigarettes on occasion, about one every 2 days. He has been smoking marijuana for about 4 years. Mr. W stated that he is more likely to smoke during times he is feeling stressed or down as an escape. He also drinks two to three glasses of wine per day in the evenings and will add scotch or beer as well if he is feeling especially stressed. He is negative (0/4) on the CAGE questions for alcohol abuse. He denied using other illicit drugs in the past or present. In terms of motivation to quit marijuana, he stated that his motivation is a 4/10 and self-efficacy is 6/10. He reported the same numbers for reducing or quitting alcohol. He indicated that he would "need something else" to help with his stress and mood if he were to quit.

Mr. W does not engage in regular exercise and stated that he has been rather sedentary since a back injury at work 5 years ago. He stated that he takes Norco PRN, which does help with the pain, but often feels that exercise would make the pain worse. He tends to eat a lot of fast food, luncheon meats, and soda. He stated he knows that with his family's cardiac history, and now his MI, he needs to make changes to his diet, and said that he is "very motivated" to do so.

Compliance With Medical Recommendations

Mr. W reported that he is compliant with taking his medications, reporting new or exacerbated cardiac symptoms, and following up with his cardiologist and primary care physician (PCP). He acknowledges that he has been told by his cardiologist and PCP that he needs to increase his physical activity and improve his diet. He cited pain and lack of motivation and education as barriers to making these changes thus far.

Psychiatric Functioning

Mr. W was cooperative, pleasant, and alert and oriented (×3) during this evaluation. Thought processes were logical and goal directed. Eye contact was appropriate. Speech was of appropriate rate and rhythm. Receptive communication and language appeared intact. No impairments in memory or concentration were noted. Affect was full and appropriate and mood is "a little down and scared."

Mr. W reported a history of depression, which started around the time of his work injury 5 years ago. He denied having experienced clinical depression symptoms prior to that. He also denied a history of anxiety. However, he describes feeling "stressed" about his finances and now his current medical situation and the need for further stenting in about 2 weeks.

Mr. W's appetite is healthy and sleep is intact. The patient currently endorses the following symptoms of depression and anxiety: sadness, anhedonia, diminished energy, increased irritability, excessive worry (about his upcoming stenting procedure), and heightened arousal.

The patient denies the following symptoms: change in sleep, change in appetite, change in weight, feelings of guilt, feelings of hopelessness, agoraphobia, repetitive behaviors, perceptual disturbances, and delusional thoughts.

The patient reports taking the following psychiatric medication: None

The patient's family history for psychiatric disorders is negative.

Assessment

This behavioral health specialist evaluation was conducted to examine the psychological, behavioral, and social factors that affect the patient's physical health and medical treatment. Mr. W presents with depression and anxiety symptoms. Specifically, he has had depressive symptoms for about 5 years, which seemed related to his work-related injury, his perceived inability to engage in physical activity, and now his MI. He also experiences "stress" (worry and heightened arousal) about his financial situation. He also expressed worry about his upcoming stent procedure. His primary methods of dealing with his depression and anxiety are maladaptive—alcohol and marijuana use, which likely further negatively impacts his mood. He is moderately motivated to quit but will need instruction on concrete adaptive stress-reduction and mood enhancement strategies to facilitate success. The patient presents with the following risk factors for heart disease: poor diet, recent smoking (marijuana), sedentary lifestyle, depression, and anxiety.

We briefly discussed the psychological and cardiac benefits of lifestyle changes, including alcohol reduction and quitting marijuana. We also discussed the importance of increasing physical activity from a mood and cardiac standpoint, and that this may be best started in a cardiac rehabilitation program. From a cognitive standpoint, he has a number of maladaptive thoughts about his current cardiac condition and prognosis (e.g., "I'll never be able to leave the house again or do things I like to do"), which warrant continued intervention.

Plan

1. Mr. W. has a long history of depression, likely exacerbated by substance use and maladaptive health behaviors. It is recommended that he continue following with this provider or another mental health provider to continue addressing his depressive symptoms and anxiety about his upcoming procedure.
2. Given that Mr. W perceives his back pain as the primary barrier to physical activity, it is recommended that his pain management regimen be reviewed. Continued education about the importance of physical activity and referral to a cardiac rehabilitation program is also recommended.
3. A follow-up appointment is recommended to discuss his financial hardship and any possible resources that may be available for him.
4. Mr. W would benefit from an appointment with a nutritional therapist to receive initial education about a heart healthy diet. All providers working with Mr. W should reinforce the importance of improved diet, regular exercise, and abstinence from substance use.
5. Mr. W would benefit from information regarding the upcoming stent procedure. He may also benefit from relaxation and diaphragmatic breathing instruction that he can utilize prior to and following the procedure to help mitigate anxiety symptoms.

REFERENCES

Ahmed, H. M., Blaha, M. J., Nasir, K., Rivera, J. J., & Blumenthal, R. S. (2012). Effects of physical activity on cardiovascular disease. *The American Journal of Cardiology*, *109*, 288–295.

Alcántra, C., Edmondson, D., Moise, N., Oyla, D., Hiti, D., & Kronish, I. M. (2014). Anxiety sensitivity and medication nonadherence in patients with uncontrolled hypertension. *Journal of Psychosomatic Research*, *77*, 283–286.

Allan, R., & Fisher, J. (2012). *Heart and mind: The practice of cardiac psychology* (2nd ed.) Washington, DC: American Psychological Association.

American Psychiatric Association. (2013). *Diagnostic and statistical manual of mental disorders* (5th ed.). Washington, DC: Author.

Barefoot, J. C., Brummett, B. H., Helms, M. J., Mark, D. B., Siegler, I. E., & Williams, R. B. (2000). Depressive symptoms and survival of patients with coronary artery disease. *Psychosomatic Medicine*, *62*, 790–795.

Beck, A. T., Epstein, N., Brown, G., & Steer, R. A. (1988). An inventory for measuring clinical anxiety: Psychometric properties. *Journal of Consulting and Clinical Psychology*, *56*, 893–897.

Beck, A. T., Steer, R. A., & Brown, G. K. (1996). *Manual for the Beck Depression Inventory-II*. San Antonio, TX: Psychological Corporation.

Bhupathiraju, S. N., & Tucker, K. L. (2011). Coronary heart disease prevention: Nutrients, foods, and dietary patterns. *Clinica Chimica Acta*, *412*, 1493–1514.

Blumenthal, J. A., Jiang, W., Babyak, M. A., Krantz, D. S., Frid, D. J., Coleman, R. E., ... Morris, J. J. (1997). Stress management and exercise training in cardiac patients with myocardial ischemia. *Archives of Internal Medicine*, *157*, 2213–2223.

Blumenthal, J. A., Lett, H. S., Babyak, M. A., White, W., Smith, P. K., Mark, D. B., ... Newan, M. F. (2003). Depression as a risk factor for mortality after coronary artery bypass surgery. *The Lancet*, *362*, 604–609.

Bonnet, F., Irving, K., Terra, J. L., Nony, P., Berthezene, F., & Moulin, P. (2005). Anxiety and depression are associated with unhealthy lifestyle in patients at risk of cardiovascular disease. *Atherosclerosis*, *178*, 339–344.

CDC, National Center for Health Statistics (2013). Compressed Mortality File, 1999–2010. (*Series 20 No 2P,* CDC *Wonder* Online Database). http://wonder.cdc.gov/cmf-icd10.html

CDC, National Center for Health Statistics: National Health and Nutrition Examination Survey, 2007–2010. CDC *Wonder* Online Database. Retrieved from www.cdc.gov/nchs/nhanes.htm

Celano, C. M., & Huffman, J. C. (2011). Depression and cardiac disease: A review. *Cardiology in Review*, *19*, 130–142.

Chida, Y., & Steptoe, A. (2009). The association of anger and hostility with future coronary heart disease. *Journal of the American College of Cardiology*, *53*, 936–946.

Clark, D. A., & Beck, A. T. (2010). *Cognitive therapy of anxiety disorders: Science and practice*. New York, NY: The Guilford Press.

Cohen, S., Kamarck, T., & Mermelstein, R. (1983). A global measure of perceived stress. *Journal of Health and Social Behavior*, *24*, 385–396.

Cohen, S., Mermelstein, R., Kamarck, T., & Hoberman, H. M. (1985). Measuring the functional components of social support. In I. G. Sarason & B. R. Sarason (Eds.), *Social support: Theory, research and applications* (pp. 73–94). Dordrecht, The Netherlands: Martinus Nijhoff Publishers.

Collins, J. A., & Rice, V. H. (1997). Effects of relaxation intervention in phase II cardiac rehabilitation. *Heart and Lung*, *26*, 31–44.

Denollet, J., & Pedersen, S. S. (2012). Type D personality in patients with cardiovascular disorders. In R. Allan & J. Fisher (Eds.), *Heart and mind: The practice of cardiac psychology* (pp. 219–247). Washington, DC: American Psychological Association.

Dixhoorn, J. V. (1998). Cardiorespiratory effects of breathing and relaxation instruction in myocardial infarction patients. *Biological Psychology*, *49*, 123–135.

ENRICHD Investigators. (2003). Effects of treating depression and low perceived social support on clinical events after myocardial infarction: The Enhancing Recovery in Coronary Heart

Disease Patients (ENRICHD) randomized trial. *Journal of the American Medical Association, 289*, 3106–3116.

Frasure-Smith, N., Lesperance, F., & Talajic, M. (1995). Depression and 18-month prognosis after myocardial infarction. *Circulation, 91*, 1819–1825.

Friedman, M., & Rosenman, R. H. (1974). *Type A behavior and your heart*. New York, NY: Knopf.

Gevirtz, R. N., & Schwartz, M. S. (2003). The respiratory system in applied psychophysiology. In M. S. Schwartz & R. Andrasik (Eds.), *Biofeedback: A practitioner's guide* (pp. 212–244). New York, NY: The Guilford Press.

Go, A., Mozaffarian, D., Roger, V., Benjamin, E., Berry, J., Blaha, M., … Turner, M. B. (2014). Heart disease and stroke statistics—2014 update: A report from the American Heart Association Statistics Committee and Stroke Statistics Subcommittee. *Circulation, 129*, 28–292.

Grenard, J. L., Munjas, B. A., Adams, J. L., Suttorp, M., Maglinone, M., McGlynn, E. A., & Gellad, M. F. (2011). Depression and medication adherence in the treatment of chronic diseases in the United States: A meta-analysis. *Journal of General Internal Medicine. 26*, 1175–1182.

Guerrero, C., & Palmero, F. (2010). Impact of defensive hostility in cardiovascular disease. *Behavioral Medicine, 36*, 77–84.

Hartley, L, Dyakova, M., Holmes, J., Clarke, A., Lee, M. S., Ernst, E., & Rees, K. (2014). Yoga for the primary prevention of cardiovascular disease. *Cochrane Database Systematic Reviews*. doi: 10.1002/14651858.CD010072.pub2

Ho, P. M., Masoudi, F. A., Spertus, J. A., Peterson, P. N., Shroyer, A. L., McCarthy, M., … Rumsfeld, J. (2005). Depression predicts mortality following cardiac valve surgery. *Annals of Thoracic Surgery, 79*, 1255–1259.

Howard, G., Prineas, R., Moy, C., Cushman, M., Kellum, M., Temple, E., … Howard, V. (2006). Racial and geographic differences in awareness, treatment, and control of hypertension: The Reasons for Geographic and Racial Differences in Stroke study. *Stroke, 37*, 1171–1178.

Engel, C., Choate, C. G., Cockfield, D., Armstrong, D. W., Jonas, W., Walter, A. G., … Miller R. (n.d.). Yoga nidra as an adjunctive therapy for PTSD: A feasibility study. Integrative Restoration Institute. Retrieved from www.irest.us/sites/default/files/WRAMH_PTSD_YN_Results_0.pdf

Juergens, M. C., Seekatz, B., Moosdorf, R. G., Petrie, K. J., & Rief, W. (2010). Illness beliefs before cardiac surgery predict disability, quality of life, and depression 3 months later. *Journal of Psychosomatic Research, 68*, 553–560.

Kessing, D., Pelle, A. J., Kupper, N., Szabó, B. M., & Denollet, J. (2014). Positive affect, anhedonia, and compliance with self-care in patients with chronic heart failure. *Journal of Psychosomatic Research, 77*, 296–301.

Kop, W. J., & Plumhoff, J. E. (2012). Depression and coronary heart disease: Diagnosis, predictive value, biobehavioral mechanisms, and intervention. In R. Allan & J. Fisher (Eds.), *Heart and mind: The practice of cardiac psychology* (pp. 153–155). Washington, DC: American Psychological Association.

Kroenke, K., Spitzer, R. L., & Williams, J. B. W. (2001). The PHQ-9: Validity of a brief depression severity measure. *Journal of General Internal Medicine, 16*, 606–613.

Kubzansky, L. D., Kawachi, I., Spiro III, A., Weiss, S. T., Vokonas, P. S., & Sparrow, D. (1997). Is worrying bad for your heart? A prospective study of worry and coronary heart disease in the normative aging study. *Circulation, 95*, 818–824.

Kubzansky, L. D., Kawachi, I., Weiss, S. T., & Sparrow, D. (1998). Anxiety and coronary heart disease: A synthesis of epidemiological, psychological, and experimental evidence. *Annals of Behavioral Medicine, 20*, 47–58.

Lesperance, F., & Frasure-Smith, N. (2000). Depression in patients with cardiac disease: A practical review. *Journal of Psychosomatic Research, 48*, 379–391.

Li, A. W., & Goldsmith, C. A. (2012). The effects of yoga on anxiety and stress. *Alternative Medicine Review, 17*, 21–35.

Magyar-Russell G., Thombs B. D., Cai J. X., Baveja T., Kuhl E. A., Singh P. P., … Ziegelstein, R. C. (2011). The prevalence of anxiety and depression in adults with implantable cardioverter defibrillators: A systematic review. *Journal of Psychosomatic Research, 71*, 223–231.

Manchanda, S. C., Narang, R., Reddy, K. S., Sachdeva, U., Prabhakaran, D., Dharmanand, S., … Bijlani, R. (2000). Retardation of coronary atherosclerosis with yoga lifestyle intervention. *Journal of Association of Physicians of India, 48*, 687–694.

Masi, C. M., Hawkley, L. C., Rickett, E. M., & Cacioppo, J. T. (2007). Respiratory sinus arrhythmia and diseases of aging: Obesity, diabetes, mellitus, and hypertension. *Biological Psychology, 74*, 212–223.

Mathers, C. D., & Loncar, D. (2006). Projections of global mortality and burden of disease from 2002 to 2030. *PLoS Medicine, 3*, 2011–2030.

Miller, T. Q., Smith, T. W., Turner, C. W., Guijarro, M. L., & Hallet, A. J. (1996). A meta-analytic review of research on hostility and physical health. *Psychology Bulletin, 119*, 322–348.

Murray, J. B. (2000). Cardiac disorders and antidepressant medications. *Journal of Psychology, 134*, 162–168.

Nasreddine, Z. S., Phillips, N. A., Bedirian, V., Charbonneau, S., Whitehead, V., Collin, I., ... Chertkow, H. (2005). The Montreal Cognitive Assessment, MoCA: A brief screening tool for mild cognitive impairment. *Journal of the American Geriatric Society, 53*, 695–699.

O'Keane, V., Dinan, T. G., Scott, L., & Corcoran, C. (2005). Changes in hypothalamic-pituitary-adrenal axis measures after vagus nerve stimulation therapy in chronic depression. *Biological Psychiatry, 58*, 963–968.

Ornish, D., Scherwitz, L. W., Billings, J. H., Gould, K. L., Merritt, T. A., Sparler, S., ... Brand, R. J. (1998). Intensive lifestyle changes for reversal of coronary heart disease. *Journal of the American Medical Association, 280*, 2001–2007.

Osman, A., Downs, W. R., Barrios, F. X., Kopper, B. A., Gutierrez, P. M., & Chiros, C. E. (1997). Factor structure and psychometric characteristics of the Beck Depression Inventory-II. *Journal of Psychopathology and Behavioral Assessment, 19*, 359–376.

Pan, A., Keum, N., Okereke, O. I., Sun, Q., Kivimaki, M., Rubin, R. R., & Hu, F. B. (2012). Bidirectional association between depression and metabolic syndrome: A systematic review and meta-analysis of epidemiological studies. *Diabetes Care, 35*, 1171–1180.

Patil, S. G., Dhanakshirur, G. B., Aithala, M. R., Naregal, G., & Das, K. K. (2014). Effect of yoga on oxidative stress in elderly with grade-I hypertension: A randomized controlled study. *Journal of Clinical and Diagnostic Research, 8*, 4–7.

Porges, S. W. (2007). The polyvagal perspective. *Biological Psychology, 74*, 116–143.

Ravven, S., Bader, C., Azar, A., & Rudolph, J. L. (2013). Depressive symptoms after CABG surgery: A meta-analysis. *Harvard Review of Psychiatry, 21*, 59–69.

Razzini, C., Bianchi, F., Leo, R., Fortuna, E., Siracusano, A., & Romeo, F. (2008). Correlations between personality factors and coronary artery disease: From type A behaviour pattern to type D personality. *Journal of Cardiovascular Medicine, 9*, 761–768.

Robinson, M. J., & Levenson, J. L. (2000). The use of psychotropics in the medically ill. *Current Psychiatry Reports, 2*, 247–255.

Rosamond, W., Flegal, K, Friday, G., Furie, K., Go, A., Greenlund, K, ... Hong, Y. (2007). Heart disease and stroke statistics – 2007 update: A report from the American Heart Association Statistics Committee and Stroke Statistics Subcommittee. *Circulation, 115*, 69–171.

Rutledge, T., Reis, V. A., Linke, S. E., Greenberg, B. H., & Mills, P. J. (2006). Depression in heart failure: A meta-analytic review of prevalence, intervention effects, and associations with clinical outcomes. *Journal of the American College of Cardiology, 48*, 1527–1537.

Sears, S. F., Matchett, M., Vazquez, L. D., & Conti, J. B. (2012). Innovations in psychosocial care for implantable cardioverter defibrillator patients. In R. Allan & J. Fisher (Eds.), *Heart and mind: The practice of cardiac psychology* (pp. 219–247). Washington, DC: American Psychological Association.

Seldenrijk, A. Vogelzangs, N., Batelaan, N. M., Wieman, I., van Schaik, D. J. F., Enninx, B. J. W. H. (2015). Depression, anxiety, and 6-year risk of cardiovascular disease. *Journal of Psychosomatic Research, 78*, 123–129.

Skowronek, I. B., Mounsey, A., & Handler, L. (2014). Clinical inquiry: Can yoga reduce symptoms of anxiety and depression? *Journal of Family Practice, 63*, 398–407.

Smith, T. W. (1994). Concepts and methods in the study of anger, hostility, and health. In A. W. Siegman & T. W. Smith (Eds.), *Anger, hostility, and the heart* (pp. 23–42). Hillsdale, NJ: Erlbaum.

Spielberger, C. D., Gorsuch, R. L., & Lushene, R. E. (1970). *Manual for the StateTrait Anxiety Inventory*. Palo Alto, CA: Consulting Psychologists Press.

Spielberger, C. D., Gorsuch, R. L., Lushene, R., Vagg, P. R., & Jacobs, G. A. (1983). *Manual for the State-Trait Anxiety Inventory*. Palo Alto, CA: Consulting Psychologists Press.

Stetler, C., & Miller, G. E. (2011). Depression and hypothalamic-pituitary-adrenal activation: A quantitative summary of four decades of research. *Psychosomatic Medicine, 73*, 114–126.

Stewart, J. C., Fitzgerald, G. J., & Kamarck, T. W. (2010). Hostility now, depression later? Longitudinal associations among emotional risk factors for coronary artery disease. *Annals of Behavioral Medicine, 39*, 258–266.

Thayer, J. F., & Lane, R. D. (2002). Perseverative thinking and health: Neurovisceral concomitants. *Psychology and Health, 17*, 685–695.

Thayer, J. F., & Lane, R. D. (2007). The role of vagal function in the risk for cardiovascular disease and mortality. *Biological Psychology, 74*, 224–242.

Thayer, J. F., & Lane, R. D. (2009). Claude Bernard and the heart-brain connection: Further elaboration of a model of neurovisceral integration. *Neuroscience and Biobehavioral Reviews, 33*, 81–88.

Tully, P. J., & Baune, B. T. (2014). Comorbid anxiety disorders alter the association between cardiovascular diseases and depression: The German National Health Interview and Examination Survey. *Social Psychiatry and Psychiatric Epidemiology, 49*, 683–691.

Tully, P. J., Baune, B. T., & Baker, R. A. (2013). Cognitive impairment before and six months after cardiac surgery increase mortality risk at median 11 year follow-up: A cohort study. *International Journal of Cardiology, 168*, 2796–2802.

Tully, P. J., Cosh, S. M., & Baumeister, H. (2014). The anxious heart in whose mind? A systematic review and meta-regression of factors associated with anxiety disorder diagnosis, treatment and morbidity risk in coronary heart disease. *Journal of Psychosomatic Research, 77*, 439–448.

Tully, P. J., Pedersen, S. S., Winefield, H. R., Baker, R. A., Turnbull, D. A., & Denollet, J. (2011). Cardiac morbidity risk and depression and anxiety: A disorder, symptom and trait analysis among cardiac surgery patients. *Psychology, Health, and Medicine, 16*, 333–345.

Vukovic, O., Tosevski, D. L., Jasovic-Gasic, M., Damjanovic, A., Zebic, M., Britvic, D., ... Ostojc, M. (2014). Type D personality in patients with coronary artery disease. *Psychiatria Danubina, 26*, 46–51.

Ware, J. E., Jr., Kosinski, M., & Keller, S. D. (1996). A 12-item short-form health survey: Construction of scales and preliminary tests of reliability and validity. *Medical Care, 34*, 220–233.

Whalley, B., Thompson, D. R., & Taylor, R. S. (2012). Psychological interventions for coronary heart disease: Cochrane systematic review and meta-analysis. *International Journal of Behavioral Medicine, 21*, 109–121.

Yogendra, J., Yogendra, H. J., Ambarkdekar, S., Lele, R. D., Shetty, S., Dave, M. (2004). Beneficial effects of yoga lifestyle on reversibility of ischemic heart disease: Caring heart project of International Board of Yoga. *Journal of the Association of Physicians of India, 52*, 283–289.

Yusuf, S., Hawken, S., Ôunpuu, S., Dans, T., Avezum, A., Lanas, F., ... Lisheng, L. (2004). Effect of potentially modifiable risk factors associated with myocardial infarction in 52 countries (the INTERHEART study): Case-control study, *Lancet, 364*, 937–952.

SIX

CHRONIC PAIN

JULIE LEWIS RICKERT, VICKI J. MICHELS, AND CHRIS HERNDON

S.O.A.P. NOTE FROM REFERRING PRIMARY CARE PROVIDER

CHIEF COMPLAINT: Chronic pain, medication refill.

S: A 46-year-old female presents to the outpatient clinic for medication refills secondary to chronic pain. PMH significant for chronic neck and back pain, fibromyalgia, anxiety, and GERD. Continues to complain of neck and back pain. Currently on Tramadol 50 mg (1 in the a.m. and 2 in the p.m.) and hydrocodone/acetaminophen 5/325 mg (1 q4h: she takes at least 2/day, occasionally 3/day on some days). Says her pain is only moderately controlled (pain level 6/10). Uses OTCs (ibuprofen) to supplement. She has been to the pain specialist and discussed epidural injections. She is frightened to pursue this route due to the risk of possible paralysis. Plans to hold off on this procedure for now.

Her fibromyalgia pain has decreased, which she relates to the change to warmer weather. Fatigue and stiffness have also improved. She was prescribed duloxetine for her fibromyalgia and anxiety but has chosen to discontinue due to worsening GERD symptoms. Wishes to wait until these symptoms improve before restarting the medication.

Anxiety is controlled with lorazepam, which she takes once or twice daily. She has not followed through with the counseling recommendation. Denies depression, hypomania/mania, substance use/abuse, or suicidality/homicidality.

GERD symptoms have worsened. She admits that over the recent holidays she ate foods that she should have avoided that caused more indigestion. She has been on conservative treatment with dietary modification and OTC ranitidine (75 mg, 2/daily). She denies nausea or vomiting. Reports normal bowel and bladder function.

O: VITAL SIGNS: Weight: 187.2 pounds. Blood pressure: 131/71 mmHg. Temperature: 98.2° F. Pulse: 82 beats per minute. Respiratory rate: 21 breaths per minute.

General: Caucasian female in no acute distress. Patient appears to be stated age. She is alert and oriented ×3. GAD-7 score of 9 (mild–moderate anxiety)

HEENT:
Head: Normocephalic, atraumatic.
Eyes: Pupils equally round and reactive to light.
Ears: Tympanic membranes were nonerythematous and nonbulging bilaterally.
Nose: Nasal mucosa pink and moist. No erythema or edema noted.
Mouth/Throat: Oral mucosa pink and moist.
Neck: Supple. Nontender. No lymphadenopathy.
Lungs: Clear to auscultation bilaterally.
Cardiovascular: S1 and S2 heard. Regular rate and rhythm. No rubs, murmurs, or gallops.
Abdomen: Soft, nontender, nondistended. Bowel sounds auscultated and normal.
Musculoskeletal: Tenderness to palpation of the paraspinal muscles in the lumbar region and sacral tenderness to palpation. Only 4 of 18 fibromyalgia tender points mildly tender.

A: Chronic neck and back pain (723.9), fibromyalgia (729.1), anxiety (300.00), gastroesophageal reflux disease (530.81)

P:
1. Chronic neck and back pain: The patient will receive refills for the following medications:
   a) Tramadol 50 mg, 1 tablet in the morning and 2 tablets in the evening, #90, zero refills.
   b) Hydrocodone/acetaminophen 5/325, 1 tab p.o. q4h p.r.n., pain, #60, zero refills.

   As the patient has not responded optimally to medication management alone, referral made to the behavioral health specialist for evaluation and treatment recommendations.
2. Fibromyalgia: Continue current treatment. Discussed importance of duloxetine for her symptoms. Patient will resume taking. Refer to behavioral health specialists for assistance.
3. Anxiety: Recommend she follow up with our behavioral health specialist re chronic pain, anxiety, and fibromyalgia. She was provided with the contact information to schedule an appointment. Renew lorazepam 0.5 mg, 1 tablet t.i.d. p.r.n., anxiety, #60, zero refills. Discussed importance of duloxetine for her anxiety and fibromyalgia symptoms. Presented again the value of CBT for anxiety. The patient reluctantly agrees to discuss with the behavioral health specialist.
4. GERD: The patient to resume GERD prevention diet and lifestyle changes. Omeprazole 20 mg, 1 tab QD, #30, two refills, started.

OVERVIEW OF CHRONIC PAIN

Chronic pain is a major contributor to the global burden of disease. An estimated 100 million American adults suffer from chronic pain (Institute of Medicine, 2011). Pain is frequently not adequately managed by our health care system (Mularski et al., 2006). Psychosocial interventions, in particular, are underutilized despite having some of the strongest evidence for reducing the burden of the condition (Keefe, Abernethy, & Campbell, 2005). The integration of psychosocial interventions into medical settings, especially primary care, is an important part of improving access to resources and outcomes for patients with chronic pain (Ehde, Dillworth, & Turner, 2014). This chapter is designed to give the behavioral health specialist (BHS) a basic understanding of pain, knowledge about how to effectively evaluate chronic pain, and a description of effective pain management techniques.

Knowledge of the biological and psychological basis of pain is important to understanding the experience of chronic pain. Pain includes both somatosensory and emotional discomfort, usually related to tissue damage, and serves a very important protective function signaling danger and encouraging behaviors to prevent future harm. Failure in the pain system is dangerous and can be associated with considerable morbidity and mortality (Nagasako, Oaklander, & Dworkin, 2003).

Pain is exceedingly complex from a neuroanatomical perspective. The pain experience involves a multidimensional distributed process incorporating many areas of the brain including the spinothalamic tract, prefrontal cortex, thalamus, somatosensory cortex, amygdala, cingulate gyrus, and other areas of the limbic system (Neugebauer, Galhardo, Maione, & Mackey, 2009). The experience of pain is also affected by genetics, learning, motivation, emotions, reasoning, and social influences. The distinction between acute and chronic pain is important as they differ in phenomenology, etiology, and the approaches to treatment. Acute pain is a sudden often sharp pain caused typically by a physical injury (cuts, broken bones, burns, childbirth). When acute pain persists beyond the healing of the injury, it is referred to as chronic pain. There are many theories about why this occurs. Some evidence suggests that the longer pain persists, the greater the proportion of the brain devoted to processing and analyzing pain (Flor, Braun, Elbert, & Birbaumer, 1997; Maihöfner, Handwerker, Neundörfer, & Birklein, 2003). While it is beyond the scope of this chapter to completely explore the nature of chronic pain, it is important to note that the very complexity of chronic pain means that the assessment and treatment of chronic pain must be equally robust.

ASSESSING THE CHRONIC PAIN PATIENT

One challenge in working with patients with pain is the lack of objective measures of pain. It is often difficult to determine how much pain a patient is experiencing because patients differ in their pain tolerance, their displays of pain, and their ability to explain their pain experiences. It is therefore critical for the BHS to perform a thorough evaluation to assess as many objective and subjective variables related to pain as possible. A thorough evaluation also aids the BHS in identifying which intervention(s) might be most efficacious. In addition to the typical demographic information gathered during an initial evaluation (social and vocational history, past medical and surgical history), the BHS should develop a thorough understanding of the patients' pain including the history of their pain, behavioral responses to the pain, impact on quality of life, comorbid mental health disorders, and health behaviors (sleep hygiene, substance use, physical activity). A guiding principle when evaluating patients is to build rapport in order to optimize both their assessment and treatment.

Building Rapport

A biopsychosocial assessment is the foundation for providing behavioral health treatment to the chronic pain patient (McGeary, McGeary, & Gatchel, 2014). Within the primary care setting the assessment will most often be brief and focused. Nevertheless, many patients will never have participated in such an evaluation and may not understand the purpose of many of the questions and details collected. It is also not uncommon for pain patients to experience ambivalence or even resistance to being referred to a "behavioral" health specialist for assessment of their "physical" pain. Patients may have inaccurate notions of the reason for seeing a BHS. They may take the referral to the BHS as indicating that their primary care provider does not believe they have pain or that the pain is psychological in nature. They may have had prior negative interactions with health care providers who communicate their inappropriate stereotyping of the chronic pain patient as "drug seekers." And lastly, the increased anxiety and irritability that often accompanies chronic pain can adversely influence patients' interpersonal behaviors, more easily eliciting negative reactions from others including their treatment providers.

Sometimes the referral to the BHS includes some degree of coercion, with the provider using continuation of opioid analgesics as a condition of participation. Patients who are referred under threat may feel angry, anxious, or mistrustful of the BHS. Any misperceptions patients have about seeing a BHS should be dispelled in order to obtain a valid assessment. Rapport building and a brief explanation about the purpose of gathering the broad range of information through the assessment are important. One possible introduction the BHS might use when first meeting a chronic pain patient is:

> Although you are experiencing some relief from your fibromyalgia, you are still experiencing pain. Chronic pain is very complicated and your pain can come from multiple sources. As you know, it influences every aspect of your life. What you may not be aware of is that there are many things about your experience of pain, the ways you coping with pain, and the stresses caused by pain or other factors that can make your pain worse. I will help you identify factors that could contribute to your pain. While you may not choose to address all of these factors, we hope to help you get some control over your pain.

Screening and Assessment Tools

Once concerns about seeing a BHS have been discussed, rapport established, and preliminary education concerning acute and chronic pain provided, the next step is the assessment. A full biopsychosocial assessment has the potential to yield a great deal of information that will direct treatment; however, the primary care evaluation of pain will likely be briefer and will utilize a number of screening tools. These tools will help the BHS explore the location and intensity of the pain, identify common comorbid psychiatric symptoms, and gauge the degree to which pain has impacted the patient's life (Cleeland & Ryan, 1994; Hooten et al., 2013). The assessment should include health behaviors such as sleep hygiene, diet, physical activity, and substance use including alcohol, tobacco, and illegal drugs.

One of the most difficult challenges when assessing patients' pain is evaluating the severity of pain. Often patients are asked to utilize a 10-point Likert scale such as a visual analog scale or a 0 to 5 scale with cartoon facial expressions such as the Faces Pain Scale (Hooten et al., 2013). The information from these scales can provide some useful information about relative pain and can assess changes following interventions but are very unidimensional and subjective. Formal instruments with published reliability and validity include the Roland–Morris Disability Questionnaire (Roland & Morris, 1983), the Brief Pain Inventory (Cleeland & Ryan, 1994), and the West Haven-Yale Multidimensional Pain Inventory (Bernstein, Jaremeko, & Hinkley, 1995). Other assessment methods including the Mankoski Pain Scale tie the pain rating to particular functional limitations and are preferred by some patients and providers (Douglas, Randleman, DeLane, & Palmer, 2014). Screening instruments for comorbid mental health disorders are part of a thorough pain evaluation and might include screening for depression with the Patient Health Questionnaire-9 (PHQ-9; Kroenke, Spitzer, Williams, 2001), the Beck Depression Inventory (BDI-2; Harris & D'Eon, 2008), and anxiety (generalized anxiety disorder-7 [GAD-7] Spitzer, Kroenke, Williams, & Löwe, 2006). The Patient Reported Outcomes Measurement Information System (PROMIS), an ultra-brief (four item) screening for depression and anxiety in chronic pain patients, is the latest in validated and reliable screening tools used with chronic pain patients (Kroenke, Yu, Wu, Kean, & Monahan, 2014). To increase efficiency when assessing chronic pain patients some BHSs may develop their own questionnaire similar to the one we use in our clinic (Exhibit 6.1).

A complete assessment should provide the BHS with an understanding of the patients' level of pain, their physical functioning, their interpersonal functioning, and their quality of life. An accurate conceptualization of the factors contributing to their pain, the impact the pain has on their life, their assets for coping with pain, and their quality of life assists the BHS in creating an effective treatment plan.

TREATMENT

Chronic pain is less responsive to treatments commonly used for acute pain such as opioid analgesia and avoiding physical activity. These approaches are sometimes deleterious, leading to physical deconditioning and escalating opioid use without improved functioning or quality of life for those with chronic pain. Ineffective treatment can leave the patient in persistent pain, leading to both financial and psychosocial stressors. Ongoing treatment for chronic pain is often expensive. Gaskin and Richard (2012) estimated that direct medical costs for treatment of chronic pain in 2010 were between $261 and $300 billion. Annual

Exhibit 6.1 Chronic Non-Cancer Pain Assessment

Name: ______________________ Date of birth: ____________

Where is your pain? (Please list all locations)

Please rate your pain on a scale of 1–10

Location	Average level	Highest in last week

How is this pain interfering with your life? ______________________

How long have you had this pain? ______________________

What do you believe caused your pain? ______________________

Has a doctor ever evaluated this pain? If so, please write his or her name and what he or she told you was the cause of your pain. ______________________

Have you noticed anything that makes your pain worse? ______________________

Please list all the things you do that seem to make the pain more bearable. ______________________

Please tell us about your sleep. ______________________

(continued)

Exhibit 6.1 Chronic Non-Cancer Pain Assessment *(continued)*

How often do you do the following?

Eat a nutritious diet ____________ Use caffeine (coffee, pop, energy drinks) ____________

Use tobacco ____________ Exercise (what and how often) ____________

Many people with pain use alcohol at times. How frequently do you drink alcohol? ____________

____

How many drinks do you typically have? ________ Highest number of drinks in the last month? ________

Do you ever use "street drugs" (like marijuana)? ____________

____

How have the other people in your life reacted to your pain?

Supportive ____________ They mostly ignore it ____________ Critical ____________

Chronic pain often causes problems with emotions. Please rate how often you were troubled by these problems in the last month.

	Daily	3–4 days/week	Weekly	Rarely
Anger or irritability				
Sadness or depression				
Anxiety, worry, or fear				
Hopelessness or helplessness				

Please list treatments prescribed in the past and rate whether you tried them and how they worked.

Method	Never tried	Side effects were too terrible	Tried briefly	Tried for a while, little or no effect	Moderately effective	Very effective

average direct medical costs for chronic low back pain in a non-Medicare eligible population was estimated to be $8,386 by Gore, Sadosky, Stacey, Tai, and Leslie (2012). From a psychosocial perspective, a chronic pain patient's significant others may not understand his or her pain, leaving the patient increasingly isolated, lonely, frustrated, and more susceptible to depression (Poleshuck et al., 2010). Pain's tendency to excite the body's fight-or-flight response can leave patients anxious, irritable, or both (Chapman, Tuckett, & Woo Song, 2008). These emotions increase the sensation of pain and resulting negative behaviors such as complaining about pain or being irritable, creating a cycle of more pain and isolation, which leads to more negative emotions (Kerns, Sellinger, & Goodin, 2011).

In contrast to many other conditions, chronic pain may cause patients to interact in ways that create conflict between them and their providers (Diesfeld, 2008). The primary cause of this conflict is the potential discrepancy between the provider's goals and the patient's goals (Allegretti, Borkan, Reis, & Griffiths, 2010). The provider's goal is often the reduction of disability, pain, and improving the patient's overall quality of life. The provider will be concerned about the iatrogenic effects of interventions (i.e., secondary problems caused by the treatments), such as addiction, sedation, and tissue damage. Often the patient's primary goal is the rapid elimination of pain because pain may be the most distressing symptom. Patients may focus on obtaining opioid analgesics and benzodiazepines as the primary method for pain control because the medications can bring immediate relief. Their providers may refuse to prescribe these medications or limit their use to avoid the consequences of long-term use of these medications. While studies suggest that some physicians may have an exaggerated fear of patients diverting their medication to others and may be unsure about when opioid prescription is medically acceptable outside of cancer treatment (Wolfert, Gilson, Dahl, & Cleary, 2010), fear of negative consequences is not unwarranted. In addition to increased regulatory scrutiny, Manchikanti et al. (2012) found that the yearly incidence of opioid-related deaths now exceed motor vehicle and suicide deaths. Opioid addiction and misuse are identified as a major public health threat (Compton & Volkow, 2006) at the same time that other studies suggest that overly conservative opioid use may be one reason for the inadequate control of pain (Wolfert et al., 2010). Awareness of the national epidemic of opioid misuse, fear of regulatory scrutiny, and difficulty discriminating "real" pain patients from those who may divert medications for recreational use create additional stress on the primary care relationship (Diesfeld, 2008). The BHS can play an important role in assisting with the screening and monitoring for misuse by patients and family members.

The Multidisciplinary Team

A multidisciplinary team approach can substantially improve outcomes in chronic pain treatment. Comprehensive chronic pain treatment programs provided by multidisciplinary teams have excellent evidence for effectiveness (American Society of Anesthesiologists Task Force on Chronic Pain Management, 2010). Comprehensive pain rehabilitation programs have been shown to lead to a significant reduction of pain, a substantial (63%) reduction in prescription pain medications, and a 62% reduction in medical costs (Turk, 2002). However, these programs may not be available to or used by many chronic pain patients due to location, cost, time, or patient preference. Working with interdisciplinary professionals both within the primary care setting and beyond may be the gold standard of care for chronic pain patients. These interdisciplinary professionals might include primary care providers, physical therapists, occupational therapists, nurse case managers, pharmacists, vocational rehabilitation specialists, and the BHS. Not all integrated care systems, however, will have all of these team members, but the goal is to maximize the involvement of as many as possible, tailoring their involvement to the particular patient. Whatever the format of service provision, utilizing multiple interventions such as physical therapy/exercise, emotional management, pacing, and medication, rather than a single modality can substantially improve outcomes for chronic pain (Williams, Eccleston, & Morley, 2012). The use of multiple modality interventions may have an additive effect and improve functioning overall. The BHS is ideally suited to provide many of these interventions or to help the patient identify other approaches to pain management, including complementary and alternative therapies. Increasing motivation to change, developing appropriate expectations, improving adherence, developing relaxation and distraction skills, improving emotional management skills, treating comorbid mental health problems, assisting with coping with grief and loss, improving relationship skills, smoking cessation, and addressing changes in identity and self-esteem are all potential goals for the BHS. The BHS can help other members of the integrated health care team understand and manage the psychosocial and behavioral problems experienced and exhibited by chronic pain patients. Clear and regular communication with the differing team members is important to provide the best possible care for patients.

Once the BHS has a comprehensive understanding of the patient's pain and its effect on his or her life, providing education to the patient about (a) the reality of the pain, (b) the complexity of chronic pain, and (c) the goals of pain management can help the patient begin to understand and manage his or her pain better.

Psychoeducation

Providing psychoeducation about chronic pain can be an important strategy. Many patients experience considerable relief when their experiences are explained and normalized. The information provides patients with a logical foundation to understanding the importance of chronic pain interventions. Psychoeducation can be provided in different formats: one-on-one, in groups, or through the use of bibliotherapy (see Other Resources for the Behavioral Health Specialist in this chapter). While some forms of treatment such as individual counseling may be more conducive for certain issues (e.g., emotional traumas believed to be involved in the experience of chronic pain), much of pain management treatment can be provided in a group format. Providing psychoeducation in a group format is more efficient and has the added benefits that come with any group intervention. Group interventions can enhance accountability, provide modeling of pain coping by more advanced participants, and provide emotional support (Spira, 1997). Being understood and understanding others can be powerful for pain patients.

The need for behavioral health services far outstrips the availability of trained mental health professionals. Groups increase the number of patients a given BHS can impact. Improving accessibility to effective treatment is an important goal of integrated primary care.

Whichever delivery method of education is provided, the following topics are useful initially in helping chronic pain patients understand pain and engage in treatment (Hooten et al., 2013).

Chronic pain is real: Patients and family members need to understand that severe pain can be experienced in the absence of acute injury or obvious damage, and that pain without an obvious source can be both severe and profoundly disabling. Patients need assurance that the pain is not "all in their head" and that their health care providers believe that their pain is real.

Pain is complex: There are multiple factors impacting the experience of pain (physical, psychological, social, cultural, etc.) and therefore multiple interventions targeting these multiple factors may be needed to help ameliorate pain.

Goals of pain management: Patients must understand that typically the complete elimination of pain is not a realistic goal for pain management. The goal of pain management is to manage pain and improve overall functioning and quality of life. Educating patients about realistic goals can improve their relationship with their medical provider. The expectation that their medical provider can give a medication or perform a procedure to eliminate all pain causes a great deal of conflict between patients and providers. Patients who expect to be pain free often become discouraged, lose motivation, and lose interest in using evidence-based, long-term, nonmedical pain management techniques when pain continues. Developing realistic goals for treatment can reduce conflicts with care providers, decrease patient treatment dissatisfaction, and improve motivation. Helping patients and their care team achieve common ground is a crucial component in successful pain management (Diesfeld, 2008).

While psychoeducation is an essential first step, patients will need to learn behavioral strategies to improve their ability to manage their pain. The best outcomes for complicated chronic pain patients are achieved when multiple self-regulatory, behavioral and cognitive techniques are used on a regular basis (Roditi & Robinson, 2011). The following section explores behavioral and cognitive techniques, which have been shown to be beneficial with chronic pain patients.

BEHAVIORAL HEALTH INTERVENTIONS FOR THE CHRONIC PAIN PATIENT

Behavioral interventions for the patient with chronic pain can be conceptualized as having five components: (a) increase patient engagement in disease management, (b) develop emotional management skills, (c) engage in long-range lifestyle strategies to resolve symptoms and prevent or minimize flare-ups, (d) develop strategies to address systems issues that impact pain, and (e) develop a large toolbox of pain self-management strategies.

Improve Engagement in Health Management

The foundation for effective treatment of chronic pain is good rapport between the patient and the health care providers. Exploring the patients' previous experiences, being aware of and reducing the BHS's own biases about chronic pain patients, and being confident that chronic pain can be managed aid the BHS in building an effective collaborative relationship with the patient. A humanistic style using strategies from motivational interviewing can help the patient assume a more active and engaged approach to pain management (Tse, Vong, & Tang, 2013). The development of a self-management approach (discussed in "Develop a toolbox of pain rescue strategies") enables chronic pain patients to take responsibility for the behavioral changes (such as physical activity) most associated with good outcomes in chronic pain (Roditi & Robinson, 2011). Adherence to skills practice and behavioral changes is correlated with improved scores on a variety of outcome measures and treatment satisfaction (Kerns et al., 2014). The BHS can use behavioral expertise to help patients develop realistic behavioral goals, identify barriers to behavior change, develop cues and rewards for specific behaviors, set up pain monitoring, and evaluate and alter plans as necessary.

Increase Emotional Management Skills

Research suggests that the development of emotional management skills is an essential part of chronic pain management (Roditi & Robinson, 2011). Emotion is an important mediator for the subjective experience of pain (Gatchel, Peng, Peters, Fuchs, & Turk, 2007). Cognitive behavioral therapy (CBT) for the treatment of chronic pain has been documented to be effective (Ehde et al., 2014). Meta-analytic studies have demonstrated small to moderate effects on pain, disability, catastrophizing, and mood, and the most robust effects are on mood improvement (Williams et al., 2012).

Patients may have difficulty understanding why emotional management is important. Sharing information about the bidirectional influence of the fight-or-flight response and pain perception can help patients recognize the relevance of stress management. Identifying the ways in which pain contributes to anxiety, irritability, depression, and hopelessness, and educating patients about the way these in turn contribute to pain and poor well-being is helpful. When the patient understands the need for emotional management, traditional cognitive behavioral techniques can be utilized. Cognitive behavioral techniques such as developing realistic expectations, increasing self-efficacy, combating catastrophizing, and reducing pain avoidance are important techniques to teach patients (Thorn, 2004). The BHS can use structured programs like the one described in *Managing Chronic Pain: A Cognitive-Behavioral Therapy Approach* (Otis, 2007) or choose a more focused and tailored approach.

Relaxation training, distraction, cognitive restructuring, and problem-solving skill training are identified as useful CBT interventions for patients with chronic pain (Kerns et al., 2011). Relaxation and distraction are covered in the section "Develop a toolbox of pain rescue strategies." Cognitive restructuring involves identifying adaptive, coping thoughts to replace exceedingly negative pain-related thoughts. For example, "This pain is terrible, I'm going crazy" might be replaced with "I am having a pain flare, by relaxing my muscles, I can make it more bearable."

Develop a Lifestyle That Minimizes Flare-ups

Living an effective pain management lifestyle is arguably the most important set of changes for long-term management of chronic pain. Patients may be reluctant to make these changes because they do not lead to immediate relief of pain, and some methods can cause a paradoxical temporary increase in pain before the relief is experienced. For example, starting a walking program for lower back pain may lead to a temporary increase in discomfort before core muscles strengthen and the positive impact on the nervous system can be realized. Developing a set of appropriate pain management techniques and reminding patients to use them as they change their lifestyle can help patients cope with their chronic and acute pain while waiting for the positive effects of the lifestyle change to occur. Passive approaches not focused on active lifestyle changes have limited evidence for effectiveness as stand-alone interventions for chronic pain (Hooten et al., 2013). The following lifestyle changes often benefit chronic pain patients.

Physical activity

Insufficient physical activity has long been identified as one of the factors that increase the risk of developing chronic pain (Sluka, O'Donnell, Danielson, & Rasmussen, 1985). Physical activity is the method most universally supported in the literature for reducing the overall morbidity of chronic pain (Hooten et al., 2013). Increasing physical activity initially causes pain, so patients may be resistant to becoming more physically active. Consequently, levels of physical activity must change slowly. Rapid increases in activity duration and/or intensity can cause pain flares that can set patients back in their recovery and threaten the trust in the therapeutic relationship.

Having a physical therapist knowledgeable in treating chronic pain patients can be very helpful. Walking, tai chi, warm water exercises, swimming, and stationary biking have all been shown to be beneficial for patients but no single modality has been shown to be more effective than another (Hooten et al., 2013). Core strengthening can be helpful particularly for back pain (Cho, Kim, & Kim, 2014). Some patients can benefit from stretching and flexibility and find that these movements help them feel good. A few patients may need assistance with balance and vestibular training to help reduce the risk of falls and injury.

Pacing

Chronic pain patients can fall into a pattern when, as soon as they feel small improvements, they overcompensate by significantly increasing their activity level. This in turn can cause them to experience a return or exacerbation of their pain. Distributing activities over the day and week with adequate rest while participating in other prevention activities can improve outcomes. Jamieson-Lega, Berry, and Brown (2013) identify "pacing" as an active self-management strategy. Individuals learn to balance time spent on activity and at rest for the purpose of achieving increased functioning and participation in meaningful activities. Another factor that pairs well with pacing is the scheduling of pleasurable activities. Pain patients can lead very restricted and isolated lives and even feel guilty about participating in pleasurable activities. Engaging in pleasurable activities has long been recommended for improving depression (Lewinsohn & Graf, 1973) and can be part of developing a healthy lifestyle for patients with pain (Otis, 2007).

Improving sleep

Sleep disturbance is a common complaint of patients with chronic pain. Pain can interfere with the amount and quality of sleep. In addition, poor sleep is associated with worsening pain (Finan, Goodin, & Smith, 2013). The association is so strong for fibromyalgia pain that some researchers have proposed that it might be better viewed as a sleep disorder (Finan et al., 2013). Improving sleep hygiene includes having a regular schedule, eliminating stimulants, increasing physical activity, using relaxation, avoiding eating when arising during the desired sleep time, minimizing napping, avoiding light exposure (especially blue spectrum light such as TVs, electronics, and fluorescents), limiting the use of the bed to sleep and sex, and identifying alternative distracting activities. CBT can be utilized to help address extremely resistant sleep (Tang, Goodchild, & Salkovskis, 2012).

Maintaining muscle warmth

Muscle tension related to cold temperatures and shivering can be uncomfortable for patients. Pain and temperature are regulated by overlapping pathways within the brain (Larson et al., 2014). Patients with fibromyalgia, in particular, have difficulties with thermoregulation and some have suggested that this is a significant factor in fibromyalgia pain (Larson, Pardo, & Pasley, 2014). While the preferred method for improving muscle warmth is increasing physical activity, patients may choose to achieve muscle warmth and minimize pain using other methods. Dressing warmly to reduce heat loss, using heating pads or heated seats, or simply warming the car in the winter are strategies that patients can use. Wearing layers of clothing is useful; patients can take off or put on pieces of clothing depending upon the temperature. The use of a sauna has been shown to improve pain, reduce anger, and increase return to work in a small study (Masuda, Koga, Hattanmaru, Minagoe, & Tei, 2005).

Posture and ergonomics

Ensuring that the activities of daily life do not irritate the patient's pain can help manage pain. For example, fitting a chair for proper height, back support, and arm support can dramatically improve the patient's ability to engage in work or pleasurable activities. Similarly, screen height and positioning of keyboards can encourage good posture and minimize pain. Slumping and crossing legs can initially feel good but can increase certain types of musculoskeletal pain. Providing occupational or workplace interventions has been shown to be effective as part of an integrated pain management intervention (Lambeek, van Mechelen, Knol, Loisel, & Anema, 2010).

Find alternatives to pain-causing activities

Develop acceptable alternatives to activities that increase pain. For example, if patients experience an increase in their pain when sitting on cold bleachers at a grandson's football games there may be several alternatives. These may range from bringing a properly supportive chair, watching only the last quarter, dressing more warmly, or bringing a battery powered heating pad. In more severe cases, having the game taped and scheduling a time to watch it with the grandson can enable the patient to feel supportive of the grandchild and not have the pain from sitting in the cold.

Impact interpersonal relationships

Pain patients describe a number of changes in interpersonal relationships that result from their pain. Changes in family roles, financial instability, use of psychoactive substances, increased irritability, and interpersonal withdrawal can all negatively impact interpersonal relationships (Snelling, 1994). Conversely, problems in relationships can cause increased anxiety, irritability, depression, and poor behavioral choices (including substance misuse, social isolation, and overdoing physical activity), which can in turn exacerbate pain.

Pain can also become the primary focus of relationships. Family members can become overly solicitous and patients with pain can become very dependent on others (Snelling, 1994). Alternately, families can become very detached, leaving pain patients feeling isolated and misunderstood (Smith, 2003). Many self-help guides, including Bruce and Hooten (2008) and Turk and Winter (2006), recommend being honest about pain yet work to develop a relationship not centered on pain. Issues related to intimacy and sexuality and may also be important to address (Smith, 2003).

Irritability may cause problems in the pain patient's relationships. Utilizing anger management strategies, relaxation, and assertiveness (see "Develop a toolbox of pain rescue strategies") can help reduce irritability. The pain patient's significant others may also have unrealistic expectations about what the pain patient is capable of doing. Patients may respond to these demands with anger or avoidance that can lead to increased pain for the patients and/or damage to their relationships. Some patients need to learn to set limits, and be more assertive with significant others about how their pain affects them and what they need from their significant others to help manage their pain. When patients are asked to do things that will make their pain worse, patients can learn to offer to do an acceptable alternative that will not increase their pain. For example, a patient asked to clear tables at a charity event may offer instead to collect tickets at the event or help the organizer make phone calls to find someone else to clear tables. Setting limits with others can prevent pain flares and ultimately help everyone involved. Patients may need to be reminded of the benefits of limit setting such as reduced pain, reduced irritability, and improvements in functioning.

Manage attitudes toward and responses to pain

Reducing catastrophizing beliefs about pain has been a core component of pain management CBT (Sullivan et al., 2001). A tendency toward catastrophizing is one of the characteristics that may make some people more prone to developing chronic pain than others (Ablin & Clauw, 2009). In addition, the ongoing fight against pain can paradoxically make pain worse. Pain acceptance can help patients focus on finding ways to engage in normal life activities despite the pain (Viane et al., 2003). The BHS can help patients develop more adaptive attitudes about pain and better manage pain through CBT.

Manage mental health disorders

Address other co-occurring mental health problems including depression, trauma, and other anxiety disorders. These may preexist, exacerbate, or in some cases, cause pain. A variety of typical psychological interventions can be used in these cases.

Although the BHS will not be prescribing medications, it is important to be aware of what psychotropic medications patients may be prescribed. Certain antidepressants can help with pain. However, patients may not understand this effect of antidepressants or, in the case of comorbid depression or anxiety, may be reluctant to try antidepressants because they may be resistant to the diagnosis or to the treatment. For reluctant patients, explaining the efficacy of medications for pain or concomitant depression and anxiety may reduce their resistance to medications.

Diet and weight control

Obesity and being overweight are correlated with chronic pain and research suggests that even modest weight loss can improve outcomes for patients with some types of pain (Messier et al., 2004). Simple interventions such as exploring ambivalence to weight control, keeping a food journal, referral to a registered dietician, initiating a pain compatible exercise program are quite appropriate for the integrated care model (Figure 6.1).

Address substance use

Caffeine is the most commonly abused psychoactive substance in the United States (Butt & Sultan, 2011). Patients with chronic pain often use caffeine to combat fatigue and elevate mood. Caffeine at therapeutic levels can have an analgesic effect and is even added to some brands of aspirin to increase analgesic effectiveness. At low doses (less than a cup of coffee), however, caffeine can inhibit the analgesic effect of some medications including some of the antidepressants, anticonvulsants, and even acetaminophen (Sawynok, 2010). Tolerance and dependence to caffeine can develop quickly and patients can

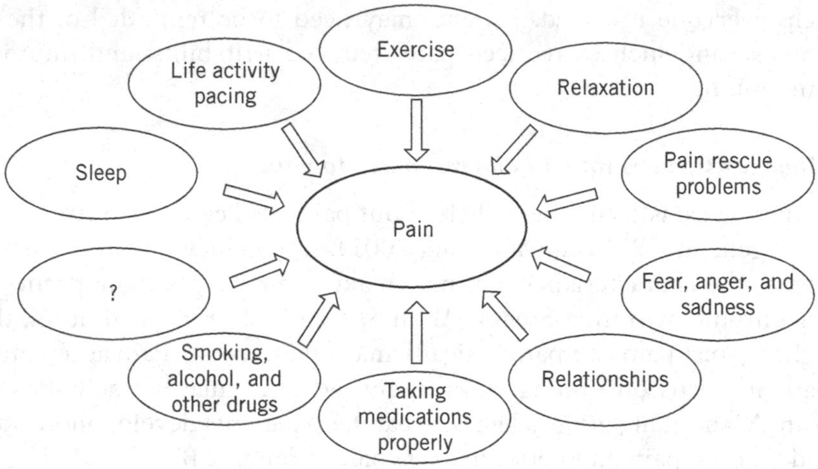

Figure 6.1 Representative integrated care menu for the treatment of chronic pain. Adapted from Sharone Abramowitz, MD; www.pcbehavioralhealth.com.

suffer withdrawal symptoms including headache if they modify their intake. Caffeine can interfere with pain management in several other ways. Because of caffeine's long half-life, if used at more than a modest level, it will still be present in the bloodstream at bedtime. This can interfere with already vulnerable sleep. In addition, caffeine can contribute to symptoms of anxiety with resulting negative effects on pain perception.

Tobacco use is strongly associated with chronic pain. The relationship between tobacco and pain is complicated. While smoking can produce a temporary analgesic effect, it is associated with increased pain and poorer functioning (Patterson et al., 2012). Nicotine cessation decreases the use of opioids in patients with chronic pain (Parkerson, Zvolensky, & Asmundson, 2013), and the BHS has a unique opportunity to assist patients with smoking cessation.

Alcohol is another problematic substance. Alcohol interacts with other medications, worsens sleep, and has abuse and addiction potential. While alcohol has a short-term analgesic effect, it is associated with long-term worsening of pain (Egli, Koobb, & Edwards, 2012).

The use of cannabis for medical purposes is controversial. In about half of our states, medical cannabis is legal; however, pain physicians have differing opinions about whether other controlled pain medications should be discontinued if patients report using cannabis (Reisfield, 2010). Cannabis may be seen as a marker of maladaptive reliance on substances, and its use has been associated with decreased adherence to opioid therapy (Reisfield, Wasan, & Jamison, 2009). Nonetheless, evidence exists to support its efficacy for pain (Rog, Nurmikko, Friede, & Young, 2005). At this time, however, there are insufficient randomized controlled trials evaluating the safety and efficacy of cannabis for sustained use in the treatment of pain.

Medication misuse, addiction, pseudoaddiction, and opioid induced hyperalgesia deserve a brief mention. Opioid analgesics and benzodiazepine medications have a high potential for misuse even in patients who have no intention of misusing their medications. Patients may require assistance in adhering to treatment plans and avoiding tolerance and dependence on these medications. Many states have prescription drug monitoring programs that help medical providers evaluate patients' use of medications by monitoring the frequency of prescription refills, number of potentially addictive medications, and number of providers prescribing pain medication reducing the potential for misuse of the drugs. Nurses and prescribing providers can access this information and identify patterns suggestive of misuse early. Misuse and aberrant drug-taking practices are not always reflective of recreational use. Pseudoaddiction is a pattern of drug-seeking behaviors in patients whose pain is poorly controlled and can be mistaken for addiction (Hooten et al., 2013). Assisting patients in appropriately managing their pain can circumvent pseudoaddiction and being labeled as "drug-seeking."

Opioid-induced hyperalgesia is a condition where opioid medications have led to a paradoxical increase in pain despite receiving escalating doses of opioids (Hooten et al., 2013). The BHS can help patients communicate more effectively with their health care team around issues of medication use to reduce misunderstandings and optimize medication management of pain.

Address Systems Issues That May Impact Pain and Coping

Pain impacts the people around the patient in pain (McCluskey, Brooks, King, & Burton, 2011). Significant others may be overly solicitous and reinforce pain behaviors, encouraging dependency on others. Alternatively significant others can isolate, neglect, or even be angry at and abuse the patient with pain. Many families will need education or even counseling to find ways to adjust to the new roles and relationships pain brings to the family. Smith (2003) recommends improving communication, including communication with family members, as necessary. The *Pain Survival Guide* (Turk & Winter, 2006) has a chapter on pain and relationships focusing on communication, assertiveness, and intimacy, which may be useful for some patients. Some patients may require help at work to identify necessary accommodations or educating employers about working with an employee with chronic pain. Finally, some patients will require assistance in accessing social services (e.g., vocational rehabilitation, social security disability) if their pain prevents them from gainful employment.

Develop a Toolbox of Pain Rescue Strategies

Lifestyle changes have the biggest impact on quality of life for pain patients but these patients also need assistance with managing acute pain as it occurs. Helping patients develop a long and varied list of coping strategies for both acute and chronic pain should be a goal for the BHS. Pain control strategies used for acute or chronic pain in the patient's toolbox include the following.

Distraction

Distraction takes advantage of the brain's filtering process, where some information is allowed to reach conscious attention while other information is ignored. The BHS can illustrate this concept by pointing out that we are usually not aware of the sound of an air conditioner or the sensation of a wedding ring on our finger until it is brought to our attention. Distraction works best at lower levels of pain and when patients do not fear pain (Johnson, 2005). Johnson (2005) identifies effective distractor characteristics as relaxing, enjoyable, absorbing/cognitively demanding, with an external sensory focus and requiring behavioral activity. Morley, Shapiro, and Biggs (2004) developed a treatment manual for attention management in chronic pain. The manual utilizes mindfulness and imagery as distraction techniques. Other practical distractors include playing games with family, completing puzzles, and doing crafts.

Relaxation

Relaxation is a key component of behavioral treatment of pain. Various relaxation techniques have been shown to be effective in managing chronic pain including diaphragmatic breathing (we use the phrase relaxed breathing with patients), progressive muscle relaxation training, mindfulness-based stress reduction, imagery, autogenic training, and hypnosis (Hooten et al., 2013). The BHS's skills with these techniques and the patient's preferences can direct the method(s) used. The key lesson for patients is that relaxation is a skill that requires regular practice to become proficient. At least some of the practice should occur when patients are not acutely anxious and when pain levels are relatively low. Using the metaphor of learning to write, ride a bike, or play an instrument can illustrate this point. When a skill is practiced often it is available even in stressful situations. There are many audio and video tapes, YouTube videos, and downloadable handouts about relaxation available on the Internet. Patients can be either provided a list of these resources or directed to perform a basic Internet search themselves for these resources. Some patients like having a recorded relaxation cue message on their smartphones so that their relaxation cue is always accessible.

Biofeedback

Biofeedback is a form of relaxation that has demonstrated efficacy for pain management (Haddock et al., 1997), particularly in the treatment of headaches (Hooten et al., 2013). Most formal biofeedback strategies require specialized equipment and training of the provider. Various physiological processes can be targeted through biofeedback. Skin conductance measured through galvanic skin response and providing feedback to patients in real time is one useful mode of biofeedback enhancing relaxation training. Muscle tension can be measured through electromyography (EMG) sensors and feedback can help patients learn to control particular muscle groups associated with pain. EMG biofeedback has been used with a variety of syndromes ranging from headaches to pelvic floor pain (Haddock et al., 1997).

Positive self-talk/CBT

Helpless and hopeless thinking, catastrophizing (thinking of the worst-case scenario), and fear of pain have been identified as particular barriers to coping with acute pain flares (Morley, Shapiro, & Biggs, 2004). Helping patients develop adaptive cognitive responses to these negative thoughts can be helpful. Making laminated cards with adaptive thoughts in response to negative thoughts can be useful in difficult situations. Examples of adaptive thoughts include: "I have survived this before and things got better. I can do it again." "I can look at my toolbox list and try something else."

Anger management

While anger management does fall within what we traditionally identify as CBT, it deserves special attention. The nature of pain as an indicator of danger and a trigger for the fight-or-flight response can predispose patients to irritability and anger when in pain. In addition, when they feel anger about external events, this can also engage their fight-or-flight system, which can negatively impact the experience of pain (Burns, Bruehl, & Quartana, 2006). Anger and hostility are strongly related to measures of pain intensity (Gatchel et al., 2007). Anger management then is important to reduce distress and the impact that pain can have on others. Using relaxation, assertiveness, improved communication, and planning for challenging situations are all appropriate interventions.

The following interventions will often be recommended by other members of the treatment team, often occupational and physical therapists. It is important for the BHS to have a basic understanding of these interventions and to help patients develop plans and cuing to use these methods when needed for pain.

Ice

The application of ice to pain-affected areas is occasionally recommended particularly for acute injury and inflammation. Precautions for its use include avoidance of damage to tissue from ice burns. If icing works for the patient, it can be put on the toolbox list and patients can make preparations so that the ice, gel packs, or bags of frozen peas are available when needed.

Heat

Although research does not support the use of heat as a stand-alone pain management strategy, many chronic pain patients report relief when applying heat to pain affected areas (Masuda et al., 2005). Hot showers/baths, hot tubs, saunas, heating pads, microwavable rice bags, and even heated car seats have all been used by chronic pain patients, often in conjunction with relaxation. Precaution and safety is a concern here as well to avoid burning tissue by overheating. Devices that provide sustained heating should have timers or active pressure switches. As with icing, the BHS can help patients plan when and how they might use these devices.

Counterpressure and self-massage

Patients can learn to use physical pressure to reduce pain (Hooten et al., 2013). Durable medical devices such as Theracanes in addition to other manual or electric massagers can be used. Ideally, instruction in the proper use of these devices will be provided by physical or occupational therapists, as using excessive force can increase pain. Again, the BHS can also assist physical or occupational therapists in instructing patients in when and how they might use these devices.

Alternative stimulation

Some pain patients are prescribed transcutaneous electrical nerve stimulation (TENS) units to assist with pain control. TENS units are small, often portable, battery-powered devices that use mild, safe electrical signals to help patients control pain. The precise mechanism of their action in improving pain control is unknown. One theory is that the electric signal produced by the TENS unit blocks the pain signals from reaching the brain. Another theory is that the stimulation may elicit neurochemicals called endorphins that reduce the sensation of pain by also blocking pain signals (Rushton, 2002). There is limited evidence supporting the TENS unit as a stand-alone pain management method (Hooten et al., 2013) but some patients find that it is helpful. In this instance it can be entered into the patient's care plan. Although TENS units can be purchased without a prescription, it is recommended that a trained professional teach patients how to use them.

Pharmacotherapy

The management of chronic pain is best conducted with a multiprofessional team using a multitude of strategies, including pharmacotherapy. It is important for today's practicing BHS to have a working knowledge of the benefits and limitations of the drugs frequently used for chronic pain. A cursory understanding of the commonly used analgesics and adjuvant medications is very important for the BHS because he or she helps patients with medication adherence and communication with the primary care provider. Due to the complex biopsychosocial nature of chronic pain, a multitude of pharmacotherapeutic treatments may be used in addition to the interventions listed previously. Medications frequently employed include opioids, antidepressants, anticonvulsants, anesthetics, nonsteroidal anti-inflammatory drugs (NSAIDs), and acetaminophen. A detailed listing of these medication classes, representative agents, and clinical pearls for the BHS may be found in Table 6.1.

Opioids are potentially the most controversial of the medications used in the primary care setting for chronic pain. The BHS may be instrumental in screening patients for risk of misusing these drugs given their significant abuse liability (addiction potential). Screening tools and interviews by the BHS will likely provide important information for the prescribing provider when deciding to start or continue these agents. Additionally, appropriate patient education surrounding safe use of these drugs, their risks, the development of agreed-upon treatment goals, and defining treatment failures are also important tasks well suited to the BHS in primary care.

The other medications used in the treatment of chronic pain are usually used as "adjuvant analgesics," although this term is likely a misrepresentation of these drugs' actual utility. While beyond the scope of this chapter, the BHS

TABLE 6.1 Representative Pharmacotherapy Utilized for the Treatment of Chronic Pain in the Primary Care Setting

Medication Class	Representative Agents	Clinical Considerations
Opioids	Fentanyl Hydrocodone Hydromorphone Methadone Morphine Oxycodone Tramadol	Risk of respiratory depression when first initiating or increasing doses. Abrupt discontinuation may lead to a withdrawal syndrome. Medications in this class may worsen depression. Oftentimes patients describe anxiolytic benefit from these agents. Misuse and abuse of these medications may be problematic and routine screening for aberrant drug-taking behaviors is paramount.
Antidepressants—selective serotonin reuptake inhibitors	Fluoxetine Sertraline Paroxetine Citalopram Escitalopram	Not frequently used for adjuvant analgesia but for comorbid depression or anxiety. Typical time of onset of activity is 2 weeks for energy, 3 to 4 weeks for mood improvement, and 6 weeks for maximum benefit. Symptoms of anxiety may worsen over first 2 weeks prior to improving with these agents. Risk of suicidal ideations is increased during first 2 weeks of treatment, especially in patients 18 to 24 years of age.
Antidepressants—serotonin–norepinephrine reuptake Inhibitors	Venlafaxine Desvenlafaxine Duloxetine Milnacipran Levomilnacipran	Typical time of onset of activity is 1 to 2 weeks for energy, 2 to 4 weeks for mood improvement, and 4 to 6 weeks for maximum benefit. Analgesic benefit seen earlier than antidepressant effect (milnacipran only indicated for fibromyalgia) Symptoms of anxiety may worsen over first 2 weeks prior to improving with these agents. Risk of suicidal ideations is increased during first 2 weeks of treatment, especially in patients 18 to 24 years of age.
Antidepressants—tricyclics	Amitriptyline Desipramine Imipramine Nortriptyline	May cause significant confusion in older adult patients. Overdose may result in cardiac arrhythmias and may be life-threatening. Questionable concern for inducing hypomania/mania in patients with Type 1 Bipolar Disorder. Significant sedation, dry mouth, constipation, and urinary retention.

(continued)

TABLE 6.1 Representative Pharmacotherapy Utilized for the Treatment of Chronic Pain in the Primary Care Setting (*continued*)

Medication Class	Representative Agents	Clinical Considerations
Anticonvulsants	Gabapentin Pregabalin Carbamazepine Topiramate	Frequently used for neuropathic pain syndromes. All agents may cause some degree of neurocognitive slowing (most pronounced with topiramate) and sedation.
NSAIDs	Celecoxib Diclofenac Ibuprofen Meloxicam Naproxen Nabumetone	Work as anti-inflammatory drugs to inhibit prostaglandins. Risk of gastrointestinal ulcer and/or bleeding. May increase risk of myocardial infarction or stroke. Take with food to decrease stomach problems.
Skeletal muscle relaxants	Baclofen Carisprodol Cyclobenzaprine Diazepam Metaxalone Orphenadrine Tizanidine	Most agents are sedating. Questionable utility long term. Carisprodol and diazepam have abuse liability.
Anesthetics	Lidocaine patch	No more than three patches at one time. Must remove after 12 hours of being applied each day.
Other	Acetaminophen	Most frequently prescribed/purchased analgesic. Risk of liver toxicity in doses over 4,000 mg each day, liver disease, or concurrent alcohol abuse. Important to consider the different prescription and over-the-counter drugs patient may be taking that contain acetaminophen.

should know several important considerations in regard to these agents when working with patients. Perhaps most concerning is the risk of increased suicidality with the anticonvulsants and antidepressants (U.S. Food and Drug Administration, 2008). The risk is more pronounced with the antidepressant medications and usually seen in the highest incidence between the ages of 18 and 24 years and within the first 2 to 3 weeks of initiation. In fact, many BHSs recommend follow-up with patients starting these medications during the early weeks to assess potential worsening of mood or appearance of suicidal or homicidal ideation and then assess for suicidality or homicidality throughout the course of treatment, particularly with patients who have a concomitant mood disorder.

Any number of the interventions reviewed previously may be appropriate for a particular patient. Addressing all interventions at once with a chronic pain patient would be surely overwhelming for the patient. Using a motivational interviewing technique to tailor or personalize treatment for a patient by focusing on a few areas and having the patient make the choice of which to work on would be ideal and may increase the likelihood that patients will be successful (Bair et al., 2009). Another option is to have a menu of interventions for pain patients such as in Figure 6.1. The patient could choose the intervention(s) they would like to address, increasing the likelihood that the patient is motivated and engaged in the intervention. Some interventions such as exercise may provide the most benefit but be the least likely to be chosen by patients. The BHS may need to actively encourage interventions that are avoided but that may provide the most benefit.

Other Resources for the Behavioral Health Specialist

There is a plethora of resources to help clinicians and patients with this challenging problem (see Table 6.2). Ehde et al. (2014) suggested exploring new technologies such as web-based and telephonic treatment in working with chronic pain patients. In addition, YouTube videos such as the one mentioned in Table 6.2 may be helpful as an adjunct to treatment. The BHS should preview and be familiar with any materials he or she makes available to patients.

TABLE 6.2 Useful Resources for the Behavioral Health Specialist

Books	*Mayo Clinic Guide to Pain Relief* (Bruce & Hooten, 2008). This book is written for patients covering many of the topics discussed in this chapter. It was designed to accompany their Chronic Pain Rehabilitation program but is written to stand alone. In addition to behavioral strategies, it discusses information about different types of chronic pain interventions including pain clinics, medications, and interventional methods.
	Managing Pain Before It Manages You (Caudill, 2009). This book is written by an internal medicine pain specialist. This book comes with a free audio download of guided relaxation exercises and has a lot of good information for the pain patient. It provides education on pain with a substantial emphasis on cognitive and behavioral interventions including coping skills, problem solving, and developing realistic goals.
	The Pain Survival Guide (Turk & Winter, 2006). This patient-education book is published by the American Psychological Association. It is a good companion for cognitive behavioral therapy. The ten lesson format is concise and accessible to patients with good medical literacy. It has less information about pain, specific syndromes, and medical treatments than the two books previously mentioned, focusing on practical interventions.

(continued)

TABLE 6.2 Useful Resources for the Behavioral Health Specialist (*continued*)	
	Managing Chronic Pain: A Cognitive-Behavioral Therapy Approach (Otis, 2007). This is a useful reference for the BHS providing structured cognitive behavioral therapy for chronic pain patients. It describes an 11-session format focusing on relaxation, stress management, cognitive restructuring, pacing, pleasurable activities, and relapse prevention. It has a companion patient workbook, *Managing Chronic Pain: A Cognitive-Behavioral Therapy Approach Workbook* (Otis, 2007), which contains more education, homework assignments, and behavior logs for use with the pain patient.
Health Care Guideline	*Assessment and Management of Chronic Pain* (Hooten et al. 2013). This is a useful reference for the BHS providing chronic pain treatment. This resource provides a great deal of the medical research on chronic pain and identifies the current state of the art in pain assessment and treatment. Of particular use is the appendix, which contains pain assessment instruments, and tools for determining opioid risk. It also contains descriptions of different types of pain syndromes and medical interventions.
Online Resources	One especially useful website with patient education videos is from painaustralia (www.painaustralia.org.au/media-news/videos.html). There is a strong focus on active approaches, thoughts and emotions, and collaboration with the treatment team.
Professional Organizations	The International Association for the Study of Pain (IASP) (www.iasp-pain.org) provides publications for clinicians and can be a good resource for the BHS. American Chronic Pain Association (www.theacpa.org) has information designed for patients and their families, but can also be useful for the BHS.

CONCLUSION

Aiding patients in managing chronic pain is multifaceted and requires working with primary care providers, subspecialty providers, pharmacists, physical therapists, and other professionals. The BHS enhances the treatment of chronic pain by his or her understanding of the interaction between pain and psychological and social factors. BHSs have unique training in assessing emotional, behavioral, and interpersonal influences on pain, mental health disorders, and pain management strategies. BHSs use their counseling skills to support patients while challenging patients' beliefs and behaviors in a manner to achieve therapeutic goals while maintaining therapeutic rapport. BHSs skills may be used to help improve collaboration between the patient and other members of the treatment team to increase treatment adherence. The BHS provides education to the patient about all aspects of pain management and education to the rest of the integrated health care team about the biopsychosocial approach to care. Finally, the BHS helps patients develop realistic goals for treatment and provides interventions to help patients improve their lives.

BEHAVIORAL HEALTH ASSESSMENT AND TREATMENT SUMMARY TO REFERRING PRIMARY CARE PROVIDER

S: Ms. Jones was referred by Dr. X for evaluation and treatment of chronic neck and back pain, fibromyalgia, and anxiety disorder. She completed a focused assessment. She identified many factors contributing to her pain and anxiety including inactivity, poor sleep, life stressors (among them conflictual relationships), and tobacco abuse. She denied symptoms of depressive disorder, bipolar disorder, and substance use disorders. She reports anxiety related specifically to episodic changes in her pain. No reports of panic attacks. No premorbid history of anxiety or panic, or of any mental illness. She denies any psychiatric hospitalizations. No significant family history of mental illness.

She is employed as an office assistant and has been happily married to the same man for 25 years. The couple is childless. The patient's mother-in-law complains that patient's pain is exaggerated and she uses it as an excuse for not visiting the mother-in-law more often. This creates some tension between the patient and her husband.

O: Ms. Jones was alert and oriented ×4. She was verbal and interactive throughout the assessment. She was initially anxious with many pain behaviors including wincing, guarding, and neck rubbing. She relaxed and her mood brightened over the course of the assessment. Thoughts were organized and logical. Judgment and insight were intact. She denied suicidal ideation.

A: Psychological factors affecting other medical conditions (moderate): Fibromyalgia and chronic neck and back pain (316); generalized anxiety disorder (300.02).

1. **Psychological factors affecting other medical conditions**: Patient education provided on acute and chronic pain. To engage her in treatment she was introduced to the following concepts: (a) that her pain is real regardless of the lack of any identifiable acute etiology, and (b) that the complexity of her pain requires multidimensional pain management. We discussed the goals of pain management, lifestyle changes, and began to explore tools/strategies she could use to better manage acute and chronic pain. She wishes to continue seeing the BHS and agreed to the following as an initial approach to pain management:

   a) Use a relaxation CD 2 to 8 times each day (with heating pad to pain affected areas).
   b) Walk 10 minutes each day.
   c) Attend fibromyalgia support group with a friend.
   d) Continue taking antidepressant for pain and anxiety control.

2. **Anxiety disorder**: The patient identified relational problems and feelings of loneliness and isolation as the cause of her anxiety. These problems are also related to her chronic pain and likely precipitate and maintain some of her chronic pain symptoms. She would be an ideal candidate for CBT to address these problems. She is ambivalent about participating in counseling at this time. We will continue to discuss a referral to CBT at her next integrated care appointment. She identified several interpersonal goals including spending more time with her nephews and church group, which she can start on immediately. I also encouraged her to follow good sleep hygiene and reduce her caffeine intake.

She is not ready to quit smoking at this time but expresses a long-range plan to quit (stage of change: contemplative). She was provided a list of bibliotherapy resources for self-help in this area. She will return in 1 week for follow-up with behavioral health.

REFERENCES

Ablin, K., & Clauw, D. (2009). From fibrositis to functional somatic syndromes to a bell-shaped curve of pain and sensory sensitivity: Evolution of a clinical construct. *Rheumatic Disease Clinics of North America*, *35*, 233–251.

Allegretti, A., Borkan, J., Reis, S., & Griffiths, F. (2010). Paired interviews of shared experiences around chronic low back pain: Classic mismatch between patients and their doctors. *Family Practice*, *27*(6), 676–683.

American Society of Anesthesiologists Task Force on Chronic Pain Management, American Society of Regional Anesthesia and Pain Medicine. (2010). Practice guidelines for chronic pain management: An updated report by the American Society of Anesthesiologists Task Force on Chronic Pain Management and the American Society of Regional Anesthesia and Pain Medicine. *Anesthesiology*, *112*, 810.

Bair, M. J., Matthias, M. S., Nyland, K. A., Huffman, M. A., Stubbs, D. L., Kroenke, K., & Damush, T. M. (2009). Barriers and facilitators to chronic pain self-management: A qualitative study of primary care patients with comorbid musculoskeletal pain and depression. *Pain Medicine*, *10*(7), 1280–1290.

Bernstein, I. H., Jaremko, M. E., & Hinkley, B. S. (1995). On the utility of the West Haven-Yale multidimensional pain inventory. *Spine*, *20*(8), 956–963.

Bruce, B., & Hooten, W. M. (2008). *Mayo Clinic guide to pain relief*. Rochester, MN: Mayo Clinic Health Solutions.

Burns, J. W., Bruehl, S., & Quartana, P. J. (2006). Anger management style and hostility among patients with chronic pain: Effects on symptom-specific physiological reactivity during anger- and sadness-recall interviews. *Psychosomatic Medicine*, *68*, 786–793.

Butt, M. S., & Sultan, M. T. (2011). Coffee and its consumption: Benefits and risks. *Critical Reviews in Food Science and Nutrition*, *51*, 363–373.

Caudill, M. A. (2009). *Managing pain before it manages you*. New York, NY: Guilford Press.

Chapman, C. R., Tuckett, R. P., & Woo Song, C. (2008). Pain and stress in a systems perspective: Reciprocal neural, endocrine and immune interactions. *Journal of Pain*, *9*(2), 122–145.

Cho, H. Y., Kim, E. H., & Kim, J. (2014). Effects of the CORE exercise program on pain and active range of motion in patients with chronic low back pain. *Journal of Physical Therapy Science*, *26*(8), 1237–1240.

Cleeland, C. S., & Ryan, K. M. (1994). Pain assessment: Global use of the Brief Pain Inventory. *Annals, Academy of Medicine, Singapore*, *23*(2), 129–138.

Compton, W. M., & Volkow, N. D. (2006). Major increases in opioid analgesic abuse in the United States: Concerns and strategies. *Drug and Alcohol Dependence, 81*(2), 103–107.

Diesfeld, K. (2008). Interpersonal issues between pain physician and patient: Strategies to reduce conflict. *Pain Medicine, 9*(8), 1118–1124.

Douglas, M. E., Randleman, M. L., DeLane, A. M., & Palmer, G. A. (2014). Determining pain scale preference in a veteran population experiencing chronic pain. *Pain Management Nursing, 15*(3), 625–631.

Egli, M., Koobb, G. F., & Edwards, S. (2012). Alcohol dependence as a chronic pain disorder. *Neuroscience and Biobehavioral Reviews, 36*, 2179–2192.

Ehde, D. M., Dillworth, T. M., & Turner, J. A. (2014). Cognitive-behavioral therapy for individuals with chronic pain: Efficacy, innovation, and directions for research. *American Psychologist, 69*(2), 153–166.

Finan, P, Goodin, B. R., & Smith, M. T. (2013). The association of sleep and pain: An update and a path forward. *Journal of Pain, 14*(12), 1539–1552.

Flor H., Braun C., Elbert T., & Birbaumer, N. (1997). Extensive reorganization of primary somatosensory cortex in chronic back pain patients. *Neuroscience Letters, 224*, 5–8.

Gaskin, D. J., & Richard, P. (2012). The economic costs of pain in the United States. *The Journal of Pain, 13*(8), 715–724.

Gatchel, R. J., Peng, Y. B., Peters, M. L., Fuchs, P. N., & Turk, D. C. (2007). The biopsychosocial approach to chronic pain: Scientific advances and future directions. *Psychological Bulletin, 133*(4), 581–624.

Gore, M., Sadosky, A., Stacey, B., Tai, K. S., Leslie, D. (2012). The burden of chronic low back pain: Clinical comorbidities, treatment patterns, and health care costs in usual care settings. *Spine, 37*(11), E668–E677.

Haddock, C. K., Rowan, A. B., & Andrasik, F., Wilson, P. G., Talcott, G. W., & Stein, R. J. (1997). Home-based behavioral treatments for chronic benign headache: A meta-analysis of controlled trials. *Cephalagia, 17*, 113–118.

Harris, C. A., & D'Eon, J. L. (2008). Psychometric properties of the Beck Depression Inventory-(BDI-II) in individuals with chronic pain. *Pain, 137*(3), 609–622.

Hooten, W., Timming, R., Belgrade, M., Gaul, J., Goertz, M., Haake, B., ... Walker, N. (2013). *Health care guideline: Assessment and management of chronic pain.* Bloomington, MN: Institute for Clinical Systems Improvement.

Institute of Medicine. (2011). *Relieving pain in America: A blueprint for transforming prevention, care, education, and research.* Washington, DC: National Academies Press.

Jamieson-Lega, K., Berry, R., & Brown, C. A. (2013). Pacing: A concept analysis of the chronic pain intervention. *Pain Research & Management, 18*(4), 207–213.

Keefe, F. J., Abernethy, A. P., & Campbell, C. (2005). Psychological approaches to understanding and treating disease-related pain. *Annual Review of Psychology, 56*, 601–630.

Kerns, R. D., Burns, J. W., Shulman, M., Jensen, M. P., Nielson, W. R., Czlapinski, R., ... Rosenberger, P. (2014). Can we improve cognitive-behavioral therapy for chronic back pain treatment engagement and adherence? A controlled trial of tailored versus standard therapy. *Health Psychology, 33*(9), 938–947.

Kerns, R. D., Sellinger, J., & Goodin, B. R. (2011). Psychological treatment of chronic pain. *Annual Review of Clinical Psychology, 7*, 411–434.

Kroenke, K., Spitzer, R. L., & Williams, J. B. (2001). The PHQ 9. *Journal of General Internal Medicine, 16*(9), 606–613.

Kroenke, K., Yu, Z., Wu, J., Kean, J., & Pasley, J. D. (2014). Operating characteristics of PROMIS four item depression and anxiety scales in primary care patients with chronic pain. *Pain Medicine, 15*(11), 1892–1901.

Johnson, M. H. (2005). How does distraction work in the management of pain? *Current Pain and Headache Reports, 9*(2), 90–95.

Lambeek, C. L., van Mechelen, W., Knol, D. L., Loisel, P., & Anema, J. R. (2010). Randomised controlled trial of integrated care to reduce disability from chronic low back pain in working and private life. *British Medical Journal, 340*, c1035.

Larson, A. A., Pardo, J. V., & Pasley, J. D. (2014). Review of overlap between thermoregulation and pain modulation in fibromyalgia. *Clinical Journal of Pain, 30*(6), 544–555.

Lewinsohn, P. M., Graf, M. (1973). Pleasant activities and depression. *Journal of Consulting and Clinical Psychology*, *41*(2), 261–268.

Maihöfner, C., Handwerker, H., Neundörfer, B., & Birklein F. (2003). Patterns of cortical reorganization in complex regional pain syndrome. *Neurology*, *6*, 1707–1715.

Manchikanti, L., Helm II, S., Fellows, B., Janata, J. W., Pampati, V., Grider, J. S., & Boswell, M. V. (2012). Opioid epidemic in the United States. *Pain Physician*, *15*, ES9–ES38.

Masuda, A., Koga, Y., Hattanmaru, M., Minagoe, S., Tei, C. (2005). The effects of repeated thermal therapy for patients with chronic pain. *Psychotherapy and Psychosomatic*, *74*(5), 288–294.

McCluskey, S., Brooks, J., King, N., & Burton, K. (2011). The influence of "significant others" on persistent back pain and work participation: A qualitative exploration of illness perceptions. *BMC Musculoskeletal Disorders*, *12*, 236.

McGeary, D., McGeary, C., & Gatchel, R. J. (2014). Managing chronic pain in primary care. In C. M. Hunter, C. L. Hunter, & R. Kessler (Eds.), *Handbook of clinical psychology in medical settings* (pp. 589–623). New York, NY: Springer Science + Business Media.

Messier, S. P., Loeser, R. F., Miller, G. D., Morgan, T. M., Rejeski, W. J., Sevick, M. A., ... Williamson, J. D. (2004). Exercise and dietary weight loss in overweight and obese older adults with knee osteoarthritis: The arthritis, diet, and activity promotion trial. *Arthritis & Rheumatism*, *50*(5), 1501–1510.

Morley, S., Shapiro, D. A., & Biggs, J. (2004). Developing a treatment manual for attention management in chronic pain. *Cognitive Behaviour Therapy*, *33*(1), 1–11.

Mularski, R. A., White-Chu, F., Overbay, D., Miller, L., Asch, S. M., & Ganzini, L. (2006). Measuring pain as the 5th vital sign does not improve quality of pain management. *Journal of General Internal Medicine*, *21*(6), 607–612.

Nagasako, E. M., Oaklander, A. L., & Dworkin, R. H. (2003). Congenital insensitivity to pain: An update. *Pain*, *101*(3), 213–219.

Neugebauer, V., Galhardo, V., Maione, S., & Mackey, S. (2009). A decade of pain research: New approaches, new targets. *Brain Research Reviews*, *60*(1), 226–242.

Otis, J. D. (2007). Managing chronic pain: *A cognitive-behavioral therapy approach*. New York, NY: Oxford.

Parkerson, H., Zvolensky, M. J., & Asmundson, G. (2013). Understanding the relationship between smoking and pain. *Expert Review of Neurotherapeutics*, *13*(12), 1407–1414.

Patterson, A., Gritzner, S., Resnick, M. P., Dobscha, S. K., Turk, D. C., & Morasco, B. J. (2012). Smoking cigarettes as a coping strategy for chronic pain is associated with greater pain intensity and poorer pain-related function. *Journal of Pain*, *13*(3), 285–292.

Poleshuck, E. L., Gamble, S. A., Cort, N., Hoffman-King, D., Cerrito, B., Rosario-McCabe, L. A., Giles, D. E. (2010). Interpersonal psychotherapy for co-occurring depression and chronic pain. *Professional Psychology: Research and Practice*, *41*(4), 312–318.

Reisfield, G. M. (2010). Medical cannabis and chronic opioid therapy. *Journal of Pain & Palliative Care Pharmacotherapy*, *24*(4), 356–361.

Reisfield, G. M., Wasan, A. D., & Jamison, R. N. (2009). The prevalence and significance of cannabis use in patients prescribed chronic opioid therapy: A review of the extant literature. *Pain Medicine*, *10*(8), 1434–1441.

Roditi, D., & Robinson, M. (2011). The role of psychological interventions in the management of patients with chronic pain. *Psychology Research and Behavior Management*, *1*(4), 41–49.

Rog, D. J., Nurmikko, T. J., Friede, T., & Young, C. (2005). Randomized, controlled trial of cannabis-based medicine in central pain in multiple sclerosis. *Neurology*, *65*(60), 812–819.

Roland, M., & Morris, R. (1983). A study of the natural history of back pain: Part I: Development of a reliable and sensitive measure of disability in low-back pain. *Spine*, *8*(2), 141–144.

Rushton, D. (2002). Electrical stimulation in the treatment of pain. *Disability and Rehabilitation*, *24*(8), 407–415.

Sawynok, J. (2010). Caffeine and pain. *Pain*, *152*, 726–729.

Sluka, K. A., O'Donnell, J. M., Danielson, J., & Rasmussen, L. A. (1985). Regular physical activity prevents development of chronic pain and activation of central neurons. *Journal of Applied Physiology*, *114*(6), 725–733.

Smith, A. A. (2003). Intimacy and family relationships of women with chronic pain. *Pain Management Nursing, 4*(3), 134–142.

Snelling, J. (1994). The effect of chronic pain on the family unit. *Journal of Advanced Nursing, 19*(3), 543–551.

Spira, J. L. (1997). Understanding and developing psychotherapy groups for medically ill patients. In J. L. Spira (Ed.). *Group therapy for medically ill patients* (pp. 3–11). New York, NY: Guilford Press.

Spitzer, R. L., Kroenke, K., Williams, J. B., & Löwe, B. (2006). A brief measure for assessing generalized anxiety disorder: The GAD-7. *Archives of Internal Medicine, 166*(10), 1092–1097.

Sullivan, M. J., Thorn, B., Haythornthwaite, J. A., Keefe, F., Martin, M., Bradley, L. A., & Lefebvre, J. C. (2001). Theoretical perspectives on the relation between catastrophizing and pain. *Clinical Journal of Pain, 17*, 52–64.

Tang, N. K., Goodchild, C. E., & Salkovskis, P. M. (2012). Hybrid cognitive-behaviour therapy for individuals with insomnia and chronic pain: A pilot randomized controlled trial. *Behaviour Research and Therapy, 50*(12), 814–21.

Thorn, B. E. (2004). *Cognitive therapy for chronic pain: A step-by-step guide.* New York, NY: Guilford Press.

Tse, M. M., Vong, S. K., & Tang, S. K. (2013). Motivational interviewing and exercise programme for community-dwelling older persons with chronic pain: A randomised controlled study. *Journal of Clinical Nursing, 22*, 1843–1856.

Turk, D. C. (2002). Clinical effectiveness and cost-effectiveness of treatments for patients with chronic pain. *Clinical Journal of Pain, 18*(6), 715–724.

Turk, D. C. & Winter, F. (2006). *The pain survival guide: How to reclaim your life.* Washington, DC: American Psychological Association.

U.S. Food and Drug Administration. (2008). Information for healthcare professionals: Suicidal behavior and ideation and antiepileptic drugs. Retrieved from http://www.fda.gov/Drugs/DrugSafety/PostmarketDrugSafetyInformationforPatientsandProviders/ucm100192.htm

Viane, I., Crombez, G., Eccleston, C., Poppe, C., Devulder, J., Van Houdenhove, B., & DeCorte, W. (2003). Acceptance of pain is an independent predictor of mental well-being in patients with chronic pain: Empirical evidence and reappraisal. *Pain, 106*, 65–72.

Williams, A. C., Eccleston, C., & Morley, S. (2012). Psychological therapies for the management of chronic pain (excluding headache) in adults. *Cochrane Database of Systematic Reviews, 11.*

Wolfert, M. Z., Gilson, A. M., Dahl, J. L., & Cleary, J. F. (2010). Opioid analgesics for pain control: Wisconsin physicians' knowledge, beliefs, attitudes, and prescribing practices. *Pain Medicine, 11*, 425–434.

SEVEN

DISORDERED SLEEP

MICHELE M. LARZELERE AND JAMES S. CAMPBELL

S.O.A.P. NOTE FROM REFERRING PRIMARY CARE PROVIDER

S: A 61-year-old man with known hypertension and diabetes mellitus type2 on lisinopril and metformin. Complains of fatigue for over a year and progressively worsening difficulty with sleep for several years. Typically retires at 10:00 p.m., sets his alarm to arise at 6:00 a.m. but virtually never sleeps continuously. He is frustrated that it takes 1 to 2 hours to doze off followed by spontaneous awakening 1 to 2 hours later. Once aroused he feels he is kept awake by constant worry related to his job as a busy attorney. Reports that a glass of bourbon before bed seems to help him nod off more quickly. Wife states he snores a lot but she denies witnessed apnea. The patient denies chest pain or dyspnea. He is gaining weight and fasting glucose today was high (211 mg/dL). Wonders if he might need sleeping pills because he can barely stay awake at work.

O: BP 161/92, pulse 92, respirations 22, temperature 98.6, height 5'11", weight 223 (BMI 31), pulse oximetry normal at 96% on room air.

General: Mildly obese and somewhat anxious. Alert and oriented to person, place, and time.
HEENT: PERRLA, TMs intact bilaterally, throat and posterior pharynx without erythema, exudate, or masses.
Neck: Without adenopathy or masses. No thyroid enlargement or asymmetry.
Lungs: Clear to auscultation bilaterally without crackles or wheezes.
Heart: RRR without murmur or gallop.
Abdomen: Soft, obese, BS+, no HSmegaly, masses, or tenderness.
Extremeties: Strong pedal pulses. No edema.
Neurologic: Motor and sensory intact. Patellar DTRs 2+ bilaterally. Gait normal. PHQ-9 depression screening reveals a score of 8, consistent with mild depression.

A: Insomnia with fatigue (780.52, 780.79), mild depression with anxiety (311), DM2 (250.02), hypertension (401.1)

P: 1) Insomnia with fatigue: Sleep hygiene instruction sheet. Avoid alcohol. CBC, CMP, and TSH level ordered. Consider sleep study. Refer to the behavioral health specialist for further assessment.
2) Mild depression with anxiety: Consider SSRI. Refer to the behavioral health specialist for further assessment.
3) DM2 (uncontrolled): Hgb A1c ordered. Will likely need increased metformin dose pending A1c level. Diet and exercise counseling recommended.
4) HTN (Uncontrolled): Increase lisinopril.

INTRODUCTION

Patients with sleep disorders tend to present with complaints of insomnia, excessive daytime sleepiness, or having recognized (or been told by a bed partner) that their intra-sleep behavior is problematic. Many sleep disorders will be primarily managed through medical intervention (e.g., continuous positive airway pressure [CPAP] for sleep apnea,[1] movement disorder medications for restless legs syndrome [RLS]; Alattar, Harrington, Mitchell, & Sloane, 2007). In the realm of sleep disorders, behavioral health specialists (BHSs) will typically find their largest role in the treatment of insomnia.

Insomnia can be a symptom or a disorder, and may evolve from one to the other. Insomnia also appears to be a risk factor for the development of depression in adults and adolescents and predicts poorer depression treatment response, as well as more frequent recurrence of major depressive episodes. Patients who are older, female patients, and those whose insomnia has been more severe are most likely to experience chronic insomnia (Morin et al., 2009). Among patients achieving remission from insomnia, almost one-third experience recurrence.

In addition to the predicted sleepiness, common sequelae of insomnia include depression, anxiety, and confusion (Bonnet & Arand, 2006). Patients often experience quality of life decrements that are comparable to other chronic medical or psychological conditions (e.g., major depression, congestive heart failure [CHF]; Katz & McHorney, 2002), and experience work disruption and absenteeism at greater rates than good sleepers (Bonnet & Arand, 2006; Léger, Massuel, Metlaine, & SISYPHE Study Group, 2006). Medical consequences of insomnia are thought to include increased cardiovascular risk (due to the sympathetic nervous system activation; Bonnet & Arand, 1998; Fernandez-Mendoza et al., 2012) and diabetes (Vgontzas et al., 2009).

[1] A positive airway pressure (PAP) or continuous positive airway pressure (CPAP) device uses mild air flow, delivered through a mask covering the nose or nose and mouth, to keep an individual's airway from collapsing or becoming blocked when the musculature of the neck becomes relaxed during sleep. The amount of pressure required to maintain the airway varies from person to person and is generally titrated during a sleep study.

ASSESSMENT

For any patient with a complaint related to sleep or wakefulness, a thorough history is the first step (Malow, 2011; Table 7.1). The history should include a detailed understanding of the patient's typical patterns of sleep (bedtime, time to sleep onset, number and duration of awakenings after sleep onset, wake time, number and duration of naps) on both weekdays (or work days) and weekends (days off). Duration of the sleep problem, as well as circumstances associated with onset, exacerbation, and amelioration of symptoms should be explored. Patients should be asked to describe their pre-sleep routines and their sleep environments. The clinician should probe for any possible disruptions by bed partners, pets, or children. Any recent travel across time zones or participation in shift work should be carefully elucidated. Patients should be questioned about how refreshed they feel upon awakening and their functioning during the day (sleepiness, situations in which patients are likely to fall asleep, memory difficulties, concentration difficulties, fatigue, irritability) and any morning symptoms they might experience (dry mouth, headaches).

Even if insomnia is the suspected diagnosis, the clinician should assess for the possible presence of other sleep disorders (see Table 7.2). Because of the genetic components to narcolepsy, sleep apnea, and other troubling sleep-related behaviors, it is very useful to inquire about the family sleep disorder history (Malow, 2011). Information should be gathered about unusual sensations before sleep onset or during the night (leg cramping, twitching or tingling, need to move the legs) and about symptoms their bed-partner might report (snoring, kicking, arousals, apneic

TABLE 7.1 Diagnostic Criteria for Insomnia *DSM-5*

Dissatisfaction with quality or quantity of sleep:

- Sleep onset difficulty
- Sleep maintenance difficulty
- Early morning awakenings

Despite adequate sleep opportunities
Producing social, occupational, or functional activity impairment
Occurring three nights per week
Occurring for 3 months
Not better explained by another sleep disorder, mental disorder, or other medical condition
Not attributable to the direct effects of a substance
Specifiers:

- Episodic (symptoms last at least 1 month, but less than 3 months)
- Persistent (symptoms >3 months)
- Recurrent (two or more episodes in 1 year)

Specifiers:

- With nonsleep disorder mental comorbidity
- With other medical comorbidity
- With other sleep disorder

Source: Adapted from American Psychiatric Association (2013).

TABLE 7.2 Common Sleep and Wakefulness Complaints

Presenting Complaint	Possible Diagnoses (*Signs and Symptoms*)	Differential Diagnostic Considerations

Difficulty with sleep onset or maintenance	*Insomnia (persistent difficulty achieving restful sleep)*	■ Shift work
		■ Psychiatric disorders
		  ■ Major depression
		  ■ Generalized anxiety disorder
		  ■ Bipolar disorder
		  ■ Posttraumatic stress disorder
		■ Medication side effect
		■ Substance use/withdrawal
		■ Medical conditions (e.g., pain)
		■ Advanced or delayed sleep phase

Excessive daytime sleepiness	*Sleep apnea (breathing cessation for 10 seconds or more with oxygen desaturation and arousal; snoring, gasping/choking sensations)* *Narcolepsy (cataplexy, sleep paralysis, hypnagogic/hypnopompic hallucinations)* *Restless legs syndrome (unpleasant aching or crawling sensation in the legs, typically worse at rest and during evening/night)*	■ Sleep deprivation/sleep fragmentation ■ Medications ■ Medical conditions ■ Psychiatric conditions ■ Substance use/withdrawal
Unusual or bothersome nighttime events	*Periodic limb movement disorder (repetitive lower extremity movements during sleep)* *Sleepwalking (partial arousals from sleep accompanied by automatic behavior, usually during the first half of the night, typically with little memory of the event)* *Sleep terrors (partial arousals marked by disorientation/confusion, accompanied by expressions of intense fear, usually during the first half of the night, typically with little memory of the event)* *Rhythmic movement disorder (stereotyped large muscle movements before sleep such as rocking, headbanging, rolling)* *Bruxism (teeth clenching or grinding during sleep, may be rhythmic)* *REM-sleep behavior disorder (lack of muscle atonia that normally accompanies REM, acting out of dreams)*	■ Sleep deprivation/sleep fragmentation ■ Medications ■ Medical conditions ■ Substance use/withdrawal

Source: Vaughn & D'Cruz (2011).

episodes/gasping). The patient and, ideally, his or her partner should be questioned about nocturia (waking at night to urinate), nocturnal enuresis (bed-wetting), sleepwalking, sleep talking, violent behavior, screaming, or automatic behaviors (e.g., eating during the night). Finally, patients should be asked about any history of muscle weakness or complete lack of muscle tone in response to surprise or strong emotions (cataplexy), intrusions of dreamlike sensory experiences at sleep onset or awakening (hypnagogic and hypnopompic hallucinations), and the experience of partial or total paralysis occurring at sleep onset or upon awakening (sleep paralysis).

The American Academy of Sleep Medicine (AASM) has established indications for sleep study in insomnia patients based on scientific review of the literature by their Standards of Practice Committee (2003). Polysomnography ("sleep study," see the following) is not recommended in the routine evaluation of all insomnia. It is, however, recommended in the face of suspected breathing disorders or periodic limb movements during sleep. It is also advocated for insomnia treatment failures, unexplained hypersomnolence (prolonged or excessive sleeping), excessive daytime sleepiness, and nonrestorative sleep, or in the face of violent/injurious arousals (AASM, 2003; Ramar & Olson, 2013). Although many patients with insomnia may misreport or misperceive the amount of sleep they are getting (Manconi et al., 2010), this alone is not sufficient cause for polysomnography prior to an intervention trial.

Polysomnography, commonly referred to as a "sleep study" is a diagnostic tool in sleep medicine in which comprehensive biophysiological recordings are taken during sleep. During a polysomnogram, a number of bodily functions are recorded, generally at night, although shift workers and individuals with certain other disorders (e.g., circadian rhythm disorders, narcolepsy) may be recorded during the daytime. Monitoring includes brain wave activity, heart rhythm, eye movements, muscle activity, nasal and oral airflow, breathing effort, and blood oxygenation. All of these parameters are used, in combination, to characterize an individual's sleep or to diagnose or rule out many sleep disorders.

The symptoms of disorders of sleep and wakefulness overlap significantly with many medical conditions, the evaluation of which is likely to have taken place prior to the patient's referral to a behavioral specialist. Sleep disorders that present with coexistent fatigue can represent diagnostic dilemmas in primary care as up to 20% of all patients presenting to a primary care office will complain of fatigue (Rosenthal, Majeroni, Pretorius, & Malik, 2008). The causes of fatigue are highly diverse, representing disease states involving virtually every organ system, some potentially serious and/or life-threatening. Extensive medical evaluation of such a broad complaint can be time consuming and costly. The dilemma may center on the extent of medical evaluation necessary for fatigue in a patient with disordered sleep. Routine initial workup for fatigue should include complete blood count (CBC), chemistry panel (CMP), thyroid function studies (TSH), erythrocyte sedimentation rate (ESR), human immunodeficiency virus (HIV) antibodies, and pregnancy test. Other additional testing has not been shown to be generally useful unless indicated by specific findings.

The referring clinician will likely have also taken a complete medication history due to the many medications that impact sleep and wakefulness through use or withdrawal (Table 7.3; Schweitzer, 2011). The behavioral clinician should

TABLE 7.3 Common Medication Types That Affect Sleep and Waking Behavior

Medication Type (Example medications are in italics.)	Effect on Sleep
Alpha-blockers (*prazosin, terazosin*)	Daytime sedation, decreased REM sleep
Analgesics (OTC)	Insomnia, some over-the-counter pain preparations (Tylenol Headache, Anacin, Excedrin) contain caffeine
Antiarrhythmics	Insomnia, daytime fatigue
Antiepileptic agents: older (*valproic acid, phenytoin*)	Increased sleep time, decreased sleep onset latency, sedation
Antiepileptic agents: newer (*lamotrigine, gabapentin*)	Sedation, increased slow-wave sleep
Antidepressants: norepinephrine and dopamine reuptake inhibitors (*bupropion*)	Vivid dreams/nightmares, insomnia, increased sleep efficiency
Antidepressants: serotonin agonist/reuptake inhibitors (*trazodone, nefazodone*)	Daytime sedation, improved sleep
Antidepressants: serotonin and norepinephrine reuptake inhibitors (SNRIs) (*venlafaxine, duloxetine*)	Vary, daytime sedation or insomnia; may increase or decrease total sleep time, REM rebound upon discontinuation
Antidepressants: selective serotonin reuptake inhibitors (SSRIs) (*citalopram, fluoxetine, paroxetine*)	Vary, daytime sedation or insomnia; may increase or decrease total sleep time, REM rebound upon discontinuation
Antidepressants: monoamine oxidase inhibitors (MAOIs) (*phenelzine, moclobemide*)	Insomnia, daytime sedation (phenelzine)
Antidepressants: Tricyclic (*amitriptyline, doxepin, clomipramine*)	Vary, some (such as amitriptyline) are very sedating, others (such as nortriptyline) may decrease total sleep time; REM rebound upon discontinuation
Antineoplastic agents: (*vincaleukoblastine, estramustine*)	Insomnia
Antiparkinsonian drugs (*carbidopa, ropinirole*)	Insomnia, disturbing dreams, increased daytime sleepiness
Antipsychotics: atypical (*risperidone, quetiapine*)	Increased sleep time, REM suppression, daytime sedation
Antipsychotics: typical (*haloperidol, chlorpromazine*)	Daytime sedation
Appetite suppressants (*methylphenidate*)	Insomnia
Benzodiazepines (*alprazolam, diazepam*)	Decreased sleep onset latency, possible increased sleep time, possible daytime drowsiness, rebound insomnia upon discontinuation
Beta-blockers (*propranolol, labetalol*)	Insomnia, nighttime awakening, nightmares, possibly daytime drowsiness
Bronchodilators (*theophylline*)	Insomnia, worse on higher doses
Cholinesterase inhibitors (*memantine, tacrine*)	Insomnia, disturbing dreams

(continued)

TABLE 7.3 Common Medication Types That Affect Sleep and Waking Behavior (*continued*)

Medication Type (Example medications are in italics.)	Effect on Sleep
Clonidine	Daytime drowsiness and fatigue, early morning awakening, nightmares
Corticosteroids (*prednisone*)	Insomnia
Decongestants (*pseudoephedrine, diphenhydramine*)	Drowsiness (diphenhydramine) or insomnia (pseudoephedrine)
Diuretics (*furosemide, chlorothiazide*)	Sleep fragmentation due to nighttime urination
Estrogen	Daytime drowsiness
Lithium (*eskalith*)	Improved nighttime sleep, increased daytime drowsiness (at least initially)
Niacin	Possibly improved sleep quality
Nicotine replacement products (*nicotine nasal, nicotine inhalant*)	Insomnia
Statins (*atorvastatin, cerivastatin*)	Insomnia, nightmares
Thyroid hormones (*levothyroxine*)	Insomnia

REM, rapid eye movement.
Source: Schweitzer (2011).

also take care to evaluate for the presence of mood disorders and anxiety disorders in the course of a complete evaluation of sleep disturbance.

Screening Measures

Unlike depression, obesity, smoking, and alcohol misuse (U.S. Preventive Services Task Force, 2010), most primary care settings do not routinely screen for sleep disorders, although sleep-related questions are becoming more common in global health assessments. For example, the Agency for Healthcare Research and Quality (AHRQ) includes a question on snoring ("Do you snore or has anyone told you that you snore?") and a question on daytime fatigue ("In the past 7 days, I was sleepy during the daytime.... Never, Rarely, Sometimes, Often, or Always") in their sample adult health assessment toolkit (AHRQ, 2013). Screening for sleep disorders is important as many patients with sleep disorders go undiagnosed and untreated (Ancoli-Israel & Roth, 1999). For pediatric patients, the BEARS sleep screening algorithm may be useful (Mindell & Owens, 2010). The BEARS provides a comprehensive screening for sleep disorders by using screening questions that vary by age for each of five domains (Bedtime problems, Excessive daytime sleepiness, Awakening during the night, Regularity and duration of sleep, Snoring). In adults, just asking about sleep and fatigue during annual exams may be a helpful start for clinicians and, in the absence of other standardized, well-validated screening questions, the BEARS mnemonic can also be used with adults. For patients suspected of having insomnia, asking about "not being able to stop thinking about work in the evening" may be a very sensitive indicator of disturbed sleep (Åkerstedt et al., 2002).

The STOP BANG screening questionnaire provides an estimation of an individual's risk of obstructive sleep apnea (OSA; Chung et al., 2012). The acronym STOP BANG refers to the eight domains assessed in the questionnaire: Snoring, Tiredness, having been Observed stopping breathing, having high blood Pressure, Body mass index greater than 35, Age over 50, Neck size larger than 17 inches (male) or 16 inches (female), and male Gender. A STOP BANG score over 5 may be suggestive of OSA.

Once a diagnosis has been made, instruments such as the Epworth Sleepiness Scale (ESS) can be used to track a patient's response to treatment (Johns, 1991). The ESS allows patients to rate their chance of falling asleep in eight different situations (e.g., "sitting quietly after a lunch without alcohol") from 0 ("would never doze") to 3 ("high chance of dozing"). Higher scores indicate greater sleepiness. Patients with insomnia average a 2.2 on the ESS, whereas scores for patients with narcolepsy, OSA, and periodic limb movement disorder are 17.5, 11.7, and 9.2, respectively. Electronic sleep diary applications that include a question on alertness can also be a useful treatment response indicator. Examining a patient's sleep diaries can also be useful in helping to distinguish individuals with sleep disorders from those who just obtain chronic insufficient sleep due to work, family or social obligations, or sleep preferences. These patients' sleep diaries will be characterized by high sleep efficiency, excessive daytime sleepiness, and the tendency to get several hours of extra sleep on weekends and holidays.

BASIC NEEDS

Most patients with insomnia do not seek consultation for sleep, and often rely on folk remedies (e.g., lavender scented pillows), herbal preparations (e.g., chamomile tea), over-the-counter medications (e.g., Tylenol PM, Unisom), and alcohol or drug (e.g., marijuana) use in order to cope with the condition (Morin, LeBlanc et al., 2006). Once sleep problems have been identified, psychoeducation can be an important component of a patient's care.

Basic Sleep Education

Some patients may benefit from an overview of normal sleep patterns, as sometimes their perception of disordered sleep is based upon an incorrect understanding of norms. The amount of sleep needed by humans varies by age and health, among other factors. Sleep need is largely genetic, but can also be influenced by recent behavioral patterns (e.g., recent sleep deprivation, voluntarily staying up late; Carskadon & Dement, 2011). Habitual sleep duration is normally distributed (Groeger, Zijlstr, & Dijk, 2004) in the adult population, and moderately heritable (Partinen et al., 1983). Not every patient requires 8 hours of sleep and an individual's sleep need can change during his or her lifetime. Each sleep event can be impacted by volitional factors, as well as circadian factors (24-hour bodily rhythms) and the pressure for sleep that builds with increased time awake (homeostatic sleep drive). Environmental input of light and dark is the primary way the circadian cycle is synchronized (Czeisler & Buxton, 2011).

Infants require the most sleep with up to 12 to 18 hours of each day devoted to sleep (Carskadon & Dement, 2011). The sleep requirement typically reduces to 12 to 14 hours per day in toddlers and to 10 to 11 hours per day by the early school years. Preadolescents and adolescents typically need 8.5 to 9.25 hours of sleep in a day, but often do not get sufficient sleep due to the demands of academics, work, and extracurricular activities (Wolfson & Carskadon, 1998). Most young adults get between 7.5 and 8.5 hours of sleep on most days, and are awake for only 5% of the time after sleep onset (Carskadon & Dement, 2011).

Recent years have seen an increased interest in characterizing the sleep of older individuals. Seniors (age 75 and older) average 9.0 hours of sleep (Basner et al., 2007). Arousals during sleep become much more frequent with age, although healthy seniors are able to return to sleep with the same speed as their youthful counterparts (Bliwise, 2011). Older individuals tend to wake at an earlier point in the circadian phase (Czeisler & Buxton, 2011). The resultant earlier exposure to light may reset their circadian cycle to an earlier time and promote ever earlier wake-up times, possibly accounting for some of the increase in insomnia frequency noted in this demographic (Czeisler & Buxton, 2011). The role of napping in the senior population has yet to be fully understood due to the multiple factors, other than purely sleep quantity and quality, which can impact an older person's tendency to nap (e.g., medical conditions, psychopathology, medications that induce sleepiness, and cultural considerations related to napping). Studies have variously shown napping to be beneficial for older persons, and to be a risk factor for morbidity and mortality.

Sleep is conventionally divided into five stages: rapid eye movement (REM) sleep and four stages of non-REM sleep (NREM stages 1, 2, 3, and 4; Carskadon & Dement, 2011). Healthy adult humans enter sleep through stage NREM 1, but it can be difficult for individuals to accurately perceive the moment their brainwave pattern transitions from wakefulness to sleep. This may contribute to the sleep state misperception of some individuals. Individuals in stage 1 are easily arousable, so an increase in stage 1 sleep is associated with disrupted sleep. Stages 2 through 4 are characterized by progressively decreased arousability. Stages 3 and 4 are together called slow-wave sleep (SWS) and can be considered deep sleep. REM sleep is when dreaming occurs. After sleep onset, individuals pass through a predictable pattern of NREM and REM sleep (sleep architecture) in 90- to 120-minute cycles. In young adults, SWS predominates during the beginning of the sleep period (first third of the night). The longest periods of REM sleep tend to occur in the early morning when core body temperature is at its lowest. The amount of SWS an individual requires decreases markedly from childhood through late adolescence and may disappear entirely by the time an individual is 60 years old. REM sleep quantity, on the other hand, is maintained in healthy old age and is correlated with preservation of intellectual functioning. Individuals whose sleep has been irregular or disrupted will often preferentially recoup SWS and REM sleep when they next sleep. Irregular sleep schedules, sleep deprivation, and chronic restriction or fragmentation of sleep can lead to a disruption in normal sleep architecture.

Sleep Hygiene Education

Although sleep hygiene instructions are not believed to be an effective single-component therapy for insomnia, they provide important general information for patients and form a basis of knowledge on which other interventions can be built. Sleep hygiene instructions generally cover four primary topics: setting regular sleep and wake times, limiting/avoiding sleep interfering substances, creating a sleep-conducive environment (physiologically and externally), and the importance of regular exercise (Stepanski & Wyatt, 2003). An example sleep hygiene instructions list is provided in Table 7.4.

A specific, growing area of concern in the domain of sleep hygiene is the impact that electronic media consumption prior to bed may have on sleep onset latency or sleep quality. Sleep may be affected by an alteration in melatonin production secondary to the light emitted by the devices (Chellappa et al., 2011; Wood, Rea, Plitnick, & Figuero, 2013). Sleep may also be fragmented by noises from devices or participation in arousing activities prior to bedtime. Storage of electronic devices outside the bedroom may be especially important for children and adolescents (Adams, Daly, & Williford, 2013) but may also be a useful sleep-facilitation tactic for adults.

Bed Partner Education/Intervention

For some patients, a partner's sleep disorder may constitute a threat to their sleep. Patients should be encouraged to consider whether their partner may need evaluation or treatment for their own sleep disorder (snoring, periodic limb movements), which may be making it challenging for their partner to get adequate rest. For partners of snorers, white noise machines and earplugs may provide a respite from the nighttime noise. Individuals disturbed by their partner's use of a CPAP device may be well-served to try to find a quieter model

TABLE 7.4 Sleep Hygiene Instructions

1. Set a regular bed time and wake-up time, 7 days a week.
2. Avoid naps.
3. Avoid caffeine, even early in the day. Absolutely eliminate caffeine in the afternoon and evenings.
4. Avoid alcohol, especially in the evenings.
5. Decrease/eliminate nicotine.
6. Make sure your bed is comfortable, and your bedroom is protected from light and noise.
7. Do not allow any clocks to be visible from your bed.
8. Make sure your bedroom is a comfortable temperature.
9. Do not go to bed hungry, but try to avoid "heavy" foods before bed.
10. Limit your fluid intake in the evening.
11. Consider removing pets and/or children from your bed.
12. Exercise regularly (but not within 3 hours of sleep).

or employ an extra-long cord so that the machine can be placed in a closet or farther away from the bed. Although not acceptable to all couples, if partner-related sleep disruption cannot be solved, some couples may wish to spend time together in the evening and then retire to separate bedrooms.

Education About Insomnia

One widely used model for helping patients understand their sleep difficulties is the 3P behavioral model (Speilman, Caruso, & Glovinsky, 1987). This model allows a clinician to easily explain how a patient's *predispositions* and *precipitating* factors may have led to an acute period of insomnia, which is now being maintained by *perpetuating* factors. Biopsychosocial predispositions may include factors such as a patient's tendency toward rumination/worry, chronic hyperarousal, or bed-partner pressure to maintain a nonpreferred (by the patient) sleep schedule. Precipitating factors are any acute biopsychosocial event that, when combined with the patient's predisposing factors, increases the likelihood of difficulty with sleep onset and maintenance. Precipitating factors can include psychiatric or medical illnesses, major life stressors, and socially necessitated changes or interruptions in sleep schedule (e.g., change in work hours, infant/elder care demands). Most patients can identify what precipitated the onset of their insomnia (Bastien, Vallieres, & Morin, 2004) with illness and worry being most common (Armstrong & Dregnan, 2014).

Perpetuating factors of insomnia are the ultimately counterproductive "solutions" individuals utilize in response to their poor sleep (Speilman et al., 1987). The most common maladaptive coping behavior utilized by patients with poor sleep is increasing their sleep opportunity (time in bed), whether through going to bed earlier, staying in bed later in the morning, or taking longer or more frequent naps. The extended time in bed often leads to fragmented sleep and poor sleep quality. When the patient's time awake in bed increases, the individual often becomes increasingly irritated about not sleeping. Repeated pairings of aggravation with sleep-related situations increase the opportunity for classically conditioned arousal (which then hampers sleep initiation). This mismatch between time in bed and time sleeping also increases the propensity for patients to engage in non-sleep-related behaviors in the bedroom (e.g., reading, watching TV, using handheld electronic devices). These non-sleep bedroom behaviors decrease the stimulus–response association between bed and sleep.

BRIEF COUNSELING METHODS

Because of growing awareness of the possible adverse effects of hypnotic drug use (Kripke, Langer, & Kline, 2012; Shuto et al., 2010), interest in nonpharmacological therapies for insomnia is on the rise. The most evidence-based of the psychological therapies for insomnia are relaxation therapy, sleep restriction, stimulus control therapy, and cognitive therapy. These methods are often implemented in combination as cognitive behavioral therapy for insomnia (CBTI). CBTI aims to alter the perpetuating factors of insomnia such as maladaptive coping behaviors and worry about sleep. CBTI has been shown to lead to significant improvement in sleep complaints, which are comparable or exceed the benefits of pharmacotherapy for both primary and secondary insomnia (Jacobs, Pace-Schott, Stickgold, & Otto, 2004; Morin, Bootzin, et al., 2006; Smith, Perlis, & Park, 2002). Because patients become adept at understanding their own sleep patterns and measures to improve their sleep, gains made through CBTI are maintained long-term, whereas the benefits of medication for insomnia end with discontinuation of the drug. Even brief (two- to four-session) primary care-based CBTI interventions have been shown to be effective (Buysse et al., 2011; Goodie, Isler, Hunter, & Peterson, 2009). CBTI can also be effectively implemented through self-help, telephone interventions, tele-health, groups, and web applications (Bastien, Morin, Ouellet, Blais, & Bouchard, 2004; Holmqvist, Vincent, & Walsh, 2014; Koffel, Koffel, & Gehrman, 2014; Siebern & Manber, 2011; Ho et al., 2015). Each component of CBTI is described, briefly, in the following sections.

Stimulus Control Therapy

Stimulus control therapy (Bootzin, 1972) is designed to help patients reestablish a regular circadian sleep–wake rhythm and to increase the association between environmental and temporal cues and sleep onset. Stimulus control instructions are relatively few in number (Table 7.5) but it is important that patients adhere to the guidelines strictly in order for them to be effective in establishing a new conditioned relationship between sleep and bed and to extinguish any conditioned arousal to the bed caused by pre-sleep anxiety or the frequent practice of sleep-incompatible behaviors in the bed. Stimulus control therapy, especially in early treatment, can also promote more rapid sleep onset by increasing a patient's sleep debt (e.g., by eliminating naps), creating a positive condition for sleep onset the following night.

Sleep Restriction

Sleep restriction therapy (SRT) attempts to limit the amount of time a patient spends in bed to the average amount of sleep he or she reports getting (Spielman, Saskin, & Thorpy, 1987). For example, if a patient reports being in bed for

TABLE 7.5 Stimulus Control Instructions

Go to bed only when you are sleepy.
If you are not able to sleep within 15 minutes of getting in bed, leave the bedroom until you are sufficiently sleepy (not just fatigued) to fall asleep.
Use your bed for sleep or sexual activity only (no TV watching, no eating, no electronics, etc.).
Get up for the day at the same time every day, no matter how much sleep you have gotten the night before.
Do not nap during the day.

10 hours each night, but sleeping only 6, time in bed would be reduced to 6 hours. The allowable sleep period is set based upon the patient's preferred wake-up time. Like stimulus control therapy, SRT prohibits napping, so if a patient has difficulty falling asleep or experiences sleep maintenance difficulties at night, the patient is still required to get out of bed at the assigned time and remain awake until the assigned sleep time, thereby increasing sleep debt. Decreasing total sleep time promotes sleep consolidation and the increased sleep debt helps counter the effect of pre-sleep conditioned arousal, which helps patients to fall asleep more rapidly (Pigeon & Perlis, 2006).

The patient's sleep time is then modified, over time, based upon the efficiency of their sleep (time asleep/time in bed × 100 = sleep efficiency; Spielman et al., 1987). For each week when sleep achieves efficiency greater than 90%, the patient is permitted to go to sleep 15 minutes earlier. If sleep efficiency is less than 85%, the permitted sleep window is reduced by 15 minutes (down to a minimum time in bed of 4.5 hours). The time in bed is adjusted in this fashion until the patient shows a consistent pattern of solid sleep efficiency (between 85% and 90%) without excessive daytime sleepiness. It is important to note that this sleep time may be different than the amount of sleep the patient believed he or she needed prior to treatment.

Sleep restriction has been found to be an effective single component therapy (Epstein, Sidani, Bootzin, & Belyea 2012; Taylor, Schmidt-Nowara, Jessop, & Ahearn, 2010) that leads to rapid improvements in sleep efficiency, decreased sleep onset latency, and decreased time awake after sleep onset (Kyle et al., 2014). One important note is that the name "sleep restriction" can sometimes be off-putting to patients who are seeing you because they feel they are not getting enough sleep. Re-branding the intervention as "sleep efficiency training," "sleep retraining," or "sleep scheduling" may help patients to be more accepting of the process.

Treatment-related adverse effects are often not considered in behavioral interventions but some life-disruptive adverse effects can occur during the initial period of SRT. These can include objectively measured decrements in performance (increased reaction time and attentional lapses), increased daytime sleepiness, and decreased overall sleep (Kyle et al., 2014). These demonstrated impairments are consistent with prior research suggesting that even relatively small decreases in allowed sleep time (1.5 hours per night) can produce performance decrements over time in previously normal sleepers (Belenky et al., 2003). Total sleep time does return to normal after further treatment, but it is important for patients to understand the possibility of short-term performance decrements (Edinger, Wohlgemuth, Radtke, Marsh, & Quillian, 2001). It is also important to continue to follow-up with patients engaged in SRT to ensure that they do not continue to restrict sleep without benefit for too long.

Sleep restriction should not be used in some populations due to its potential to exacerbate existing conditions (Morin, 2011). Manic episodes may be precipitated by sleep restriction in patients diagnosed with bipolar disorder. Sleep restriction is also contraindicated in patients with a known seizure disorder. When undertaking sleep restriction protocols with patients who have a known sleepwalking disorder, patients should be educated about the possible increased risk of sleepwalking episodes when sleep-deprived. A cost–benefit analysis of SRT should be conducted and carefully documented when working with patients whose employment or other daytime responsibilities require frequent driving or working with heavy machinery.

Cognitive Therapy

While there is no evidence that cognitive therapy is an effective monotherapy for insomnia, many patients have a pattern of counterproductive cognitive activity prior to sleep onset, so cognitive interventions are often included in CBTI treatment packages. The "cognitive" portion of the CBTI seeks to change faulty beliefs and excessive worrying about sleep, both of which can lead to increased difficulty with sleep onset (Perlis, Jungquist, Smith, & Posner, 2005). Patients may have catastrophically negative beliefs about the consequences of poor sleep or sleep deprivation (e.g., "If I don't get enough sleep I will perform poorly at work tomorrow and get fired") and may exhibit performance anxiety regarding their ability to get to sleep. The same type of self-challenging dialogue as is used frequently in CBT interventions for depression (Beck, Rush, Shaw, & Emery, 1979) can be helpful in altering these thoughts (Perlis et al., 2005). Patients also need to be taught that although they can, to some extent, force themselves to stay awake (by consuming stimulants, engaging in stimulating mental activity, being physically uncomfortable), efforts to force sleep are unlikely to work and are counterproductive. Adopting a more accepting outlook on their sleep may be most useful. Other helpful interventions might include paradoxical intention (trying not to fall asleep; Shoham-Salomon, Rosenthal, 1987) and teaching patients to use specific imagery techniques to provide cognitive content as an alternative to worry prior to sleep onset (Harvey & Payne, 2002).

Relaxation Techniques

For patients who have difficulty with physiological arousal at bedtime, relaxation training may be a useful adjunct to other interventions. There are a number of different types of relaxation techniques that can be helpfully targeted to the patient's primary presenting difficulty. For patients who complain of muscle tension or who have pain complaints, progressive muscle relaxation may be helpful. Those patients experiencing somatic symptoms (such as chest tightness or breathing changes) due to anxiety at bedtime may find diaphragmatic breathing to be a good option. Imagery-based relaxation scripts can be useful for patients who have difficulty "shutting off" their minds when going to sleep. Although teaching these relaxation techniques can be time consuming, doing the exercise for the first time in session can be a helpful way to increase the likelihood that a patient will be adherent to a relaxation training recommendation. If the clinic's setup or time demands will not permit relaxation training during a visit, training apps for all of these relaxation techniques can be readily found for any type of mobile platform and a patient can be assisted in downloading them prior to leaving the clinic. For less technologically savvy patients, books or CDs describing relaxation techniques may be recommended (Davis, Eshelman, & McKay, 2000; Fanning & McKay, 2008). Patients should be educated that relaxation is a skill that must be practiced in order to become useful. Encouragement to practice these techniques daily, at a time other than bedtime, helps patients focus on mastering the skill. When patients become comfortable with the technique, they can begin to incorporate it into their nighttime routine.

Exercise

Increasing exercise is a frequent recommendation for patients experiencing insomnia. There is some evidence that increased exercise may be beneficial; however, several weeks of exercise adherence may be required before the patient perceives a benefit (Yang, Ho, Chen, & Chien, 2012). In addition to possibly assisting patients to decrease physiological arousal prior to their sleep attempt, afternoon or early evening exercise may also promote sleep through the effect of declining core body temperature postexercise (Horne & Staff, 1983). For those patients physically unable to exercise, a similar effect may be possible to achieve through taking a hot bath several hours before attempted sleep onset.

BEHAVIORAL FACTORS IN DISEASE MANAGEMENT AND ADHERENCE

Insomnia has, in the past, often been viewed as a symptom of other conditions (major depression, generalized anxiety disorder) or medication side effect rather than an independent condition (Katz & McHorney, 2002). Regardless of cause, however, once insomnia becomes persistent there are typically behavioral and psychological elements that help maintain the condition. These perpetuating behaviors are the primary targets of the behavioral interventions described previously. As with most therapies, improved adherence to the treatment interventions (e.g., time in bed restrictions, strict wake-up time) is predictive of improved outcomes (Riedel & Lichstein, 2001). This is particularly problematic for CBTI, as rates of therapy adherence (Matthews, Arendt, McCarthy, Cuddihy, & Aloia, 2013) and completion are rather low (14%–40% in one estimate; Ong, Kuo, & Manber, 2008). Adherence to CBTI instructions can be enhanced by a strong, noncritical alliance with the treatment provider (Constantino et al., 2007), and with motivational support, especially for patients burdened by depression (Lancee, Sorbi, Eisma, van Straten, & van den Bout, 2014). Motivational interviewing strategies (Rollnick, Miller, & Butler, 2008; as described in Chapter 3) can also be a useful way to help patients become more committed to the short-term behavioral changes required to improve sleep in the long run. Support of a bed partner for behavioral changes and limits on the use of alcohol while implementing behavioral insomnia therapies may also be important promoters of adherence (Ruiter Petrov, Lichstein, Huisingh, & Bradley, 2014). Patients may also be more likely to implement the intervention with fidelity if the primary side effect of early treatment (daytime sleepiness) is directly targeted (e.g., through stimulant prescription; Perlis et al., 2004). Not surprisingly, as patients receive benefit from the interventions, they are increasingly likely to be adherent to the behavioral restrictions encouraged by the intervention (Ruiter Petrov et al., 2014).

Unfortunately, although nonpharmacological interventions for insomnia are recommended as the first-line treatment for insomnia (National Institute of Health, 2005), many patients presenting to a behavioral specialist will already have been started on medication, will be taking over-the-counter sleep aids (Bertisch, Herzig, Winkelman, & Buettner, 2014), or may have a strong preference to begin pharmacotherapy for insomnia at the time of their clinic visit.

In the past, benzodiazepines (e.g., diazepam [Valium], clonazepam [Klonopin]) were frequently used for sleep promotion although they are currently used more frequently to treat anxiety. The most prescribed sleep aids at the present time are the nonbenzodiazepine so-called "z-drugs" (e.g., zolpidem [Ambien], zaleplon [Sonata], eszopiclone [Lunesta]; Bertisch et al., 2014). Some antidepressant medications (e.g., trazodone [Desyrel], mirtazapine [Remeron]) are also used to treat insomnia, as are antihistamines (e.g., hydroxyzine [Vistaril]). The melatonin antagonist ramelteon (Rozerem) and reformulations of the tricyclic antidepressant doxepin (Silenor) are more recent additions to the sleep medication armamentarium.

If patients are initiating medication, it is preferable to initiate both pharmacotherapy and CBTI at the same time as this appears to be more effective than introducing CBTI after medications have been initiated (Vallières, Morin, & Guay, 2005). When patients have been on hypnotics, even for a short period of time, it is important to anticipate rebound insomnia and increased anxiety upon discontinuation (Greenblatt, Harmatz, Zinney, & Shader, 1987). Rebound insomnia, and the prompt relief of this symptom experienced by patients if they return to use of the hypnotic, promotes tremendous psychological reliance on these medications by patients. Importantly, a growing body of literature supports the benefits of CBTI in patients gradually tapering from pharmacological interventions (Belleville, Guay, & Morin, 2007; Lichstein et al., 2013).

BEHAVIORAL HEALTH ASSESSMENT AND TREATMENT SUMMARY TO REFERRING PRIMARY CARE PROVIDER

Chief Complaint: Joseph Franklin is a 61-year-old married African American male with a 2- to 3-year history of sleep difficulty.

Subjective/Objective

- **Behavioral observations:** Mr. Franklin was on time for the assessment session and was accompanied by his wife. He was alert and oriented ×4. Mood was dysphoric, affect was within normal limits. The patient was sad but fully cooperative throughout the interview. Answers to questioning were open, and appeared honest. Eye contact was within normal limits. Mr. Franklin was casually dressed and appropriately groomed. He appeared to be of above average intelligence and was well-spoken. He was an adequate historian. The patient's insight into his behavior and the behavior of others was average. The patient reports subjective difficulty with attention and concentration, but these difficulties were not evident during the session. The patient denied symptoms suggestive of psychosis and did not appear to be responding to internal stimuli during the interview. The patient reported no suicidal ideation. The patient willingly signed a consent form for treatment and limits of confidentiality were explained in this context.

- **Overview of psychological history**: Mr. Franklin has never been treated as an inpatient or outpatient for psychological or psychiatric reasons. He has never been treated for the overuse or abuse of drugs or alcohol. When asked about a family history of psychiatric conditions, the patient reported his mother and sister have struggled with depression and are currently being treated with antidepressants (both on citalopram).

  A number of disorders and conditions were reviewed with the patient at the time of intake. He denies any history of mania or psychosis. He is not troubled by obsessions, compulsions, or uncontrollable worry. He does not meet criteria for social or specific phobias. He denies any history of trauma or abuse.
- **Social situation**: Mr. Franklin lives with his wife in his own detached home. He and his wife have two adult children living out of state. His wife's mother currently also lives with them due to financial crisis. The patient has been married for 32 years. He describes the relationship as "up and down but currently up." Mr. Franklin's mother lives independently near his home and is in good health. His father is deceased. He has two siblings living locally and reports they are close. He has several long-time friends whom he sees weekly. He is the managing partner of a law practice (36 years). He describes his job as "much too busy." He does not participate in any clubs, hobbies, or regular activities. He states he "used to be religious" but does not currently attend church. He reports no financial or legal stressors.
- **Medical problems/health behaviors**: The patient has been diagnosed with hypertension and DM2. He is also overweight (BMI = 31). He consumes 6 to 8 oz of bourbon most nights but no other alcohol. He denies the use of illegal/illicit drugs or tobacco. He consumes two caffeinated colas each day (one at lunch, one mid-afternoon), two servings of caffeinated tea at dinner (around 7 p.m.), and multiple cups of coffee while at work ("at least a pot"). He does not exercise regularly.
- **Insomnia:** Mr. Franklin reports sleep onset latency of 1 to 2 hours due to psychological agitation/worry at bedtime. He goes to bed around 10 p.m. on weekdays and 12 p.m. on Friday and Saturday nights. His sleep onset latency is 1 to 2 hours (better on nights before weekends). He reports waking one to two times each night and has difficulty falling back asleep. On weekdays he sets his alarm for 6 a.m. but often falls back asleep until 7 a.m. when he is prompted by his wife to get up. On weekends he typically sleeps until 9 a.m. or later. He typically falls asleep while watching

TV on weekday evenings (approximately 30 minutes). He does not nap on weekends. He estimates that on weekdays he gets about 6 hours of sleep. On weekend days he gets 8 hours of sleep.

Mr. Franklin's sleep difficulties began 2.5 years ago when his law firm merged with another small firm. As managing partner he found himself constantly thinking about organizational matters and plans for the new firm. He would frequently wake at night to make lists of tasks that needed to be handled. He experienced significant anxiety and worry about the merger and admits, "I tend to be rather high strung." Now that the merger is complete he states he has trouble shutting off his thoughts at bedtime but they tend to be more mundane thoughts about work and progress in his cases rather than true worries. When having difficulty falling asleep, he will often watch TV from the bed with the sound off to keep from waking his wife. When he wakes during the night, he states, "I just lie in bed and watch the clock and wait for morning." Mr. Franklin states that prior to the merger he had no difficulty with sleep and would arise without difficulty in the morning before his alarm. When he was sleeping well, he usually got 7.5 hours of sleep each night. He is not aware of any family history of sleep disturbance.

Mr. Franklin snores, but his wife has not witnessed any apneic events nor has she observed excessive limb movements from the patient while he sleeps. Mr. Franklin does not experience odd sensations in his legs at night nor has he ever experienced cataplexy, sleep paralysis, or hypnagogic/hypnopompic hallucinations. His sleep environment is comfortable and conducive to sleep. He is not bothered by environmental stimuli other than his dog who will often wake him by jumping on the bed during the night. The patient does not typically wake to urinate. His prior treatment attempts have included the use of Tylenol PM and Unisom, both of which left him "feeling hung over" in the morning. He has tried OTC melatonin supplements, but they were not effective for him. He currently takes "energy supplements" every afternoon at work. His Epworth Sleepiness Scale score was 9 (slight chance of dozing sitting and reading, sitting in a public place, or lying down in the afternoon; high chance of dozing while watching TV or as a passenger in a car).

- **Dysphoric mood (PHQ-9 = 8):** Mr. Franklin denies depressed mood but states that he often has no interest in engaging in activities he formerly enjoyed because of his sleep problems. He has given up several hobbies (e.g., golfing, fishing) and going to church on weekends because he does not want to commit to getting up early in case he sleeps poorly. He reports feeling fatigued or low in energy on most days due to his poor sleep. He states he is used to being a "driven, high energy person," so he is quite bothered by this change in activity level. He denies other symptoms of depression.

Assessment

Insomnia (780.52), dysphoric mood secondary to insomnia (780.79)

Plan

Mr. Franklin appears to be experiencing insomnia precipitated by a stressful work event currently perpetuated by a number of sleep-interfering behaviors. He is positive for nighttime alcohol use, excessive caffeinated beverages, and ingestion of "nutrition supplements" (containing additional caffeine, yerba mate, green tea extract, B vitamins), all of which can disrupt sleep. He also keeps an inconsistent sleep schedule, naps, and extends his time in bed. He remains in bed while awake, clock watches, and experiences pet-related sleep disruption. The "depressive" symptoms noted by his physician appear to be secondary to sleep disruption.

The nature and treatment of insomnia were discussed with Mr. Franklin. Predisposing, precipitating, and perpetuating factors were discussed. Sleep hygiene information was reviewed with particular emphasis on gradual reduction of caffeine (and other stimulant) intake. He was also encouraged to discontinue nighttime use of alcohol as this can lead to sleep fragmentation. The importance of aligning homeostatic and circadian drivers of sleep was stressed.

Mr. Franklin set the following goals:

1. Set a consistent bedtime and wake-up time (12 p.m. to 6 a.m.), leave the bed if awake for more than 20 minutes; monitor sleep using a sleep diary app with alertness feature.
2. No naps during the day. Watch TV in a less comfortable chair to prevent dozing.
3. Decrease/eliminate alcohol, caffeine, "energy" supplements.
4. Discontinue use of TV in the bedroom and cover alarm clock to prevent clock watching.
5. Purchase and begin using a guided imagery app for his phone.
6. Begin daily moderate exercise, as per primary care physician's recommendation
7. Return to clinic in 1 week to discuss sleep diary results and implement sleep scheduling intervention.

REFERENCES

Adams, S. K., Daly, J. F., & Williford, D. N. (2013). Adolescent sleep and cellular phone use: Recent trends and implications. *Health Services Insights*, 6, 99–103.

Agency for Healthcare Research and Quality. (2013). *Health assessments in primary care: A how-to guide for clinicians and staff*. Retrieved from www.ahrq.gov/professionals/prevention-chronic-care/improve/system/health-assessments/index.html

Åkerstedt, T., Knutsson, A., Westerholm, P., Theorell, T., Alfredsson, L., Kecklund, G. (2002). Sleep disturbances, work stress, and work hours: A cross-sectional study. *Journal of Psychosomatic Research*, *53*, 741–748.

Alattar, M., Harrington, J. J., Mitchell, M., & Sloane, P. (2007). Sleep problems in primary care: A North Carolina Family Practice Research Network (NC-FP-RN) study. *Journal of the American Board of Family Medicine*, *20*(4), 365–374.

American Psychiatric Association. (2013). *Diagnostic and statistical manual of mental disorders* (5th ed.). Arlington, VA: American Psychiatric Publishing.

Ancoli-Israel, S., & Roth, T. (1999). Characteristics of insomnia in the United States: Results of the 1991 National Sleep Foundation Survey I. *Sleep*, 22(Suppl. 2), S347–S353.

Armstrong, D., & Dregnan, A. (2014). A population-based investigation into the self-reported reasons for sleep problems. *PLoS One, 9*(7). e101368.

Basner, M., Fomberstein, K. M., Razavi, F. M., Banks, S., William, J. H., Rosa, R. R., ... Dinges, D. E. (2007). American time use survey: Sleep time and its relationship to waking activities. *Sleep, 30*, 1085–1095.

Bastien, C. H., Morin, C. M., Ouellet, M. C., Blais, F. C., & Bouchard, S. (2004). Cognitive-behavioral therapy for insomnia: Comparison of individual therapy, group therapy, and telephone consultations. *Journal of Consulting and Clinical Psychology, 72*(4), 653–659.

Bastien, C. H., Vallieres, A., & Morin, C. M. (2004). Precipitating factors of insomnia. *Behavioral Sleep Medicine*, 2(1), 50–62.

Beck, A. T., Rush, A. J., Shaw, B. F., & Emery, G. (1979). *Cognitive Therapy of Depression*. New York, NY: Guilford Press.

Belenky, G., Wesensten, N. J., Thorne D. R., Thomas, M. L., Sing, H. C., Redmond, D. P. ... Balkin, T. J. (2003). Patterns of performance degradation and restoration during sleep restriction and subsequent recovery: A sleep dose-response study. *Journal of Sleep Research, 12*(1), 1–12.

Belleville, G., Guay, C., & Morin, C. M. (2007). Hypnotic taper with or without self-help treatment of insomnia: A randomized clinical trial. *Journal of Consulting and Clinical Psychology, 75*, 325–336.

Bertisch, S. M., Herzig, S. J., Winkelman, J. W., & Buettner, C. (2014). National use of prescription medications for insomnia: NHANES 1999–2010. *Sleep, 37*(2), 343–349.

Bliwise, D. L. (2011). Normal aging. In M. H. Kryger, T. Roth, & W. C. Dement (Eds.), *Principles and Practice of Sleep Medicine* (5th ed., pp. 27–41). St. Louis, MO: Elsevier Saunders.

Bonnet, M. H., & Arand, D. L. (1998). Heart rate variability in insomniacs and matched normal sleepers. *Psychosomatic Medicine, 60*(5), 610.

Bonnet M. H., & Arand D. L. (2006). Consequences of insomnia. *Sleep Medicine Clinics, 1*, 351.

Bootzin, R. R. (1972). Stimulus control treatment for insomnia. *Proceedings, 80th Annual Convention, APA*, 7, 395–396.

Buysse, D. J., Germain, A., Moul, D. E., Franzen, P. L., Brar, L. K., Fletcher, M. E., ... Monk, T. H. (2011). Efficacy of brief behavioral treatment for chronic insomnia in older adults. *Archives of Internal Medicine, 171*(10), 87–95.

Carskadon, M. A., & Dement, W. C. (2011). Normal human sleep: An overview. In M. H. Kryger, T. Roth, & W. C. Dement (Eds.), *Principles and practice of sleep medicine* (5th ed., pp. 16–26). St. Louis, MO: Elsevier Saunders.

Chellappa, S. L., Steiner, R., Blattner, P., Oelhafen, P., Gotz, T., & Cajochen, C. (2011). Non-visual effects of light on melatonin, alertness, and cognitive performance: Can blue-enriched light keep us alert? *PLoS One, 6*(1), e16429.

Chung, F., Subramanyam, R., Liao, P., Sasaki, E., Shapiro, C., & Sun, Y. (2012). High STOP BANG score indicates a high probability of sleep apnoea. *British Journal of Anaesthesia, 108*(5), 768–775.

Constantino, M. J., Manber, R., Ong, J., Kuo, T. F., Huang, J. S., & Arnow, B. A. (2007). Patient expectations and therapeutic alliance as predictors of outcome in group cognitive-behavioral therapy for insomnia. *Behavioral Sleep Medicine, 5*(3), 210–28.

Czeisler, C. A., & Buxton, O. M. (2011). The human circadian timing system and sleep-wake regulation. In M. H. Kryger, T. Roth, & W. C. Dement (Eds.), *Principles and practice of sleep medicine* (5th ed., pp. 402–419). St. Louis, MO: Elsevier Saunders.

Davis, M., Eshelman, E. R., & McKay, M. (2000). *The relaxation and stress reduction workbook* (5th ed.). Oakland, CA: New Harbinger.

Edinger, J. D., Wohlgemuth, W. K., Radtke, R. A., Marsh, G. R., & Quillian, R. E. (2001). Cognitive behavioural therapy for treatment of chronic primary insomnia: A randomized controlled trial. *JAMA, 258*, 1856–1864.

Epstein, D. R., Sidani, S., Bootzin, R. R., & Belyea, M. J. (2012). Dismantling multicomponent behavioral treatment for insomnia in older adults: A randomized controlled trial. *Sleep, 35*(6), 797–805.

Fanning, P., & McKay, M. (2008). *Progressive relaxation and breathing* (audio CD). Oakland, CA: New Harbinger.

Fernandez-Mendoza, J., Vgontzas, A. N., Liao, D., Shaffer, M. L., Vela-Bueno, A., Basta, M., & Bixler, E. O. (2012). Insomnia with objective short sleep duration and incident hypertension: The Penn State Cohort. *Hypertension*, *60*(4), 929.

Groeger, J. A., Zijlstra, F. R. H., & Dijk, D. J. (2004). Sleep quantity, sleep difficulties and their perceived consequences in a representative sample of 2000 British adults. *Journal of Sleep Research*, *13*, 359–371.

Goodie, J. L., Isler, W. C., Hunter, C., & Peterson, A. L. (2009). Using behavioral health consultants to treat insomnia in primary care: A clinical case series. *Journal of Clinical Psychology*, *65*(3), 294–304.

Greenblatt, D. J., Harmatz, J. S., Zinney, M. A., & Shader, R. I. (1987). Effect of gradual withdrawal on the rebound sleep disorder after discontinuation of triazolam. *New England Journal of Medicine*, *317*, 722–728.

Harvey, A. G., & Payne, S. (2002).The management of unwanted pre-sleep thoughts in insomnia: Distraction with imagery versus general distraction. *Behaviour Research and Therapy*, *40*(3), 267–277.

Ho, F. Y., Chung, K. F., Yeung, W. F., Ng, T. H., Kwan, K. S., Yung, K. P., & Cheng, S. K. (2015). Self-help cognitive-behavioral therapy for insomnia: A meta-analysis of randomized controlled trials. *Sleep Medicine Reviews*, *19*, 17–28.

Holmqvist, M., Vincent, N., & Walsh, K. (2014). Web- vs. telehealth-based delivery of cognitive-behavioral therapy for insomnia: A randomized controlled trial. *Sleep Medicine*, *15*, 187–195.

Horne, J. A., & Staff, L. H. (1983). Exercise and sleep: Body-heating effects. *Sleep*, *6*(1), 36–46.

Jacobs, G. D., Pace-Schott, E. F., Stickgold, R., & Otto, M. W. (2004). Cognitive behavior therapy and pharmacotherapy for insomnia: A randomized controlled trail and direct comparison. *Archives of Internal Medicine.*, *164*(17), 1888–1896.

Johns, M. W. (1991). A new method for measuring daytime sleepiness: The Epworth Sleepiness Scale. *Sleep*, *14*, 540–545.

Katz, D. A., & McHorney, C. A. (2002). The relationship between insomnia and health-related quality of life in patients with chronic illness. *Journal of Family Practice*, *51*(3), 229.

Koffel, E. A., Koffel, J. B., & Gehrman, P. R. (2014). A meta-analysis of group cognitive behavioral therapy for insomnia. *Sleep Medicine Reviews*, *16*, 6–16.

Kripke, D. F., Langer, R. D., & Kline, L. E. (2012). Hypnotics' association with mortality or cancer: A matched cohort study. *British Medical Journal Open*, 2, 1–8.

Kyle, S. D., Miller, C. B., Rogers, Z., Siriwardena, A. N., Macmahon, K. M., & Espie, C. A. (2014). Sleep restriction therapy for insomnia is associated with reduced objective total sleep time, increased daytime somnolence, and objectively impaired vigilance: Implications for the clinical management of insomnia disorder. *Sleep*, *37*(2), 229–237.

Lancee, J., Sorbi, M. J., Eisma, M. C., van Straten, A., & van den Bout, J. (2014). The effect of support on internet-delivered treatment for insomnia: Does baseline depression severity matter? *Behavior Therapy*, *45*(4), 507–516.

Léger, D., Massuel, M. A., Metlaine, A., & SISYPHE Study Group. (2006). Professional correlates of insomnia. *Sleep*, *29*(2), 171.

Lichstein, K. L., Nau, S. D., Wilson, N. M., Aguillard, R. N., Lester, K. W., Bush, A. J., & McCrae, C. S. (2013). Psychological treatment of hypnotic-dependent insomnia in a primarily older adult sample. *Behavior Research and Therapy*, *51*(12), 787–796.

Malow, B. A. (2011). Approach to the patient with disordered sleep. In M. H. Kryger, T. Roth, W. C. Dement (Eds.), *Principles and practice of sleep medicine* (5th ed., pp. 641–646). St. Louis, MO: Elsevier Saunders.

Manconi, M., Ferri, R., Sagrada, C., Punjabi, N. M., Tettamanzi, E., Zucconi, M., ... Ferini-Strambi, L. (2010). Measuring the error in sleep estimation in normal subjects and in patients with insomnia. *Journal of Sleep Research*, *19*(3), 478–486.

Matthews, E. E., Arendt, J. T., McCarthy, M. S., Cuddihy, L. J., & Aloia, M. S. (2013). Adherence to cognitive-behavioral therapy for insomnia: A systematic review. *Sleep Medicine Reviews*, *17*(6), 453–464.

Mindell, J. A., & Owens, J. A. (2010). *A clinical guide to pediatric sleep. Diagnosis and management of sleep problems* (2nd ed.). Philadelphia, PA: Lippincott Williams & Wilkins, Wolters Kluwer.

Morin, C. M. (2011). Psychological and behavioral treatments for insomnia 1: Approaches and efficacy. In M. H. Kryger, T. Roth, & W. C. Dement (Eds.), *Principles and practice of sleep medicine* (5th ed., pp. 866–883). St. Louis, MO: Elsevier Saunders.

Morin, C. M., Bélanger, L., LeBlanc, M., Ivers, H., Savard, J., Espie, C. A., ... Grégoire, J. P. (2009). The natural history of insomnia: A population-based 3-year longitudinal study. *Archives of Internal Medicine*, *169*(5), 447.

Morin, C. M., Bootzin, R. R., Buysse, D. J., Edinger, J. D., Espie, C. A., & Lichstein, K. L. (2006). Psychological and behavioral treatment of insomnia: An update of the recent evidence (1998–2004). *Sleep*, *29*(11), 1398–1414.

Morin, C. M., LeBlanc, M., Daley, M., Gregoire, J. P., Merette, C. (2006). Epidemiology of Insomnia; prevalence, self-help treatments, consultations, and determinants of help-seeking behaviors. *Sleep Medicine*, *7*, 123–130.

National Institute of Health. (2005). NIH State-of-the-Science Conference statement on manifestations and management of chronic insomnia in adults. *NIH Consensus and State-of-the-Science Statements*, *22*(2), 1–30.

Ong, J. C., Kuo, T. F., & Manber, R. (2008). Who is at risk for dropout from group cognitive-behavior therapy for insomnia? *Journal of Psychosomatic Research*, *64*, 419–425.

Partinen, M., Kaprio, J., Koskenvuo, M., Putkonen, P., & Langinvainio, H., (1983). Genetic and environmental determination of human sleep. *Sleep*, *6*, 179–185.

Perlis, M. L., Jungquist, C., Smith, M. T., & Posner, D. (2005). *Cognitive behavioral treatment of insomnia: A session-by-session guide*. New York, NY: Springer.

Perlis, M. L., Smith, M. T., Orff, H., Enright, T., Nowakowski, S., Jungquist, C., & Plotkin, K. (2004). The effects of modafinil and cognitive behavior therapy on sleep continuity in patients with primary insomnia. *Sleep*, *27*(4), 715–725.

Pigeon, W. R., & Perlis, M. L. (2006). Sleep homeostasis in primary insomnia. *Sleep Medicine Reviews*, *10*(4), 247–254.

Ramar, K., & Olson, E. J. (2013). Management of common sleep disorders. *American Family Physician*, *88*(4), 231–238.

Riedel, B. W., & Lichstein, K. L. (2001). Strategies for evaluating adherence to sleep restriction treatment for insomnia. *Behavior Research and Therapy*, *39*, 201–212.

Rollnick, S., Miller, W. R., & Butler, C. C. (2008). *Motivational interviewing in health care*. New York, NY: Guilford Press.

Rosenthal, T. C., Majeroni, B. A., Pretorius, R., & Malik, K. (2008). Fatigue: An overview. *American Family Physician*, *78*(10), 1173–1179.

Ruiter Petrov, M. E., Lichstein, K. L., Huisingh, C. E., & Bradley, L. A. (2014). Predictors of adherence to a brief behavioral insomnia intervention: Daily process analysis. *Behavior Therapy*, *45*(3), 430–442.

Schweitzer, P. K. (2011). Drugs that disturb sleep and wakefulness. In M. H. Kryger, T. Roth, & W. C. Dement (Eds.), *Principles and practice of sleep medicine* (5th ed., pp. 542–560). St. Louis, MO: Elsevier Saunders.

Shoham-Salomon, V., & Rosenthal, R. (1987). Paradoxical interventions: A meta-analysis. *Journal of Consulting and Clinical Psychology*, *55*, 22–28.

Shuto, H., Imakyure, O., Matsumoto, J., Egawa, T., Jiang, Y., Hirakawa, M., ... Yanagawa, T. (2010). Medication use as a risk factor for inpatient falls in an acute care hospital: A case crossover study. *British Journal of Clinical Pharmacology*; *69*, 535–542.

Siebern, A. T., & Manber, R. (2011). New developments in cognitive behavioral therapy as the first line treatment of insomnia. *Psychology Research and Behavior Management*, *4*, 21–28.

Smith, M. T., Perlis, M. L., Park, A., Smith, M. S., Pennington, J., Giles, D. E., & Buysse, D. J. (2002). Comparative meta-analysis of pharmacotherapy and behavior therapy for persistent insomnia. *American Journal of Psychiatry*, *159*(1), 5–11.

Speilman, A., Caruso, L., & Glovinsky, P. (1987). A behavioral perspective on insomnia treatment. *The Psychiatric Clinics of North America*, *10*, 541–553.

Spielman, A. J., Saskin, P., & Thorpy, M. J. (1987). Treatment of chronic insomnia by restriction of time in bed. *Sleep*, *10*, 45–56.

Standards of Practice Committee of the American Academy of Sleep Medicine. (2003). Practice parameters for using polysomnography to evaluate insomnia: An update for. *Sleep*, *26*(6), 754–760.

Stepanski, E. J., & Wyatt, J. K. (2003). Use of sleep hygiene in the treatment of insomnia. *Sleep Medicine Reviews*, *7*(3), 215–225.

Taylor, D. J., Schmidt-Nowara, W., Jessop, C. A., & Ahearn, J. (2010). Sleep restriction therapy and hypnotic withdrawal versus sleep hygiene education in hypnotic using patients with insomnia. *Journal of Clinical Sleep Medicine*, *6*(2), 169–175.

U.S. Preventive Services Task Force. (2010). USPSTF A and B recommendations. Retrieved June 24, 2015, from http://www.uspreventiveservicestaskforce.org/Page/Name/uspstf-a-and-b-recommendations

Vallières, A., Morin, C. M., & Guay, B. (2005). Sequential combinations of drug and cognitive behavioral therapy for chronic insomnia: An exploratory study. *Behaviour Research and Therapy*, *43*(12), 1611.

Vaughn, B. V., & D'Cruz, O. F. (2011). Cardinal manifestations of sleep disorders. In M. H. Kryger, T. Roth, & W. C. Dement (Eds.), *Principles and practice of sleep medicine* (5th ed., pp. 647–657). St. Louis, MO: Elsevier Saunders.

Vgontzas, A. N., Liao, D., Pejovic, S., Calhoun, S., Karataraki, M., & Bixler, E. O. (2009). Insomnia with objective short sleep duration is associated with type 2 diabetes: A population-based study. *Diabetes Care*, *32*(11), 1980–1985.

Wolfson, A. R., & Carskadon, M. A. (1998). Sleep schedules and daytime functioning in adolescents. *Child Development*, *69*, 875–887.

Wood, B., Rea, M. S., Plitnick, B., & Figuero, M. G. (2013). Light level and duration of exposure determine the impact of self-luminous tablets on melatonin suppression. *Applied Ergonomics*, *44*(2), 237–240.

Yang, P. Y., Ho, K. H., Chen, H. C., & Chien, M. Y. (2012). Exercise training improves sleep quality in middle-aged and older adults with sleep problems: A systematic review. *Journal of Physiotherapy*, *58*(3), 157–163.

EIGHT

GERIATRIC CONDITIONS

TRACY WHARTON AND DENISE GAMMONLEY

S.O.A.P. NOTE FROM REFERRING PRIMARY CARE PROVIDER

S: Patient is an 80-year-old man presenting to the family practice with his wife for his scheduled 3 month f/u visit for HTN, angina, and hyperlipidemia. Patient's spouse expressed concern about his memory and mood. Spouse indicates the patient is sluggish and slow moving at times, irritable and argumentative at other times, and frequently refuses to drive or claims to be uncertain about directions when he is driving. Patient expresses frustration with wife's characterizations of his behavior but also acknowledges: "I'm old; what do you expect is going to happen? Why should I be any different than my friends who are all on their way out?" Both the patient and his spouse admit to currently experiencing stress that is affecting their relationship.

Blood pressures at home are at goal. The patient denies chest pain, shortness of breath, headache, or dizziness. No dyspnea on exertion or paroxysmal nocturnal dyspnea. No complaint of abdominal pain or new muscle pain or discomfort. Denies fever or pain. No problems with sleep, appetite, or bowel/bladder. Tolerating all medications. No changes in medications. Current medications include:

Hydrochlorothiazide 12.5 mg daily
Valsartan 80 mg qd
Amlodipine 5 mg daily
Atorvastatin 10 mg at bedtime
Metoprolol 25 mg BID
Aspirin 325 mg daily
Calcium 500 mg bid
Vitamin D 1000 units daily
Multivitamin with multiminerals daily

O: Height: 5'9", weight: 175 (BMI 25.8), BP 125/83, pulse 73, respirations 20, temperature 98.6.
General: Pleasant gentleman; alert and oriented to person, place, and time.
Heent: PERRLA, TMs clear. Nares patent. Oropharynx clear.
Neck: Supple. No lymphadenopathy. No thyromegaly.
Lungs: Clear to auscultation bilaterally.
Heart: RRR without murmur, rubs, or gallop. No clubbing/cyanosis/edema
Abdomen: Soft, nontender, +BS, no HSM
Extremities: 2+ distal pulses bilaterally.
Neurologic: DTRs 2+ and equal bilaterally. Gait normal. PHQ-2 positive, PHQ-9 with a score of 4 consistent with borderline mild depression.

Mini-Cog screen of memory and executive functioning revealed normal recall of three of three items on the memory test but inaccuracies in the clock drawing (clock face numbers in incorrect sequence; clock hands placed incorrectly) suggesting possible cognitive impairment. Spouse's results on the Short Form of the Informant Questionnaire on Cognitive Decline in the Elderly (Short-IQCODE) are suggestive of potential impairment.

A: R/O cognitive disorder (294.9), HTN (401.1), angina (413.9), HLD (272.2)

P: Mr. Dale presents a complex pattern of behavioral symptoms associated with potential cognitive impairment and/or geriatric depression. There is inconsistency in the patient's report of symptoms with the pattern of symptoms reported by his spouse. Results from formal cognitive and depression screening are suggestive of possible dementia and/or a depressive illness. The couple also acknowledges stress within the dyadic relationship. A more comprehensive geriatric biopsychosocial assessment inclusive of psychosocial issues associated with marital concerns and grief and loss is recommended. Refer to the behavioral health specialist for a comprehensive behavioral health assessment.

Hypertension, angina, and HLD are all stable on current medications. The patient is to continue current medication regimen as well as lifestyle recommendations discussed previously.

SCREENING AND REFERRAL IN PRIMARY CARE

Scientific literature generally considers gerontology the study of adults over the age of 60, with individuals over the age of 85 being considered the "oldest old" (U.S. Department of Health and Human Services [HHS], 2009). Gerontology has become more visible as a practice and research field over the last decade as the "baby boomers" have begun to fit this definition. Metabolic and psychosocial changes happen in the later parts of people's lives. Although Americans may live to be over 100 years old, there are distinct and important differences between young adults (aged 18–60) and older ones, particularly in terms of medical care and pharmacy. Recent research has identified genetic and lifestyle factors that may contribute to the development of cognitive impairment in later life (HHS, 2009), and has identified a range of different forms of dementia including Alzheimer's type, frontotemporal type, vascular type, and Lewy body type.

Organizations such as the Alzheimer's Association have raised awareness about dementias in older adults. With increasing information moving into mainstream culture, it has become increasingly common for primary care providers (PCPs) to hear complaints and concerns about memory from their patients. Similar to cancer, the specter of the disease compels people to scrutinize every potential sign that may appear as they age. However, also similar to cancer, not every memory problem heralds the onset of a dementia. Figure 8.1 shows some of the potential causes for cognitive impairment in older adults that providers must balance in their assessment. While it is important to note that memory lapses, confusion, and affective dysregulation are not a normal part of aging, neither are they necessarily heralds of irreversible diseases. Proper assessment is required to adequately address the patient's concerns and those of worried family members.

Approximately 1% to 2% of older adults in the United States develop a dementia each year (Mayo Clinic, 2012) and aging remains the greatest risk factor for development of cognitive impairment. While Alzheimer's disease accounts for 90% of all diagnosed dementias, not all dementias are Alzheimer's disease. Known for the hallmark "plaques and tangles" that are evident in the brain of someone who has this disease, Alzheimer's type dementia presents a different type of neurological development than other types of dementia. "Frontotemporal dementia" involves degeneration of the anterior (forward) parts of the brain,

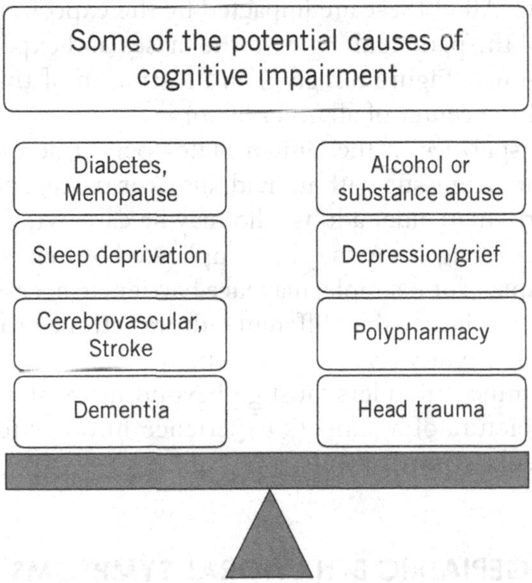

For more information, visit these sources:
- The UK's Patient website: http://www.patient.co.uk/doctor/mild-cognitive-impairment
- The Mayo Clinic online: http://www.mayoclinic.org/diseases-conditions/mild-cognitive-impairment/basics/causes/con-20026392

Figure 8.1 Potential Causes of Cognitive Impairment.

for example. The importance of diagnosing the causes for memory concerns is critical since treatments available to slow the progression of Alzheimer's disease are quite different from treatments available for other diseases. For example, the commonly prescribed medication for Alzheimer's disease donepezil does not help someone suffering from depression, just as the antidepressant medication bupropion does nothing to slow the progression of dementia.

The number of older adults in the United States is rapidly expanding. Current projections indicate that the 13% of the 65+ population as of 2014 will expand to at least 19% of the total population by 2030 (Federal Interagency Forum on Aging-Related Statistics [FIFARS], 2012). With nearly one fifth of the U.S. population in this group, the demand for health care will expand. Already the frequency of skilled nursing facility stays has doubled since 1994. While the number of hospital stays for older adults has remained fairly stable, the number of days per stay has declined, suggesting that patients are discharged more quickly and potentially with more fragile health status than their normal baseline (FIFARS, 2012). Rates of home health care visits and visits to health care providers have steadily increased since 2000 and individuals with multiple chronic conditions have expenses that tend to be four times higher than those who suffered no chronic illnesses (FIFARS, 2012). Aging-related health concerns will continue to be a growing part of primary care practice for years to come with care for chronic diseases a substantial part of that practice.

Health care providers must consider a wide range of information when assessing patients, not simply physical findings but also psychosocial well-being and stressors related to aging. Health and well-being lie at the intersection of biological health, functional capacity, social network support, and psychological well-being. All of these are impacted by the expectations and perceptions of the culture of the patient along with the biases and expectations of our broader American culture. Figure 8.2 gives an illustration of this idea with health and well-being at the center of all other factors.

Health disparities in the United States persist across demographic groups and are as much an issue with individuals over the age of 65 as in any other age group. In particular, older adults who may be caregiving for another adult often face unique challenges that may be complicated by demographics. Unmarried or same sex couples, for example, may face barriers to accessing resources and support. Research indicates that different cultural-ethnic groups access information and support differently (HHS, 1999; Dunlop, Manheim, Song, & Chang, 2002). With this in mind, providers must go beyond medical assessment and examine the broader picture of a patient's experience in order to truly understand and address presenting impairments.

EPIDEMIOLOGY OF GERIATRIC BEHAVIORAL SYMPTOMS PRESENTED IN PRIMARY CARE

According to a report by the Surgeon General (1999), one in five adults in the United States over the age of 65 will be diagnosed with a mental health disorder yet only 50% of those who receive a diagnosis will receive appropriate mental health

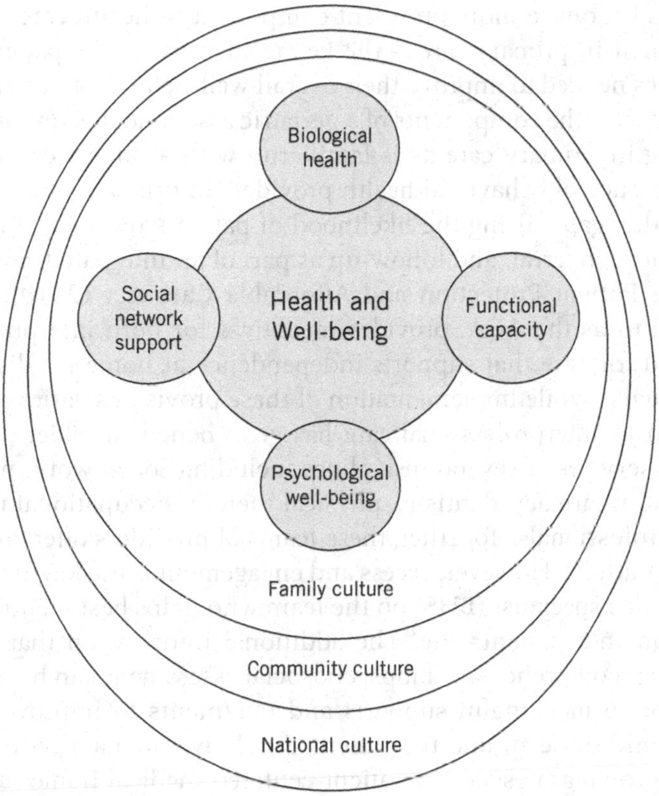

Figure 8.2 Impacts on Health and Well-Being for Older Adults.

treatment, and in some demographic groups, such as Native American older adults, rates of help seeking are even lower (HHS, 1999). While mental health interventions are gaining more acceptance in younger cohorts, older Americans continue to grapple with a perception of stigma related to help-seeking (Bartels et al., 2004). In some groups, it is common for psychiatric symptoms to be expressed somatically—in the body—and this can create challenging diagnostic pictures that often lead to inappropriate or missed opportunities for intervention. Long-term consequences in aging adults can be much more complex than in younger groups, as untreated issues such as depression or substance use can exacerbate chronic physical conditions, leading to decreased quality of life (QOL), increased levels of morbidity and mortality, and higher health care utilization and costs.

ASSESSMENT OF GERIATRIC BEHAVIORAL SYMPTOMS IN PRIMARY CARE

Patient Presentations in Primary Care Settings

For adults struggling with mental health issues including memory loss concerns, substance issues, or limiting chronic physical ailments, primary care is the most likely place for them to seek help (Bartels et al., 2004). PCPs often assess for complex needs and refer to specialty geriatric clinics focused on the unique needs of older adults. As the aging population in the United States has grown, specialty care has become a more prevalent component in health care. However, the first assessment in primary care is the key to identifying the patient's needs and the resources needed to improve their overall well-being and functional status. Being familiar with the components of a geriatric assessment is important for providers working in primary care as is familiarity with available community resources. The presence of behavioral health providers in primary care settings often helps bridge this gap, raising the likelihood of patients receiving a thorough geriatric assessment, referral, and follow-up as part of an integrated care plan.

The Patient Protection and Affordable Care Act (2010), more commonly referred to as the ACA, provides incentives for both interprofessional primary care and for care that supports independence at home for disabled and elderly individuals. While implementation of these provisions varies across the country, the shift to interprofessional care has great benefit to older patients who often use the services of several disciplines including social work, nursing, case management, pharmacy, dentistry, physical therapy, occupational therapy, and other allied professionals. Together, these teams of providers offer comprehensive care for older adults. However, access and engagement is the key. It is often the behavioral health specialist (BHS) on the team who helps best identify what is actually going on in a patient's life. The additional information that the BHS can add through a comprehensive biopsychosocial assessment can be the key to opening the door to meaningful supports and treatments to improve the QOL for the patient and those around the patient. Similarly, care navigators or care managers have a growing presence in patient-centered medical homes and are invaluable for coordination of care for older adults who often have multiple health care providers. The kind of support that care managers can provide not only raises level of care plan compliance by helping identify barriers to care such as transportation or scheduling issues, but also reduces the risks of polypharmacy and overtreatment (Manderson, McMurray, Piraino, & Stolee, 2012). Care management, usually provided by a nurse or a social worker, may also lead to fewer hospital visits and help optimize the use of available insurance resources.

Among the most significant concerns for the treatment of older adults in primary care settings are the long-term effects of chronic conditions. Chronic medical conditions that may begin earlier in life, such as diabetes or arthritis, can limit function and decrease QOL. Chronic mental health conditions such as depression, anxiety, or trauma-related stress may have long-term consequences, particularly if the mental health symptoms are suboptimally treated. Depression, grief, and loss are common in the elderly and may present as a range of symptoms including physical impairment, memory complaints, mental health concerns, or overall decrease in global functioning. Evidence suggests that depression is highly comorbid with decreased mobility in later life, which can lead to problems with balance and gait and subsequent quality-of-life concerns (Zivin, Wharton, & Rostant, 2013). Similarly, vision and hearing problems are not uncommon with aging and if not properly assessed in an independent manner (i.e., separate from a depression screen and physical exam) may become the root of more complex problems. Additionally, polypharmacy causes many problems that may present as mental health symptoms, so regular reviews of medications are critically important in older patients.

Although each of these issues is common in the lives of older adults, they should not be considered a part of "normal aging." While it is certainly "normal" for aging adults to experience role changes, grief at losses, sensory changes, long-term physical decline and mobility limitations, and overall functional status changes, it is not acceptable to dismiss these as simply a part of life of the elderly and fail to provide options that may alleviate these experiences. There are often options for treatment, although sometimes providers must be creative in accessing interventions in geographical areas such as communities where resources may be limited. Non pharmacological interventions are becoming a first-line standard of care for older adults.

Assessment Procedures and Considerations for Primary Care Settings

Facilitating effective referrals and coordinating services for geriatric patients is one of the primary interventions available to BHSs in primary care settings. As discussed previously, a comprehensive assessment is needed when working with the geriatric patient. The American Geriatrics Society (2012) advocates that a comprehensive geriatric assessment should include investigation of the following:

- A full medical workup including special attention to tests of hearing and vision, and assessment of mobility and continence, as well as screening for potential delirium
- Pharmacy review for polypharmacy—a common problem among older adults and one that can often masquerade as another medical problem
- Nutrition and access to appropriate food choices
- Functional assessment of activities of daily living (ADLs—bathing, dressing, toileting) and instrumental activities of daily living (IADLs—cooking, driving, shopping, and particularly housecleaning, as that has recently been shown to correlate with decline of function)
- Psychological/psychiatric assessment, including past and present perception of functioning, family history of mental illness or dementia, and personal and family history of substance use
- Assessment of formal support systems, including access to sufficient finances to pay for necessary care, options for community-based supports for transportation and nutrition, and the availability of case management services to help with complicated medication regimens and appointment scheduling
- Assessment of interpersonal relationships including current and past relationships and functioning, both socially and intimately with partner(s)/spouse(s)
- Community engagement and social interaction with individuals or groups outside of the home
- Assessment of the physical environment in which the patient and family live, including:
  - Living arrangements and layout of the home
  - Safety issues such as lighting, stability of flooring, carpeting that may impede ambulation
  - Ability to access the bathtub/shower, toilet, and sink with minimal risk of falling or slipping

- Heating/cooling
- Presence of stairs, outside or inside the home
- Safe access in the kitchen, with minimal fall risk and adequate reach and lighting to complete tasks
- Neighborhood safety and the presence or absence of sidewalks
- Availability of emergency services or supports

Although this list seems long and specific, many of these domains can be assessed fairly rapidly in a primary care setting with a brief interview. By approaching the family with a conversational, rapport-building approach, a great deal of insight can be gained into all of these areas. Simply having patients describe where they live; what they do during the day or week; and where they receive their social, financial, and physical support can be a quick way to assess many of these areas. Engagement of clinical skills to build rapport and engage with both patients and caregivers is the best way to obtain critical information that will shape the care plan.

In addition to a good interview, the use of validated screening tools can be important. When screening for depression in older adults the Geriatric Depression Scale (Sheikh & Yesavage, 1986) may be used. The Quality of Life Inventory (Frisch, 2009) is often used to examine domains related to perceived life satisfaction and value. There are a number of instruments that may be used to assess both cognitive functioning of an individual and caregiver burden, as well as screens for delirium (an acute medical crisis involving the rapid onset of confusion and disorientation as hallmark features). The most common of these are the Mini Mental Status Exam (MMSE), the Montreal Cognitive Assessment (MoCA), the Zarit Burden Scale, and the Confusion Assessment Measure (CAM; Folstein, Folstein, & McHugh, 1975; Inouye et al., 1990; Nasreddine et al., 2005; Zarit, Reever, & Bach-Peterson, 1980). A few cautions are appropriate, however, for the use of cognitive screening instruments with older adults. For example, the MMSE is a brief screening instrument of basic cognitive function but is copyrighted and should be used with permission only and is not very accurate or useful for screening individuals with high levels of education. The MoCA, also a screening instrument for cognitive function but more involved and time consuming than the MMSE, is not appropriate for individuals with low literacy. There are wide variations in the literacy level of older adults in particular that may not be easily apparent due to compensatory skills but should be considered before using cognitive screening instruments that require reading skill. Many instruments have a recommended adaptation for literacy and education levels and adjustments should always be made in order to avoid either false-positive or false-negative results.

Considerations in Assessing Geriatric Patients

Geriatric assessments require that the BHS remember that patients have *autonomy*. While we have a responsibility to act when a vulnerable older adult may be in danger or at risk of harm, adults who are cognitively able have the right to make decisions that we may feel are not in their best interest. How the assessment is performed is important to obtaining a complete and accurate picture of the patient and to making helpful recommendations. Geron, Andrews, and Kuhn (2005) outline the following process:

- Establishing rapport
- Explaining the purpose of the assessment
- Using observation and clinical judgment
- Maintaining confidentiality
- Honoring the person assessed
- Handling difficult situations

An important issue to consider when assessing an older adult is that there may be a very close relationship with a caregiver, particularly if the caregiver is a partner/spouse. When two individuals have built a life together they may be more appropriately viewed as a dyad. Some of these relationships may become symbiotic where the two individuals function well together but struggle when either is impaired in any way. Because health care interventions and care planning in the United States are "patient focused" and not "family focused," it is not unusual to encounter situations in which necessary care is unavailable or unobtainable because of restrictive insurance criteria involving family dynamics. For example, in the case presented at the beginning of this chapter, the patient's ability to function safely and maintain his life in his home depends heavily on the presence and functional capacity of his wife. However, home care providers and respite care options are often based on the patient's capacity and do not consider or provide billable supports that depend on whether his wife is in need of support in order to continue facilitating his success. Interventions that fail to consider this patient's wife will likely be unsuccessful as it is his wife who may be managing his medications, ensuring his nutrition, and helping him plan his daily activities. While there is growing awareness in the therapeutic community and among geriatric researchers about this issue, there are currently no evidence-based clinical practice guidelines for dyadic caregiver interventions, and relatively few pilot interventions specifically targeted to dyads.

COMMUNITY TREATMENT APPROACHES FOR GERIATRIC MENTAL HEALTH SYMPTOMS

Older adults with mental health symptoms receive mental health care in a variety of community-based outpatient health and social care settings. These include traditional PCP offices and health clinics, and from both public and not-for-profit specialty mental health provider agencies. Occasionally, programs are offered by senior centers and organizations affiliated with the aging services network, although these vary from state to state (HHS, 2014). Significant attitudinal and system of care barriers limit the use of specialty mental health services by older adults. Byers, Arean, and Yaffe (2012) found that 70% of older adults with anxiety or depressive disorders failed to access treatment. When older adults do access behavioral health services, they report these services are beneficial at similar rates reported by younger adults (Karlin, Duffy, & Gleaves, 2008).

Primary care remains a preferred location where older adults seek treatment for mental health issues and can lead to improved access to mental health care (Bartels et al., 2004). The BHS in primary care plays an essential role in screening for impairments, consulting with PCPs and other providers, referring for specialty care, and delivering interventions for common problems such as depression, anxiety, cognitive impairment, and grief and loss. Recent changes to Medicare requirements requiring risk screening for depression and cognitive functioning during a patient's annual wellness visit highlight the increasing importance of the BHS in delivering care to geriatric patients in primary care (HHS: CMS, 2014).

Geriatric depression is frequently comorbid with anxiety and often complicated further by the presence of comorbid physical illness or cognitive impairment that may limit pharmacological treatments and interfere with recommended behavioral interventions (Wolitzky-Taylor, Castriotta, Lenze, Stanley, & Craske, 2010). Despite the importance of addressing these symptoms, older adults with depression remain undertreated in the community (Barry, Abou, Simen, & Gill, 2011; Garrido, Kane, Kaas, & Kane, 2011).

Community treatments may be delivered by private practitioners using psychotropic medications, outpatient brief individual and/or group therapies, through partial hospitalization, and within inpatient psychiatric hospitals. Access to publically funded specialty mental health services for older adults who lack the resources to pay for private services has historically been limited. The implementation of the ACA is expected to alter this trend, but ongoing shortages in the availability of specialist geriatric mental health providers are expected to continue and may limit access to specialty mental health services (Institute of Medicine, 2012).

Selecting the appropriate community treatment approach for an older adult with depression or anxiety requires careful consideration of their comorbid physical illnesses, medication used, personal preferences, and ability to access services in the community (Arean & Niu, 2014). The Substance Abuse and Mental Health Services Administration (SAMHSA, 2011) recognizes the following interventions as evidence-based practices to treat geriatric depression:

- Psychotherapy including cognitive behavioral therapy (CBT), behavioral therapy, problem-solving treatment, interpersonal therapy, reminiscence, and bibliotherapy
- Antidepressant medications
- Collaborative and integrated physical and mental health services
- Geriatric mental health outreach services

Cognitive Behavioral Interventions

An extensive range of treatment studies including randomized controlled trials (RCTs) support the efficacy of mental health therapies (Samad, Brealey, & Gilbody, 2011) and CBT approaches for both geriatric anxiety and depression (Chand & Grossberg, 2013; Nordhus & Pallesun, 2003). Efforts have also been made to identify strategies to adapt the delivery of CBT to accommodate sensory impairments or physical limitations often found with geriatric patients. Pasterfield et al. (2014) describe strategies to modify and adapt behavioral activation for older adults. They recommend careful assessment of four domains of functioning when considering the use of behavioral activation: physical health limitations, cognitive impairment, the availability of social support, and risk of suicide. To address issues of physical limitations, the assessment should include collaboration with the patient and any involved caregivers to identify activities appropriate for the functional abilities of the patient. If cognitive impairment is present, the clinician should simplify the use of language and distribute homework activities across more sessions. The BHS should assess available social support provided by friends and family and provide referrals to community organizations that offer socialization when the patient is socially isolated. As risk of suicide is a concern, clinicians should also include a careful assessment of passive suicidal ideation (desire to die without a specific plan) prior to using behavioral activation. As general modifications to behavioral activation, Chand and Grossberg (2013) recommend the use of repetition, a slower pace, and using alternate formats for psychoeducational materials to promote use of CBT with older adults. Jameson and Scully (2011) recommend adapting CBT delivered to older adults in primary care by reducing the number of sessions delivered and focusing on symptom self-management skills as a primary goal.

Recent research has also sought to enhance the translation of CBT and behavioral activation interventions within integrated and collaborative care services in order to increase access to treatment for older adults. The Improving Mood-Promoting Access to Collaborative Treatment (IMPACT) approach is an evidence-based model incorporating medication, behavioral activation, and problem solving that has been translated successfully for use with older adults having a wide range of comorbid medical conditions. Central to the intervention is the depression care manager (DCM), often a clinical social worker, nurse, or psychologist, who conducts a focused assessment and develops an initial 10- to 12-week treatment plan in collaboration with the PCP. Using a stepped-care approach, the IMPACT model incorporates consultation from psychiatry to evaluate new patients and to revise treatment plans for those patients having suboptimal response to treatment. Over time, the DCM gradually tapers contact with the patient through periodic telephone contacts. Outcomes of RCTs indicate that IMPACT produces improvements in depression severity and functional impairments over an 18- to 24-month period. It has also been successfully used across primary care settings and across a range of health systems (Administration for Community Living, 2014). For a patient who presents with a combination of symptoms suggestive of depression and cognitive impairment such as the one in the case at the beginning of this chapter, the IMPACT model may be particularly helpful. Outcome studies indicate improvements in depression for older adults served by IMPACT who had both depression and cognitive impairment (Steffens et al., 2006).

Before symptoms associated with cognitive impairment may be addressed within primary care settings, careful assessment of the nature of impairments, identification of the etiology, potential for reversibility, long-term prognosis, and understanding of the environmental context and functional capacities surrounding the patient are required. Temporary impairments such as a delirium caused by a urinary tract infection or some similar acute medical condition must be ruled out, and it is important to note that no further assessment for dementias can be done in the presence of delirium. If available, such detailed assessment is best accomplished through referral to a comprehensive multidisciplinary geriatric assessment program. For primary care patients who are exhibiting mild cognitive impairment due to traumatic brain injury or post-stroke, cognitive rehabilitation approaches are an important treatment strategy. More recently, cognitive training models for memory symptoms associated with mild cognitive impairments, Alzheimer's, and vascular dementias have emerged. Unfortunately, early systematic reviews of cognitive training and rehabilitation for these disorders have found limited or inconsistent evidence to support their efficacy and further investigation is needed (Martin, Clare, Altgassen, Cameron, & Zehnder, 2011; Alves et al., 2013; Bahar Fuchs, Clare, & Woods, 2013).

An important role for the BHS in primary care is to conduct periodic re-screening to assess the progression of cognitive impairments over time. Screening for symptoms of impairment is now mandated for older adults as part of the Medicare annual wellness visit. This should include both screening of memory and executive functioning. A variety of screening tools are widely in use; however, as mentioned previously, practitioners must be careful in selecting the appropriate tool(s). Recent recommendations include using specific screening tools such as the MoCA as well as conducting assessments of functional impairments and caregiver functioning when indicated (Nasreddine et al., 2005; Smith, Gildeh & Holmes, 2007; Petersen, 2011).

Grief and Loss

Responding to grief and loss among aged primary care patients is another role for the BHS. Significant symptoms associated with acute grieving include intense yearning and wishing to be reunited with the deceased, sadness and feelings of remorse, intense images or hallucinatory experiences involving the deceased, somatic symptoms similar to those associated with major depression, and feeling disconnected (Shear et al., 2011). Patients who have experienced recent bereavement exhibit more physical health problems, use more medication, have more disabilities, and are more likely to be hospitalized (Stroebe, Schut, & Stroebe, 2007). One important risk factor associated with poor health outcomes and complicated grief reactions is poor health prior to the loss (Utz, Caserta, & Lund, 2012). Stahl and Schulz (2014), in a systematic review of risk and health behaviors among older bereaved spouses, note the importance of maintaining nutritional status and body weight as well as addressing sleep difficulties and alcohol use to promote adjustment following a loss. For bereaved primary care patients who had been engaged in hospice services as part of end-of-life care for their loved one, referral to follow-up hospice bereavement services may be indicated. This may be particularly helpful for those experiencing complicated grief reactions (Bergman, Haley, & Small, 2011). Bereavement counseling offered through hospice organizations may include group treatment, peer support groups, individual grief counseling and, increasingly, Internet-based support groups (Litz et al., 2014).

Complicated grief reactions arise when patient experiences transcend the normative processes associated with bereavement. Some suggest that symptoms of acute grief that persist beyond 6 to 12 months are reflective of complicated grief (Shear et al., 2011). Symptoms of complicated grief are characterized by sadness and prolonged yearning for the deceased (Shear et al., 2011). Recommended interventions include implementing health promotion efforts, training in the use of self-care approaches, and cognitive behavioral therapies (Boelen, de Keijser, van den Hout, & van den Bout, 2007). One model that has been tested with promising results incorporates both behavioral activation and therapeutic exposure treatment. This model uses a five-session format delivered by peer counselors. This model consists of using video education, two face-to-face treatment sessions with a bereavement counselor, and two phone consultations, and has achieved reductions in self-reported depression symptoms and improved perceptions of physical health status (Acierno et al., 2011).

Recent evaluations of model programs integrating primary care and geriatric mental health treatment hold promise for engaging difficult-to-reach geriatric patients in need of behavioral health interventions. Early efforts such as the Primary Care Research in Substance Abuse and Mental Health for the Elderly (PRISM-E) intervention achieved beneficial outcomes in outreach, screening, and engagement of geriatric patients (Bartels et al., 2004). Older adults in the PRISM-E integrated care condition attended more visits for mental health concerns compared to peers referred to specialty mental health providers. The Bridging Resources of an Interdisciplinary Geriatric Health Team via Electronic Networking (BRIGHTEN) program adapted this model to address challenges in establishing behavioral health services colocated with medical clinics (Emery, Lapidos, Eisenstein, Ivan, & Golden, 2012). The BRIGHTEN program successfully established a virtual electronic team capable of engaging patients and providers across geographically dispersed clinics using e-mail and phone communications. Reported patient outcomes for the BRIGHTEN intervention include a significant reduction in depressive symptoms and a significant reduction in symptoms of mental distress.

Challenges in Treating Homebound Patients

Primary care geriatric patients who are homebound due to physical health conditions or those who suffer from long-term mental illnesses face special challenges in accessing mental health care.

Targeted outreach and home-based interventions have been developed to provide services to this often vulnerable and physically frail population. Using community gatekeepers (e.g., postal delivery personnel, bank tellers) to identify at-risk elders is a strategy that has some empirical support (van Critters & Bartels, 2004). The programs and services of the Administration for Community Living (ACL), which are funded through the Older Americans Act and delivered through organizations affiliated with local Area Agencies on Aging (AAA; Older Americans Act of 1965, 1965), also offer home-based programming to support the behavioral health needs of older adults. Nonspecialist providers from ACL programs have also been trained to engage elders at home and successfully assess and treat depression comorbid with chronic medical conditions using self-management and behavioral activation techniques (Quijano et al., 2007). Homebound patients with depression symptoms and serious COPD or heart failure have achieved reductions in depression symptoms and emergency department use with a self-management tele-health intervention (Gellis et al., 2012) and this technology provides promising options for critical access to care for the aged.

For older adults with long-standing serious mental illnesses, interventions to promote sustained engagement in both medical and behavioral health treatment are essential due to the high prevalence of serious medical comorbidities in this population such as respiratory illnesses, diabetes, cardiovascular disease, and risks for poor care transitions (Bartels, 2004; Hendrie et al., 2013). Illness self-management training addressing both medical and psychiatric conditions is a promising approach for BHSs treating this vulnerable group of elders in primary care. A recent effort integrating psychiatric and medical illness self-management techniques has achieved promising benefits for this complex patient population (Bartels et al., 2014). Patient education was provided by a nurse and resulted in positive outcomes in self-reported and clinician-rated self-management of diabetes and psychiatric symptoms.

ADDRESSING NEEDS TO PROMOTE DISEASE MANAGEMENT, MEDICAL ADHERENCE, AND WELL-BEING

Results from a comprehensive geriatric assessment should include a detailed analysis and set of recommendations for meeting basic needs as well as referrals to promote effective chronic disease management through supporting medical treatment adherence and promotion of optimal well-being. Referrals for financial issues, accessing transportation, and educational and legal issues associated with advance directives are often also indicated for geriatric patients in order to ensure adherence to treatment regimens.

Financial Considerations

Costs of care play an especially important role in promoting medication adherence among older adults with chronic disease and comorbid mental health concerns (Campbell et al., 2014). Cost sharing requirements for health plans can lead to the accumulation of medical debt for middle- and low-income elders reliant on fixed incomes (Grande, Barg, Johnson, & Cannuscio, 2013). Medicare prescription drug plan choices (Medicare Part D) are complex and the older adult must also understand how existing Veterans Affairs or pension insurance programs influence their choices. Many older adults will benefit from the assistance of a specialist to review their options. Each state offers a federally funded State Health Insurance Assistance Program (National SHIP Resource Center, 2014) providing free counseling and assistance to help select appropriate insurance carriers. Financial issues play a role in every aspect of an older adult's well-being. Financial resources are often critical in determining housing options when the individual's residential environment no longer meets his or her needs due to declining health circumstances or functional abilities. Access to supportive services or to programs that enhance socialization for the elderly such as those offered through senior centers can also be limited for older adults with modest incomes.

Access to Transportation

Absence of a broad range of accessible transportation services limit opportunities for out-of-home socialization and restrict access to medical care offices for many older adults. The problem is particularly acute in, though not exclusive to, geographically dispersed rural communities. Even in densely populated urban centers, transportation may be inaccessible due to poorly designed environments that make walking to transportation access points hazardous. Public transport routes are generally designed for commuter trips in cars rather than the types of walking routes preferred by older persons (AARP Public Policy Institute, 2010). Transportation resources for older adults include Area Agency on Aging sponsored services providing trips to medical appointments and community aging organizations, private providers providing transportation services, and not-for-profit organizations offering transportation through volunteer networks (Wacker & Roberto, 2014). The local Area Agency on Aging is usually the place to start when trying to identify this type of resource.

Advance Care Planning

Incorporating patient preferences into medical decision making takes on special importance when a comprehensive geriatric assessment reveals the presence of a disorder such as a dementia or another debilitating condition that may impair capacity. An advance directive is a legal document outlining patient preferences for medical care in the event of incapacity, and is an important part of managing such situations (National Institute on Aging, 2012). Advance directives provide specific instructions to guide decision making about life-sustaining treatment when an older adult at the end-of-life lacks the capacity to make his or her wishes known. There is considerable variation across states in the required content and forms of legally executed advance directive documents, so BHSs should research local requirements and recommend legal consultation if needed for completing advance directives. Advance directives include attention to preferences for end-of-life care as well as choices for who will be involved in making end-of-life care decisions on behalf of an incapacitated patient. The living will is a document designating preferences for medical treatments to be received and to be avoided at the end of life. Documentation of a health care proxy, sometimes referred to as health care "surrogate" or agent, allows the older adult to select an individual to represent his or her interests and make decisions regarding medical treatments at the end of life. A variety of model forms have been developed and disseminated to encourage completion of advance directives. Helpful resources for professionals engaged with older adults considering advance directives can be found at the Institute for Healthcare Improvement and its Conversation Project initiative (theconversationproject.org/) and Caring Connections from the National Hospice and Palliative Care Organization (caringinfo.org).

Over the past 10 years the overall proportion of older adults in the population completing advance directives has increased (Silveira, Wiitala, & Piette, 2014). Being female, White, literate, and of an advanced age is associated with higher rates of completing an advance directive (Alano et al., 2010; Waite et al., 2013). Advance directives are less likely to be completed among minority patients and patients with low literacy (Alano et al., 2010; Waite et al., 2013). Educational interventions have been effective in encouraging the completion of an advance directive among older adults (Bravo, Dubois, & Wagneur, 2008; Kossman, 2014). Providing patients with written educational materials through resources such as the American Hospital Association's "Put it in Writing" brochure or the Administration on Community Living's "Advance Care Planning for Serious Illness" could help introduce the topic within a primary care practice setting (Administration for Community Living, n.d.; American Hospital Association, 2012).

One of the most challenging aspects to geriatric primary care is consistency in follow-up. Older adults sometimes need help identifying ways to facilitate issues like medication schedules for complicated drug regimens, transportation to appointments, and remembering unusual appointments such as those to specialists. Primary care teams must make sure that patients receive periodic pharmacy reviews to avoid polypharmacy issues, and that recommendations from consultations are integrated into the care plan and followed. It is important that information from consultants is relayed back to the referring provider to enable the provider to tailor the best possible care options for the patient. For example, in our case study, it is critical that the BHS provide a comprehensive report back to the PCP so that the primary care team can follow up with periodic reassessment of functional status, behavioral symptoms, psychosocial needs, and medication management for the patient.

Patient Autonomy

Biases about older adults, as well as our own educational limitations, can easily cloud our perceptions of competency and safety. It is incumbent upon ethical providers to remember that our patients have lived entire lives filled with many experiences and have managed to survive to the point of arriving at our door. They are office workers, teachers, nurses, parents, engineers, and sometimes even doctors. They are from all over the world, all types of spiritual paths, gay, straight, transgendered, scholarly, eccentric, and everything in between. They have families that may include biological family as well as family by marriage and family by choice. We must always respect preferences for privacy, living arrangements, type of care, decision making, spirituality, and life choices, and not impose—either intentionally or otherwise—our own biases. Competency for decision making is situational and contextually based and depends heavily on the question at hand; we must never take away the rights of any individual without deep consideration of all factors involved and consults from other providers. Additionally, we must remember that although care for older adults is often dyadic or family oriented in nature (particularly including married partners), our patients have had a lifetime to develop what may be complicated relationships and families do not always communicate and partner with providers as easily as we might wish. Except in extreme situations of safety, communication with family members, regardless of relationship, is governed by very strict rules of confidentiality and privacy. By keeping the principle of autonomy in mind, providers may more easily navigate these complicated waters, and engage support from the extended social network of their patients, for the best possible team care.

BEHAVIORAL HEALTH ASSESSMENT AND TREATMENT SUMMARY TO REFERRING PRIMARY CARE PROVIDER

S: Patient is an 80-year-old Caucasian male referred with his wife for concerns about memory, anxiety, and stress.

O/A: Patient appears his stated age, was appropriately dressed and groomed, and presented to the clinic with his wife of 57 years. Both were ambulatory without any assistance, and the patient did not appear to have issues with balance or gait, although he was somewhat slow rising from a chair, and pushed down on the armrests to stand. He passed a Get-Up-and-Go assessment with little difficulty. Patient denied continence issues. He manages his own medications with no assistive aid. He denied any medication errors or missed doses, although his wife believes that he occasionally misses doses. Patient does operate a motor vehicle. The couple described daily challenges, such as confusion about whether the patient's morning medications had been taken, misplacing items, and forgetfulness about plans that had been made. They also described inattention, particularly when driving, and forgetting where he was going. Patient's wife described constant anxiety about her husband's condition. This couple is highly interdependent—she does not drive and relies on him for transportation; it appears that she is the organizer and planner for the couple, and he is the one who figures out how to get things done and makes sure that they get where they need to be. They share most everyday tasks and functions.

Psychosocial history: No family history of dementia, substance abuse, or known mental illness. Patient had a career in business administration, and his wife worked as a secretary in a factory until leaving to raise their children. Patient is retired and collects a pension and Social Security. He served in the army at the age of 18, and was honorably discharged after several years of service. He served briefly in the Korean War in 1952, and has a shrapnel injury to his left leg. He has a 40% disability rating with the Veterans Administration. They have two male adult children who reside out of state. Both children are married, and the older child has a daughter in grade school. The couple sees their children and granddaughter about once a year. They speak weekly by phone with each of their sons. The family members are all on good terms. The children are financially independent, and (per the patient's wife) are not at this time aware of their parents' concerns for the patient's memory. The couple owns their home—a two-story, four-bedroom house, with a large backyard and basement, and has lived in this home since their second child was born. They have long-term care insurance, but have not talked about their wishes for long-term care needs, nor do either of them have a living will or a health care proxy document.

The couple has maintained contact with three long-term friends. One of these friends died of cardiac disease 2 years ago, and one is in advanced stages of cancer and nearing the end of life. They both became tearful when discussing their friends. There remains a great deal of unresolved grief and there appears to be a significant issue of anticipatory grief related to the impending death of their friend of cancer. The patient's wife has family history of cancer, and there is fear for themselves, although neither of them has been diagnosed with cancer. There appear to be some complicated grief issues that are impacting the patient's functioning, his wife's functioning, and subsequently the marital dyad. As the patient's grief has deepened he has begun to struggle with depression and his functioning has become increasingly impaired over the last 7 to 8 months, with sleep and eating disruption in addition to memory concerns. As his functioning has become impaired, his wife's anxiety has increased concurrently. This has created a feedback loop where he is forgetful, she becomes anxious, her anxiety triggers feelings of guilt and shame for the patient, conflict arises between the couple, and subsequently, both his symptoms and her anxiety become increasingly worse.

Safety and assessment of risk: The couple lives in a two-story house, with a staircase to the upper floor, and three steps to the front door. Bedrooms are upstairs. Laundry is in the basement, as is their freezer. Although they claim that the stairs are not a problem, the patient has fallen twice on the basement stairs, and his wife admits that carrying laundry baskets up and down requires her husband's help. Although the stairs may not currently be a barrier for them, it is clear that the risk for falls is high in this situation. Additionally, although the couple still clean their home and maintain the lawn and garden without help, procurement of some assistance or supervision in the near future will be necessary.

The patient's wife does the cooking for the couple, and insists that she has no difficulties with forgetfulness or difficulty preparing their meals. They eat at least twice a day every day. They grocery shop together at the nearest store about ¾ mile from their home. There are limited sidewalks in their neighborhood, so walking involves being in the road. As the patient's inattention has increased, his wife has become concerned about riding with him in the car, although since she does not drive, this is her only means of transportation currently. They are unaware of public transportation or elder transport services in their area.

As the patient manages his own medications without a pill box or other structured aid, he is at high risk for accidental overdose or missed medication.

Depression, anxiety, and quality of life (QOL) assessment: The patient had a high score on the Geriatric Depression Scale-Short Form (GDS-15). High scores indicate substantial impact of depression on functioning. The patient also had a low score on the Quality of Life Inventory (QOLI), a validated measure of positive mental health, life satisfaction, and well-being. This low score is indicative of poor perception of QOL. Such scores are highly correspondent to both clinical depression and poor functional status, often related to poor treatment adherence and unsuccessful coping. There was no suicidal ideation but apathy to life was high. He became frustrated during assessment. Memory problems are a well-documented symptom of geriatric depression. He may benefit from a low-dose antidepressant, along with behavioral activation, mental stimulation, and supportive counseling for depression and complicated bereavement/grief. An antidepressant that stimulates appetite could have a beneficial impact on his nutritional status, as he has had substantial loss of appetite comorbid to the depression. The couple does not leave the house much, and their social life has suffered since the death of their friend.

Recommendations

1. The patient's memory problems appear to be related to psychosocial stress and emotional well-being. Neuropsychological testing should be done and ongoing monitoring for vascular depression and dementia that may appear in the future would be beneficial.
2. The patient would benefit from an antidepressant—preferably one with appetite stimulation effects. A pharmacy consult is needed to examine possible polypharmacy issues.
3. The patient's depression is exacerbated by what appears to be complicated grief. Supportive counseling that includes behavioral activation is strongly recommended for both the patient and his wife.
4. The patient should be encouraged to refrain from driving until his symptoms alleviate and he is able to remain focused on task appropriately. Depression and complicated grief are impacting his functioning; these may alleviate with treatment, so it is not necessary to assess for removal of his driver's license at this time, as it is hard to reverse this action. However, if his symptoms do not improve in 6 months with depression and grief intervention and supportive counseling, he should be referred to the Department of Motor Vehicles for a driver's safety assessment. In the meanwhile, alternate transportation options will need to be explored with assistance for shopping, appointments, and social activities.
5. The patient will receive a pill box for his weekly medications and will fill it on Sundays. This will allow him to maintain control of his medications and avoid dosage accidents.
6. The patient and his wife have been provided with the following information:
   a. Referral to a grief support group for older adults.
   b. Information about their local Area Agency on Aging and the possible resources that may be available, both for immediate support and

future needs. The AAA should be able to connect them to Meals on Wheels, providing both reliable nutrition and external contact and observation on a regular basis. Additionally, the AAA will have information about local transportation options.

c. Information about their local community senior center. They have been encouraged to engage with events at the center, to support the goals of behavioral activation, mental stimulation, and social interaction for both of them.

7. Contact with the adult children could provide additional insight into the challenges and opportunities for support. The couple will need support from their PCP to initiate this conversation with their children.
8. Ongoing support is needed to identify future planning needs regarding long-term care options and financing, and end-of-life choices that should be identified by obtaining living wills from both. Planning for a change of living arrangements is best done in advance, rather than in the situation of a crisis.
9. Referral to a VA social worker would be helpful, to assess for the possibility of unclaimed VA pension, access to the VA pharmacy for inexpensive prescriptions, access to a range of mental health resources, and ability to access Aid and Attendance benefits in the future. Aid and Attendance benefits are paid to qualified veterans or their spouses for care required to maintain an individual in his or her home. The VA has a range of caregiving supports, such as support groups, educational information, and crisis lines that may be supportive to the couple.
10. This couple will need to be assessed as a dyad in the future, as they are closely symbiotic in the course of their daily life.

REFERENCES

AARP Public Policy Institute. (2010). *Linking transportation and housing solutions for older adults*. Retrieved from www.nhc.org/media/documents/fs170-transportation-housing.pdf

Acierno, R., Rheingold, A., Amstadter, A., Kurent, J., Amella, E., Resnick, H., ... Lejuez, C. (2011). Behavioral activation and therapeutic exposure for bereavement in older adults. *American Journal of Hospice and Palliative Medicine*, *29*, 13–25.

Administration for Community Living. (2014). *Aging and disability evidence-based programs and practices intervention summary*. Retrieved from www.acl.gov/Programs/CDAP/OPE/docs/IMPACT_summary.pdf

Administration for Community Living. (n.d.). Advance care planning for serious illness. Retrieved from www.eldercare.gov/eldercare.NET/Public/Resources/Advanced_Care/docs/AdvancedCarePlanning.pdf

Alano, G. J., Pekmezaris, R., Tai, J. Y., Hussain, M. J., Jeune, J., Louis, B., ... Wolf-Klein, G. P. (2010). Factors influencing older adults to complete advance directives. *Palliative and Supportive Care*, *8*(3), 267–275.

Alves, J., Magalhaes, R., Thomas, R. E., Gonçalves, Ó. F., Petrosyan, A., & Sampaio, A. (2013). Is there evidence for cognitive intervention in Alzheimer disease? A systematic review of efficacy, feasibility, and cost-effectiveness. *Alzheimer Disease & Associated Disorders*, *27*(3), 195–203.

American Geriatrics Society Expert Panel on the Care of Older Adults with Multimorbidity. (2012). Guiding principles for the care of older adults with multimorbidity: An approach for clinicians. *Journal of the American Geriatric Society*, *60*(10), E1–E25. doi:10.1111/j.1532-5414.2012.04188.x

American Hospital Association. (2012). Put it in writing. Retrieved from www.aha.org/advocacy-issues/initiatives/piiw/index.shtml

Arean, P. A., & Niu, G. (2014). Choosing treatment for depression in older adults and evaluating response. *Clinics in Geriatric Medicine*, *30*(3), 535–551.

Bahar-Fuchs, A., Clare, L., & Woods, B. (2013). Cognitive training and cognitive rehabilitation for mild to moderate Alzheimer's disease and vascular dementia. *The Cochrane Database of Systematic Reviews*, *6*. doi: 10.1002/14651858.CD003260.pub2

Barry, L. C., Abou, J. J., Simen, A. A., & Gill, T. M. (2012). Under-treatment of depression in older persons. *Journal of Affective Disorders*, *136*(3), 789–796.

Bartels, S. J., Coakley, E. H., Zubritsky, C., Ware, J. H., Miles, K. M., Areán, P. A., ... Levkoff, S. E. (2004). Improving access to geriatric mental health services: A randomized trial comparing treatment engagement with integrated versus enhanced referral care for depression, anxiety, and at-risk alcohol use. *American Journal of Psychiatry*, *161*(8), 1455–1462.

Bartels, S. J. (2004). Caring for the whole person: Integrated health care for older adults with severe mental illness and medical comorbidity. *Journal of the American Geriatrics Society*, *52*(s12), S249–S257.

Bartels, S. J., Pratt, S. I., Mueser, K. T., Naslund, J. A., Wolfe, R. S., Santos, M., ... Riera, E. G. (2014). Integrated IMR for psychiatric and general medical illness for adults aged 50 or older with serious mental illness. *Psychiatric Services*, *65*(3), 330–337.

Bergman, E. J., Haley, W. E., & Small, B. J. (2011). Who uses bereavement services? An examination of service use by bereaved dementia caregivers. *Aging & Mental Health*, *15*(4), 531–540.

Boelen, P. A., de Keijser, J., van den Hout, M. A., & van den Bout, J. (2007). Treatment of complicated grief: A comparison between cognitive-behavioral therapy and supportive counseling. *Journal of Consulting and Clinical Psychology*, *75*(2), 277.

Bravo, G., Dubois, M. F., & Wagneur, B. (2008). Assessing the effectiveness of interventions to promote advance directives among older adults: A systematic review and multi-level analysis. *Social Science & Medicine*, *67*(7), 1122–1132.

Byers, A. L., Arean, P. A., & Yaffe, K. (2012). Low use of mental health services among older Americans with mood and anxiety disorders. *Psychiatric Services*, *63*(1), 66–72.

Campbell, D. J., King-Shier, K., Hemmelgarn, B. R., Sanmartin, C., Ronksley, P. E., Weaver, R. G., ... Manns, B. J. (2014). Self-reported financial barriers to care among patients with cardiovascular-related chronic conditions. *Health Reports*, *25*(5), 3–12.

Chand, S. P., & Grossberg, G. T. (2013). How to adapt cognitive-behavioral therapy for older adults. *Current Psychiatry*, *12*(3), 10.

Dunlop, D., Manheim, L., Song, J., & Chang, R. (2002). Gender and ethnic/racial disparities in health care utilization among older adults. *Journals of Gerontology Series B: Psychological and Social Science*, *57*(4), S221–S233. doi:10.1093/geronb/57.4.S221

Emery, E. E., Lapidos, S., Eisenstein, A. R., Ivan, I. I., & Golden, R. L. (2012). The BRIGHTEN Program: Implementation and evaluation of a program to bridge resources of an interdisciplinary geriatric health team via electronic networking. *Gerontologist*, *52*(6), 857–865.

Federal Interagency Forum on Aging-Related Statistics (FIFARS). (2012, July). *Older Americans 2012: Key indicators of well-being*. Washington, DC: U.S. Government Printing Office. Retrieved from www.agingstats.gov/Main_Site/Data/Data_2012.aspx

Folstein, M. F., Folstein, S. E., & McHugh, P. R. (1975). "Mini-mental state": A practical method for grading the cognitive state of patients for the clinician. *Journal of Psychiatric Research*, *12*(3), 189–198.

Frisch, M. (2009). *The quality of life inventory (QOLI) handbook: A practical guide for laypersons, clients, and coaches*. Minneapolis, MN: Pearson Assessments.

Garrido, M. M., Kane, R. L., Kaas, M., & Kane, R. A. (2011). Use of mental health care by community-dwelling older adults. *Journal of the American Geriatrics Society*, *59*(1), 50–56.

Gellis, Z. D., Kenaley, B., McGinty, J., Bardelli, E., Davitt, J., & Ten Have, T. (2012). Outcomes of a telehealth intervention for homebound older adults with heart or chronic respiratory failure: A randomized controlled trial. *The Gerontologist*, *52*(4), 541–552.

Geron, S., Andrews, C., & Kuhn, K. (2005). Infusing aging skills into the social work practice community: Strategies for continuing professional education. *Families in Society*, *85*(3), 431–440.

Grande, D., Barg, F. K., Johnson, S., & Cannuscio, C. C. (2013). Life disruptions for midlife and older adults with high out-of-pocket health expenditures. *Annals of Family Medicine*, *11*(1), 37–42.

Hendrie, H. C., Lindgren, D., Hay, D. P., Lane, K. A., Gao, S., Purnell, C., ... Callahan, C. M. (2013). Comorbidity profile and healthcare utilization in elderly patients with serious mental illnesses. *American Journal of Geriatric Psychiatry*, *21*(12), 1267–1276.

Inouye, S., van Dyck, C., Alessi, C., Balkin, S., Siegal, A., & Horwitz., R. (1990). Clarifying confusion: The confusion assessment method. *Annals of Internal Medicine*, *113*(12), 941–948.

Institute of Medicine. (2012). *The mental health and substance use workforce for older adults: In whose hands?* Washington, DC: The National Academies Press.

Jameson, J. P. & Scully, J. A. (2011). Cognitive behavioral therapy for older adults in the primary care setting. In K. H. Sorocco & S. Lauderdale (Eds.). *Cognitive behavior therapy with older adults* (pp. 291–316). New York, NY: Springer Publishing.

Karlin, B. E., Duffy, M., & Gleaves, D. H. (2008). Patterns and predictors of mental health service use and mental illness among older and younger adults in the United States. *Psychological Services*, *5*(3), 275–294.

Kossman, D. A. (2014). Prevalence, views, and impact of advance directives among older adults. *Journal of Gerontological Nursing*, *40*(7), 44–50.

Litz, B. T., Schorr, Y., Delaney, E., Au, T., Papa, A., Fox, A. B., ... Prigerson, H. G. (2014). A randomized controlled trial of an internet-based therapist-assisted indicated preventive intervention for prolonged grief disorder. *Behaviour Research and Therapy*, *61*, 23–34.

Manderson, B., McMurray, J., Piraino, E., & Stolee, P. (2012). Navigation roles support chronically ill older adults through healthcare transitions: A systematic review of the literature. *Health and Social Care in the Community*, *20*(2), 113–127.

Martin, M., Clare, L., Altgassen, A. M., Cameron, M. H., & Zehnder, F. (2011). Cognition-based interventions for healthy older people and people with mild cognitive impairment. *Cochrane Database of Systematic Reviews*, *1*(1). Retrieved from www.update software.com/BCP/WileyPDF/EN/CD006220.pdf

Mayo Clinic Online. (2012). Mild cognitive impairment. *Diseases and conditions*. Retrieved from http://www.mayoclinic.org/diseases-conditions/mild-cognitive-impairment/basics/definition/con-20026392

Nasreddine, Z. S., Phillips, N. A., Bédirian, V., Charbonneau, S., Whitehead, V., Collin, I., ... Chertkow, H. (2005). The Montreal Cognitive Assessment, MoCA: A brief screening tool for mild cognitive impairment. *Journal of the American Geriatrics Society*, *53*(4), 695–699.

National Institute on Aging. (2012). *Advance care planning: Tips from the National Institute on Aging*. Retrieved from www.nia.nih.gov/sites/default/files/advance_care_planning_tipsheet_0.pdf

National SHIP Resource Center. (2014). *SHIP talk*. Retrieved from www.shiptalk.org/default.aspx

Nordhus, I. H., & Pallesen, S. (2003). Psychological treatment of late-life anxiety: An empirical review. *Journal of Consulting and Clinical Psychology*, *71*(4), 643.

Older Americans Act of 1965, Pub. L. No. 109-365, 42 U.S.C. § 3001 et seq., as amended or reauthorized 1967, 1968, 1972, 1973, 1974, 1975, 1977, 1978, 1984, 1987, 1992, 1997, 2000, 2006.

Pasterfield, M., Bailey, D., Hems, D., McMillan, D., Richards, D., & Gilbody, S. (2014). Adapting manualized behavioural activation treatment for older adults with depression. *The Cognitive Behaviour Therapist*, *7*, e5.

Patient Protection and Affordable Care Act and Reconciliation Act of 2010 (ACA), 42 U.S.C. § 18001 *et seq*.

Petersen, R. C. (2011). Mild cognitive impairment. *New England Journal of Medicine*, *364*(23), 2227–2234.

Quijano, L. M., Stanley, M. A., Petersen, N. J., Casado, B. L., Steinberg, E. H., Cully, J. A., & Wilson, N. L. (2007). Healthy IDEAS: A depression intervention delivered by community-based case managers serving older adults. *Journal of Applied Gerontology*, *26*(2), 139–156.

Samad, Z., Brealey, S., & Gilbody, S. (2011). The effectiveness of behavioural therapy for the treatment of depression in older adults: A meta analysis. *International Journal of Geriatric Psychiatry*, *26*(12), 1211–1220.

Shear, M. K., Simon, N., Wall, M., Zisook, S., Neimeyer, R., Duan, N., ... Keshaviah, A. (2011). Complicated grief and related bereavement issues for DSM5. *Depression and Anxiety*, *28*(2), 103–117.

Sheikh, J., & Yesavage, J. (1986). Geriatric Depression Scale (GDS): Recent evidence and development of a shorter version. *Clinical Gerontologist*, *5*(1–2), 165–173.

Silveira, M. J., Wiitala, W., & Piette, J. (2014). Advance directive completion by elderly Americans: A decade of change. *Journal of the American Geriatrics Society*, *62*(4), 706–710.

Smith, T., Gildeh, N., & Holmes, C. (2007). The Montreal Cognitive Assessment: Validity and utility in a memory clinic setting. *Canadian Journal of Psychiatry*, *52*(5), 329.

Stahl, S. T., & Schulz, R. (2014). Changes in routine health behaviors following late-life bereavement: A systematic review. *Journal of Behavioral Medicine*, *37*(4), 736–755.

Steffens, D. C., Snowden, M., Fan, M-Y., Hendrie, H., Katon, W. J., & Unützer, J. (2006). Cognitive impairment and depression outcomes in the IMPACT study. *American Journal of Geriatric Psychiatry*, *14*(5), 401–409.

Stroebe, M., Schut, H., & Stroebe, W. (2007). Health outcomes of bereavement. *The Lancet*, *370*(9603), 1960–1973.

Substance Abuse and Mental Health Services (SAMHSA) SHHS Pub. No. SMA-11-4631, Rockville, MD: Center for Mental Health Services, SAMHSA, U.S. Dept of Health and Human Services.

U.S. Department of Health and Human Services (1999). *Mental health: A report of the Surgeon General*. Washington, DC: U.S. Public Health Service.

U.S. Department of Health and Human Services. (2009). *Progress report on Alzheimer's disease: Translating new knowledge*. Washington, DC: HHS.

U.S. Department of Health and Human Services. (2014). *Tips and resources for caregivers: What resources are available in my area?* Washington, DC: Medicare.

U.S. Department of Health and Human Services: CMS. (2014). Medicare Learning Network: Quick reference information: The ABCs of providing the annual wellness visit. Washington, DC: CMS. Retrieved from www.cms.gov/Outreach-and-Education/Medicare-Learning-Network-MLN/MLNProducts/downloads/AWV_chart_ICN905706.pdf

Utz, R. L., Caserta, M., & Lund, D. (2011). Grief, depressive symptoms, and physical health among recently bereaved spouses. *The Gerontologist*, *52*(4), 460–471.

Van Critters, A. D., & Bartels, S. J. (2004). A systematic review of the effectiveness of community-based mental health outreach services for older adults. *Psychiatric Services*, *55*(11), 1237–1249.

Wacker, R. R., & Roberto, K. A. (2014). *Community resources for older adults: Programs and services in an era of change*. Los Angeles, CA: Sage.

Waite, K. R., Federman, A. D., McCarthy, D. M., Sudore, R., Curtis, L. M., Baker, D. W., ... Paasche-Orlow, M. K. (2013). Literacy and race as risk factors for low rates of advance directives in older adults. *Journal of the American Geriatrics Society*, *61*(3), 403–406.

Wolitzky-Taylor, K. B., Castriotta, N., Lenze, E. J., Stanley, M. A., & Craske, M. G. (2010). Anxiety disorders in older adults: A comprehensive review. *Depression and Anxiety*, *27*(2), 190–211.

Zarit, S., Reever, K., & Bach-Peterson, J. (1980). Relatives of the impaired elderly: Correlated feelings of burden. *The Gerontologist*, *20*, 649–655.

Zivin, K., Wharton, T., & Rostant, O. (2013). The economic, public health, and caregiver burden of late-life depression. *Psychiatric Clinics of North America*, *36*, 631–649.

NINE

CANCER-RELATED CONDITIONS

MARY ANN BURG AND GAIL ADORNO

S.O.A.P. NOTE FROM REFERRING PRIMARY CARE PROVIDER

S: The patient is a 59-year-old woman, 5 years s/p right breast lumpectomy and radiation for DCIS tumor HER2/Neu positive, who recently completed tamoxifen therapy. She complains of episodic lymphedema of the right upper extremity. Comorbid DM2 is poorly controlled (last A1c: 8.3, recent fasting glucose 193) using glyburide and metformin. She reports occasional polyuria. She also complains of fatigue and some mild anxiety related to her previous diagnosis of breast cancer (illness worry). She denies suicidality. She experiences no chest pain, shortness of breath, headache, or dizziness. She denies fever/chills, or nausea/vomiting. She reports sleep disorder (early morning awakening) related to illness worry. She reports a good appetite but 10 pound weight gain in the last 6 months. Bowel functioning is at her baseline.

O: Vital signs are stable. BP 121/76, pulse 68, temperature 98°F, height 5′4″, weight 194 pound

General: Patient is alert, interacting appropriately, in no distress

Heent: PERRLA. Sclerae and conjunctivae clear. TMs clear bilaterally. Nares patent. Oropharynx clear without erythema or exudate. No lymphadenopathy

Neck: Supple, no thyromegaly

Lungs: Clear without rales, rhonchi, or wheezing

Heart: RRR without murmurs, rubs, or gallops

Abdomen: +BS, no HSM, no hernia

Breast: Mild asymmetry with slightly reduced volume on the right secondary to lumpectomy and subsequent radiation. Healed surgical scar on the right without masses or tenderness in either breast. No dimpling, fibrocystic changes, or nipple discharge. No axillary adenopathy

Extremities: DTRs 2+ and equal bilaterally, strength 5/5, no clubbing/cyanosis, 1+ nonpitting edema right distal arm/wrist/hand

Neuro: Depression screen negative. Anxiety reported related to concerns about cancer recurrence

A: Neoplasm of right breast (233.0), DM2 (250.02), obesity (BMI 34.9)

P: 1. Neoplasm of right breast—5 years s/p cancer treatment. Refer to physical therapy for assistance with episodic right lymphedema. Has illness worry and insomnia not uncommon in recovering patients. Refer to behavioral health specialist to address.
2. DM2—Uncontrolled, without complications. The patient prefers not to change her medications. Would like to work on lifestyle changes to improve A1c. Refer to behavioral health specialist to assist with diet and exercise behaviors.
3. Obesity—BMI 33.3. Refer to behavioral health specialist to assist with weight management, exercise, and education.

THE PATIENT'S EXPERIENCE: CANCER SURVIVORSHIP IN THE PRIMARY CARE SETTING

The phrase "cancer survivorship" describes a broad experience on the cancer continuum—living with, through, and beyond a cancer diagnosis (National Coalition for Cancer Survivorship [NCCS], 2014). Consequently, *cancer survivor* encompasses all cancer patients and cancer-related conditions from the moment of diagnosis through treatment, recurrence, and end-of-life care. Cancer survivors encompass persons newly diagnosed who are undergoing active cancer treatments, persons who are post-cancer treatment for any length of time, and persons who are living with advanced cancer but not currently receiving any cancer-directed treatments. Collectively, early detection, improved cancer treatments, and an aging population will contribute to the increasing numbers of cancer survivors in the coming decades. Cancer survivors compose the approximately 14 million people who are post-cancer treatment and the more than 1.6 million people who are newly diagnosed with cancer each year. By 2022 the post treatment cancer survivor population in the United States is projected to be 18 million and by 2030, 2.3 million people are expected to be newly diagnosed with cancer each year (Institute of Medicine, 2013).

Cancer surveillance has always been a primary care task and cancer is often first detected in the primary care setting. Nearly one third of all cancer-related care occurs in the primary care setting (Hewitt, Greenfield & Stovall, 2005); therefore, the burden of cancer care will be increasingly visible in primary care practices. While cancer care has not traditionally been considered something that is dealt with in the realm of primary care, the numbers of cancer survivors using primary care as their primary medical home is increasing (Nekhlyudov & Wenger, 2014).

Older adults constitute the greatest percentage of cancer survivors in the country, with 61% being aged 65 years and older. The number of older cancer survivors will nearly double by the year 2030. While the number of older persons in the population increases, aging is also one of the greatest risk factors for developing a cancer. Thus, more and more older adults will be diagnosed with a first, second, and in some cases even a third primary cancer as they age. Furthermore, it is becoming more common for octogenarians who are relatively fit to receive aggressive cancer-directed therapies for an advanced cancer diagnosis, thus prolonging lives beyond what was possible in the past (Scott et al., 2011; Sequist & Lynch, 2003).

A patient's experience with a cancer diagnosis and subsequent treatment is often complicated by the presence of preexisting conditions that require management and vigilance throughout the treatment of cancer. This is particularly salient for older cancer survivors with preexisting conditions. Aging physiology coupled with comorbidities, whether related to cancer or its treatment, contributes to the complexity of cancer care across the cancer continuum.

Although cancer treatments have improved the survival time for cancer patients, some cancer-directed therapies can cause adverse side effects, also known as late effects, which may appear a few months to years after cancer treatment has been completed. Many cancer survivors have a risk of developing long-term side effects with the type and severity associated with the specific cancer treatments received. Hence, the evaluation for and treatment of late and long-term effects are an important part of survivorship care. Late effects can come from any of the primary types of treatments available for cancer (i.e., surgery, pharmacotherapy, or radiation). Late effects associated with the cancer experience may range from physical concerns to functional and cognitive changes to psychological and emotional problems such as anxiety and depression. For example, cytotoxic systemic chemotherapies such as anthracyclines used in the treatment of some breast cancers can result in serious cardiovascular complications (Broder, Gottlieb, & Leport, 2008). For persons with brain metastases or at high risk for brain metastases, whole brain irradiation is generally initiated; however, long-term effects can involve severe cognitive and neurological problems and diminished quality of life (Shaw & Ball, 2013). Moreover, the constellation of side effects can be challenging and complex in the primary care setting (Wikman, Johar, & Lagergren, 2014). For example, survivors of esophageal cancer or oral, head, and neck cancer often experience problems with swallowing, eating difficulties, reflux and cough, and dry mouth, which collectively impact overall survival and quality of life. Another example is men who have undergone treatment for prostate cancer and often experience temporary or permanent incontinence and impotence, a situation that can severely interfere with quality of life and relationships. Many of these side effects may bring a patient specifically to see the primary care provider and behavioral health specialist (BHS). So, although the cancer itself is not treated in primary care, cancer can—and should—become a focus of primary care and behavioral health management in primary care.

According to the Institute of Medicine (2007) report, *Cancer Care for the Whole Patient: Meeting Psychosocial Health Needs*, cancer survivors require focused and coordinated psychosocial services to meet their specialized needs. Needed services include facilitating self-management and adoption of behavioral strategies to reduce risk for new and recurrent cancers; support for coping psychologically with the ongoing need for medical and personal surveillance for the spread of cancer, its recurrence, and second cancers; psychosocial support in dealing with the adverse medical and psychosocial late effects of cancer and its treatment; and helping survivors meet the challenges of navigating the complex treatment and disease-management information needed to facilitate informed decision making across the survivorship trajectory.

Types of Cancer and Cancer Treatments

Treating cancer is a complex process that often includes one or more therapeutic approaches, and from the patient's point of view, the decision making about treatment is often a time of confusion and charged with emotion. Patients often experience acute anxiety at this stage, particularly during the lag time between detection/biopsy and diagnosis, and may request psychosocial support at this phase of cancer care. The BHS can assist in helping the patient and caregiver(s) sift through the clinical information and deal with concerns about treatment.

The most common forms of cancer treatment include surgery, chemotherapy, radiation therapy, targeted therapy, and stem cell transplant. The choice of cancer treatment is dependent on a variety of factors, most importantly the type of tumor (e.g., blood-borne tumor vs. hard tissue tumor), the staging of the tumor, and whether the cancer has metastasized (spread beyond the primary site). Once a screening test or the patient's report of symptoms indicates that cancer may be present, patients are then given diagnostic tests that aim to make determinations about the specific site of the cancer tumor and to stage the tumor. Typically, these tests will involve one or more of the following: biopsies, imaging tests (chest x-ray-computed tomography [CT], or positron emission tomography [PET] scan), blood tests, and bone marrow aspiration and biopsy (especially for the blood-borne tumors). In some cases, the patient's diagnostic workup may include genetic testing to select specific cancer therapies that target abnormal genes and subsequent carcinogenesis, that is, personalized cancer therapy.

Tumor stage is also important for determining the severity of a patient's cancer diagnosis and the decision of how to treat a cancer. Staging not only helps to identify the extent to which the tumor has grown but is also critical for the prognosis of the patient's survival from the cancer. Staging systems can be specific for certain types of cancer; however, some cancers do not have a staging system. The TNM classification system is a numerical approach to staging that is widely used in cancer facilities for classifying many malignant solid tumors. "T" refers to the size or direct extent of the tumor, "N" refers to the degree of regional spread to the lymph nodes, and "M" refers to the presence of spread to other organs beyond the regional lymph nodes. Staging of some cancers such as leukemias and diffuse lymphomas, cancers of the brain and spinal cord, and ovarian cancer utilize different staging systems. For example, leukemias are classified across three stages, as either low, intermediate, or high risk based on blood cell counts and the accumulation of leukemia cells in other organs such as the liver or spleen. Summary staging is generally used to classify *all* cancers by grouping cancers into one of five categories. Stage 0 refers to cancer in situ, or cancer in a primary site with no spread beyond that site. Stage 1 generally refers to localized disease. Stages 2 and 3 refer to more extensive disease and spread of the cancer to nearby sites. Stage 4 usually indicates a tumor that has spread to distant tissues or organs (National Cancer Institute [NCI]; www.cancer.gov/cancertopics/factsheet/Detection/staging).

- **In situ**: Abnormal cells are present only in the layer of cells in which they developed.
- **Localized**: Cancer is limited to the organ in which it began, without evidence of spread.
- **Regional**: Cancer has spread beyond the primary site to nearby lymph nodes or tissues and organs.
- **Distant**: Cancer has spread from the primary site to distant tissues or organs or to distant lymph nodes.
- **Unknown**: There is not enough information to determine the stage (NCI; www.cancer.gov/cancertopics/factsheet/Detection/staging).

The NCI defines the common components of all tumor staging systems as follows:

- Site of the primary tumor and the cell type (e.g., adenocarcinoma, squamous cell carcinoma)
- Tumor size and/or extent (reach)
- Regional lymph node involvement (the spread of cancer to nearby lymph nodes)
- Number of tumors (the primary tumor and the presence of metastatic tumors, or metastases)
- Tumor grade (how closely the cancer cells and tissue resemble normal cells and tissue)

Potential Physical Side Effects of Cancer

Once the cancer is staged the oncologist and/or surgeon discusses treatment options with the patient. Sometimes the treatment decisions are very specific given the type of cancer diagnosis. Often, however, treatment decisions are more complex and a source of anxiety for the patient and the caregiver(s). There are many variables to consider in choosing cancer treatment options and decisions often must be made quickly, contributing to patients' sense of confusion about treatment choice and overall distress. One of these sources of potential confusion is the side effect profile associated with different treatment approaches. For the most part, all types of systemic cancer treatments, that is, treatment using substances that travel through the bloodstream, reaching and affecting cells all over the body (cancer cells, healthy cells), can have significant side effects. While varying in severity, these side effects may have short-term and long-term impacts on a patient's physical and psychological quality of life. Table 9.1 is a summary of potential physical side effects of cancer that may impact patients during or after cancer treatment.

Survivors of childhood cancers have an especially high risk for late effects of cancer and its treatment as well as higher risks for comorbid chronic conditions. Estimates indicate that more than 60% of childhood cancer survivors

TABLE 9.1 Potential Physical Side Effects of Cancer

Side Effect Types	Specific Problems
Fatigue	Fatigue is the most common complaint of cancer survivors. Cancer-related fatigue results from the cancer, its treatment, and treatment side effects. Survivors often complain that they cannot get over feeling tired, regardless of how much sleep they get.
Cancer Recurrence or Secondary Cancers	All cancer patients live with the possibility that their cancer will recur or spread (metastasize). Some patients also may develop secondary cancers, some of which may be a result of treatments used for their original cancer.
Dental Problems	Chemotherapy may affect tooth enamel and increase the risk of long-term dental problems. High-dose radiation to the head and neck area can change tooth development and cause gum disease. It may also cause tooth decay or loss. Soreness or ulcers in the mouth or throat may result from cancer treatment. These side effects can be painful and make it difficult to eat, talk, and swallow. Xerostomia (dry mouth) is common in head and neck cancer survivors because salivary glands are susceptible to radiation damage. Xerostomia makes it harder to swallow, sleep, and speak, and is associated with loss of appetite due to altered taste.
Diabetes	Steroid drugs used to treat certain cancers may increase blood glucose levels (hyperglycemia) in some patients who do not have diabetes. Although it is unclear if these patients will develop diabetes, they are at higher risk because their glucose levels may remain elevated after treatment stops.
Endocrine Changes	Men and women whose cancer treatments are designed to eliminate the sex hormones that many cancers need to grow may experience the following side effects: ■ Decreased sex drive ■ Memory loss ■ Anemia ■ Decreased muscle mass ■ Depression ■ Weight gain ■ Loss of body hair
Hypothyroidism	Survivors of cancer to the head and neck, and Hodgkin's lymphoma who were treated with radiation therapy often suffer from hypothyroidism, a condition in which there is too little thyroid hormone. Symptoms include weight gain, constipation, dry skin, and sensitivity to cold. Hypothyroidism can be treated with medication.
Incontinence	Removal of the prostate or bladder increases the possibility of incontinence or urine leakage depending on the type of surgery performed. Survivors with continent urinary diversion after the removal of the bladder can gain an element of bladder control through special exercises, but incontinence while sleeping is inevitable.

(continued)

TABLE 9.1 Potential Physical Side Effects of Cancer (*continued*)

Side Effect Types	Specific Problems
Infertility	Either chemotherapy or radiation may cause infertility in both sexes. In women, chemotherapies with alkylating agents such as cyclophosphamide can damage the ovaries, resulting in irregular or absent menstrual periods. Men with colorectal or genitourinary cancers who have had chemotherapy and radiation therapy are at increased risk of infertility. Chemotherapies that affect male fertility include alkylating and methylating agents, vinca alkaloid, antimetabolite, and platinum.
Learning and Memory Problems	Many cancer patients have problems with learning and memory during and immediately after treatment. Researchers have also discovered that the cancer itself may affect verbal learning and memory functions. The good news is that memory loss is one side effect that improves in long-term survivors. Cognitive problems resulting from chemotherapy is called "chemobrain."
Lymphedema	Lymphedema occurs when lymph nodes under the arm are damaged by radiation or surgically removed as part of breast cancer treatment. Lymphatic fluid accumulates in the tissue, causing painful inflammation and limited arm function. It is estimated that 12%–25% of breast cancer patients develop lymphedema, mostly in the first year after treatment. However, lymphedema can occur many years later.
Neuropathy	One of the most difficult treatment side effects is neuropathy, a tingling or burning sensation in the hands and feet due to nerve damage. Neuropathy can be caused by radiation, surgery, and chemotherapies such as taxanes, platinum, vincristine, and thalidomide. Neuropathy is generally thought to be irreversible and can progress.
Organ Damage	Certain types of cancer treatment can age or damage the heart, lungs, liver, or kidneys. This damage may cause long-term health problems. These problems may appear as you age or have other health problems. Some cancer treatments cause heart failure. Certain types of chemotherapy medicine are harmful to the heart. Heart failure symptoms include shortness of breath, feeling weak and tired after regular activity or while at rest, chest discomfort, or feeling the heart beat fast. Certain drugs damage the lungs and airways. These drugs include some antibiotics, chemotherapy medicines or some types of biotherapies. Common symptoms of lung damage include problems breathing, coughing, or pneumonia. It is important that the health care provider is informed if any of these symptoms occur. Some chemotherapy medicines damage the liver. Symptoms of liver damage may include dark urine, pale stools, yellowing of the eyes or skin, swelling or pain in the abdomen (stomach area), flu-like symptoms, or severe fatigue. When taking some chemotherapy drugs, the patient will have regular blood tests to check how the liver is working. Other chemotherapy medicines damage the kidneys. Symptoms of kidney damage include decreased urine flow or bladder irritation and bleeding. A change in urine color or a burning sensation may occur when urinating. The health care provider will check kidney function regularly.

(*continued*)

TABLE 9.1 Potential Physical Side Effects of Cancer (*continued*)

Side Effect Types	Specific Problems
Osteoporosis	Bone loss is a common side effect for survivors of lymphoma, leukemia, breast and prostate cancers. Osteoporosis can be caused by the cancer itself, cortisone-type drugs, treatment-induced menopause, cancer cells in the bone marrow, and treatments that affect testosterone, which is crucial to bone health.
Pain	Pain can be a side effect of treatment or from the cancer itself. While pain management in patients undergoing active cancer treatment has improved significantly in recent years, little is known about long-term pain among disease-free survivors, which can be severe and affect quality of life.
Premature Aging	Cancer patients treated with certain chemotherapies and radiation may experience health conditions normally seen in older people. One of the most common long-term side effects for women is early menopause, which also increases the risk for osteoporosis. The effects of cancer treatment on men include osteoporosis, incontinence, infertility, and erectile dysfunction or impotence.
Sexual Dysfunction	Many men and women treated for cancer experience sexual side effects. Problems getting or keeping erections can occur in men, especially when the cancer begins in the pelvic organs. In women, cancer treatment can lead to sudden menopause or can worsen the vaginal dryness that occurs gradually after natural menopause. If sex becomes painful the health care provider should be notified.

Source: Retrieved May 15, 2014 from www.cancer.net/survivorship/long-term-side-effects-cancer

have at least one chronic condition and over one quarter have a severe chronic condition (Oeffinger et al., 2006). These disorders are associated with the type of cancer, the types and combinations of cancer treatments received (e.g., chemotherapy agents and radiation), and patient-related factors (e.g., gender, age at diagnosis). Childhood cancer survivors, especially those who had bone cancers, central nervous system (CNS) tumors, and Hodgkin's disease, are especially at risk for second cancers, cardiovascular disease, renal dysfunction, severe musculoskeletal problems, cognitive dysfunction, seizure disorders, and fertility problems. Although children who have had cancer are usually treated and followed clinically by pediatric oncology specialists, there is a growing awareness of the need for specialty survivorship care for adult survivors of childhood cancer since many of these chronic problems manifest in adulthood. Yet, since these patients currently are seen in primary care settings, their care requires intensive risk-based surveillance for second cancers and late effects of cancer treatments (physical, developmental, psychosocial), and their care needs to include primary, secondary, and tertiary prevention approaches.

Psychosocial Side Effects of Cancer

Even though cancer treatments have improved the survival rates of most cancers so much so that many cancers are now characterized as a type of chronic illness, the experience of cancer is considered by most people as a distinctively different illness than other chronic diseases (Adorno, 2015). Perhaps more feared than any other disease, cancer is imbued with historical and sociocultural meanings that still equate a cancer diagnosis with death. In the book *The Emperor of All Maladies*, oncologist Siddhartha Mukherjee tells the unique story of how cancer was first described in a 1600 BCE hieroglyphic record and how it continues to be perceived as a disease unlike any other (Mukherjee, 2010). In the last century we discovered that cancer emerges from the disturbance or mutation of one cell, a microscopic accident, which may result from a genetic or an environmental trigger that starts a cascade of cells growing out of control and, if left unchecked, will invade and destroy other organs in the body. In our culture we view cancer as an invader and this view has invoked a "war on cancer." The language of cancer is full of militaristic metaphors that can invoke fear in the patient. For some patients the diagnosis of cancer is heard as the beginning of the dying process. The bellicose language of cancer treatment is often used to inspire cancer patients to respond to the cancer journey as their own vendetta to conquer and destroy the invader, thus contributing to a mythic narrative about the heroic cancer patient. This response can actually serve to help the patient withstand the often painful and debilitating treatments for cancer. However, each cancer patient's journey is unique and should be respected. Imposing expectations on cancer patients about how to be a cancer patient, while well intentioned, may inadvertently diminish the cancer patient's sense of control (Adorno, 2015).

The diagnosis of cancer is such a significant milestone in most patients' lives that many cancer survivors define their life as "before and after diagnosis." The experience of cancer can be a traumatic event and as with any traumatic event, it may trigger intense distress affecting the patient and those close to the patient. Furthermore, the point at which the patient completes cancer treatment and is discharged back to his or her usual source of care in the community can be an especially difficult emotional transition for cancer survivors. Finally, the likelihood of psychological distress is high when patients experience milestones in their post treatment care, routine follow-up surveillance (e.g., imaging studies), and anniversaries of diagnosis and treatment.

Although the epidemiological data show that most cancer survivors will not experience a major depressive disorder (see Chapter 2), post traumatic stress disorder, or other acute psychiatric disorder, many cancer survivors will cycle in and out of a variety of distressed emotions and thoughts. Fear of recurrence is the most frequent type of distress that survivors experience and this may be a persistent feature manifesting as psychosocial morbidity even years after diagnosis and can be especially critical at the time of follow-up appointments, anniversaries of diagnosis, or in response to media triggers (Koch, Jansen, Brenner, & Arndt, 2013).

SCREENING AND ASSESSMENT OF THE CANCER SURVIVOR

It is important to realize that the research indicates that many cancer survivors do not seek out professional psychosocial support (Forsythe et al., 2013). More often, cancer survivors are not offered any psychological support or counseling services since many oncology treatment settings, apart from comprehensive and academic cancer centers, are not staffed to provide these services. Historically the needs of cancer survivors were mostly invisible. Within the medical community and in lay circles, an implicit message existed that simply to survive a diagnosis of cancer was a sufficient goal. As many cancer survivors live well beyond the standard 5-year post treatment milestone for "cure," many cancer survivors with late effects from cancer and or cancer treatments may not readily identify their concerns to health professionals or identify their concerns as having to do with their history of cancer. The broader health community's understanding of the unmet needs of cancer survivors is only recently finding its way into clinical practice. Thus, as a BHS in a primary care setting you may find that your referrals specifically for supportive care of cancer survivors are infrequent. Referrals may be made for a behavioral consult for diabetes management including lifestyle changes, medication adherence, sexual dysfunction, chronic fatigue, depression, or anxiety, and with screening you may discover that the referred patient has had cancer treatment and is not sure if his or her problems are connected to the cancer treatment. The BHS is in the best position to consider the needs of the "whole patient" and therefore may be the first provider encountered by the cancer survivor who engages in comprehensive screening of cancer-related concerns. Psychosocial care delivery to cancer survivors can be vastly improved if it becomes standardized as a routine component of care in the primary care setting. Thorough and comprehensive behavioral health screening of the cancer survivor is imperative for improving the quality of care and clinical outcomes of the cancer survivor in primary care.

First, we review the components of an initial consultation visit with a cancer survivor that has been prompted through routine screening for behavioral health needs or by direct referral from a primary care provider. Depending on how behavioral health services are implemented in your clinical setting, your work with referred patients may be open-ended so that you can complete an initial assessment and then plan one or more follow-up visits with the patient in person and/or by telephone, or you may be limited to one visit for assessment and referral to other providers. The information you obtain in an initial consultation may also vary by how much time you are allowed in your setting for a consultation visit. In some settings consultations may be scheduled as 30-minute visits, in others it may be 50- or 60-minute visits.

An ideal model for newly diagnosed cancer patients engaged in cancer treatment is an oncology–primary care partnership to support transitions in care, attend to preventive care needs and comorbid conditions during cancer treatment, and provide supportive care (i.e., psychosocial, informational) (Sussman & Baldwin, 2012). However, its implementation in clinical practice is rare despite improvements in quality of cancer care that such a model would provide across the cancer continuum. More likely, the BHS may encounter the newly diagnosed cancer patient in the primary care setting on an acute, episodic basis. Nevertheless, the patient's link to the primary care provider and BHS during this early stage on the cancer continuum can lay a valuable foundation for post-treatment survivorship care.

Assisting in cancer recovery also ideally involves ongoing screening of the psychosocial needs of the patient across the years of survivorship since cancer patients may experience emergent and/or persistent side effects even years after cancer treatment. Cancer patients who have access to psychosocial care have better quality of life, show better medical adherence, and report better satisfaction with their care (Epstein & Street, 2007; Forsythe et al., 2012). The types of psychosocial care that cancer patients need depends on their stage in the cancer care continuum, their personal experiences with cancer, the type and stage of their cancer diagnosis and treatment modalities received, and modifiable (lifestyle behaviors) and non modifiable (age, gender, relationship status, race/ethnicity, education, and income) personal characteristics.

First Steps in Assessment: Biopsychosocial Assessment

The first focus of assessment of the cancer survivor in primary care is the problem for which the referral was made. For example, if the primary care provider made the referral for diabetes and weight management and lifestyle changes, then the BHS will focus the initial parts of the assessment on identifying the patient's knowledge of, beliefs about, and personal barriers to optimal diabetes and weight management and their relationship to lifestyle factors and the patient's goals and level of confidence and motivation in achieving better management. If the patient acknowledges, for example, that he or she is more concerned about cancer returning than about diabetes, the BHS can then embark on helping the patient identify how the cancer anxiety and diabetes management may be interconnected, and how working on both problems will enable the patient to regain a sense of personal control and quality of life. Importantly, this initial assessment will also focus on assessing the patient's understanding of the association among diabetes, obesity, and cancer recurrence. The link between the primary referral for diabetes management and cancer is complex and important to untangle in working with your patient. Obesity, energy intake, and increased activity are modifiable risk factors with respect to diabetes management but are also tied to cancer recurrence and survival among cancer survivors (Demark-Wahnefried et al., 2012). As a result of the collective impact of T2DM, obesity, and cancer, the American Diabetes Association and the American Cancer Society have published a consensus report providing guidelines for clinical care (Giovannucci et al., 2010). As in this chapter's case example, the BHS is compelled to address the presenting referral for diabetes and weight management, but must understand the implications of such within the context of the patient's history of cancer.

Behavioral health needs will vary depending on whether the patient is newly diagnosed, in treatment, treatment-complete and cancer free, in recurrence and in the chronic cancer phase, or at the end-of-life. Consequently, one of the first tasks in assessment is to determine where the patient is in the cancer continuum or stage of survivorship. In transitioning from cancer treatment, recovery from the side effects of cancer treatment becomes a focus for the cancer survivor and the focus of behavioral health interventions in primary care. Based on what is known about the experience of having had cancer and the late effects and psychosocial needs of all cancer survivors, identifying where the cancer survivor is in relation to the survivorship trajectory can help establish a baseline from which to begin a person-centered assessment. For example, cancer survivors who are within their first year post treatment may have very different concerns and needs than another survivor who is 10 years from the last treatment and is now experiencing a recurrence. Childhood cancer survivors who reach late adolescence and young adulthood represent another unique facet of survivorship with respect to growth and development problems resulting from treatment and the late physical and emotional effects of cancer that can continue into adulthood. In particular, issues of identity, independence (e.g., financial, emotional, self-management), fertility/sexuality, and negotiating relationships may surface anew as childhood cancer survivors reach specific developmental milestones. Adolescents and young adults (AYAs) diagnosed with cancer represent another population of cancer survivors who face unique stressors from coping with their developmental stage and concurrently dealing with a life-limiting illness. Research suggests that 44% of AYAs experience at least moderate levels of post traumatic stress symptoms (PTSS) 1 year following their cancer diagnosis with 3% suffering from severe PTSS (Kwak et al., 2013).

Aging cancer survivors are another subset of survivors reaching primary care who may live with late effects of cancer and cancer-related treatments but also new morbidities associated with senescence. For older cancer survivors, comorbidities (e.g., hypertension, arthritis, sensory deficits, osteoporosis) may be present before a cancer diagnosis, exacerbated during and following cancer treatment, or be a consequence of that treatment (Economou, Hurria, & Grant, 2012). The intersection of aging and late and long-term effects of having had cancer is not well understood at this time, though we do know that cancer and its treatment may increase the older cancer patient's functional and cognitive limitations (e.g., mobility, activities of daily living). Thus, the BHS must understand that the increased risk for depression and anxiety with respect to loss of independence and increased dependency, limited social support, and even perhaps cognitive decline among older adults may be intertwined with the older adult's experience of having had cancer.

The second task of assessment with respect to the cancer survivor's psychosocial and behavioral health is determining severity of risk. This task can be conceptualized through three pathways that delineate risk severity according to the following criteria: (a) patients with physical side effects, (b) patients with psychiatric and/or psychological side effects, and (c) patients with subdromal syndromes and existential concerns (Holland & Reznik, 2005). The first group refers to those cancer survivors who may be at high risk for psychosocial distress with respect to treatment-related concerns such as cognitive and neuropsychological problems, sexuality and infertility, functional disability or amputation, body/facial image due to surgical procedures or lymphedema, and chronic fatigue. The second group of survivors may be physically healthy but suffer psychological problems with respect to post traumatic stress disorder, anxiety and other mood disorders, and persistent or exacerbated psychiatric disorders. The third group of survivors may be healthy as well without overt psychological or psychiatric effects, yet their quality of life is compromised. These survivors may experience a crisis of meaning, purpose, and direction in life as a result of having had cancer. Their level of distress may not reach that of a psychiatric condition but nevertheless symptoms of depression or anxiety dampen fully productive engagement with relationships, employment, and overall well-being following their cancer experience. This third group may find their way to the BHS though there are nonspecific complaints or other tangential concerns.

Assisting cancer patients in recovery requires a wide breadth of knowledge of the potential side effects of cancer treatment and the research on evidence-based interventions (Alfano & Rowland, 2006). Physical side effects (e.g., pain, functional disability, speech or swallowing problems, incontinence, fatigue), body image problems (e.g., due to surgical excisions such as mastectomy or head and neck cancers, swelling due to lymphedema), sexuality problems (e.g., impotence due to prostate treatment, vaginal dryness, and/or pelvic pain secondary to gynecological cancers), and chemotherapy-induced cognitive problems (e.g., "chemobrain") are important items for inclusion in behavioral health screening. Social and emotional side effects of cancer should also be included in the behavioral health screening (Table 9.2).

TABLE 9.2 Potential Social and Emotional Side Effects of Cancer

Side Effect Types	Specific Problems
Fear of Recurrence	Many survivors live in fear that their cancer will come back at some point. For some, a milestone event like the anniversary of their diagnosis or the end of care by their cancer doctor can trigger these feelings and worries. Fear can be positive if it motivates the patient to discuss health changes with their health care provider, or it can cause unnecessary worry. It is important to distinguish between normal changes and more serious symptoms.
Grief	Grief is a natural result of loss. With cancer, such losses may include health, sex drive, fertility, and physical independence. To get past the grief, it is important for the patient to experience all these feelings. Support groups and counseling can help the patient work through these issues.
Depression	It is estimated that 70% of cancer survivors experience depression at some time. Depression can be hard to diagnose in cancer survivors because the symptoms are so similar to the side effects of cancer treatment, including weight loss, fatigue, insomnia, and inability to concentrate. A 10-year follow-up study has found that symptoms of depression were associated with a shorter survival time, so it is crucial to seek treatment for depression.
Body Image and Self-Esteem	Cancer survivors who have experienced amputations, disfigurement, and loss of organs like the colon or bladder often grapple with how they relate to themselves and other people. A negative body image and low self-esteem can affect a survivor's ability for intimacy with a partner, which has a major impact on quality of life. Good communication is essential to retaining or regaining intimacy after cancer. Patients should seek medical advice if problems continue.

(continued)

TABLE 9.2 Potential Social and Emotional Side Effects of Cancer (*continued*)

Side Effect Types	Specific Problems
Spirituality	Many survivors find that life takes on new meaning after cancer, and will renew their commitment to spiritual practices or organized religion. Research suggests that spirituality improves quality of life through a strong social support network, adaptive coping, lessened depression, and better physiological function.
Survivor Guilt	Some people feel guilty for surviving cancer when others do not. The patient may wonder "Why me?" or begin to reevaluate life goals and ambitions. If the patient suffers from a prolonged sense of guilt, a psychotherapist, clergy member, or support group may help.
Relationships	How other people react to cancer patients' illness is perhaps the biggest challenge faced by cancer survivors. Friends, coworkers, and family members may feel awkward about discussing the cancer diagnosis. They may remain silent, avoid the survivor, or pretend nothing has happened. Others may use humor in an effort to take the survivor's mind off the situation, instead of being someone with whom issues can be discussed. Because cancer can be a long-term illness, overcoming communication barriers early is crucial.
Life and the Workplace	Re-entering social and professional life can be accompanied by many fears: worry about being out in the world with an increased risk of infection; not having enough energy to get through a workday; and anxiety about not being able to think clearly because of "chemobrain" or memory loss. After struggling with life-and-death questions, many cancer survivors feel apart from peers who have not had the same experience and may turn to other survivors for support and friendship.

Source: Retrieved May 15, 2014 from www.mdanderson.org/patient-and-cancer-information/cancer-information/cancer-topics/survivorship/ side-effects-of-cancer-treatment/social-impact.html

Screening and Assessment for Depression and Anxiety

Depending on the screening process established in your primary care clinic (e.g., universal, targeted), cancer survivors may be referred to you based on their initial brief screening for depression such as the Patient Health Questionnaire-2 (PHQ-2) (Arroll et al., 2010). Further specific screening of the nature of the cancer-related distress should be undertaken by the BHS. The American Society of Clinical Oncology (ASCO) has developed a thorough set of guidelines for screening, assessment, and care of anxiety and depressive symptoms in cancer survivors across the continuum of cancer care with the target audience including providers in primary care settings (Anderson et al., 2014). First, ASCO recommends that all cancer survivors be screened for depressive symptoms at transition from cancer-specific treatment to primary care and when other changes in disease or treatment status occur including recurrence or progression of cancer, at checkups, or when other stressors occur (Table 9.3). Second, the ASCO guidelines recommend using valid and reliable screening measures and to observe validated scoring criteria for recommending further professional treatment (pharmacological intervention, counseling).

TABLE 9.3 Vulnerable Times for Cancer Survivors
Cancer survivors may be especially vulnerable for distress at certain times across the cancer care continuum: ■ Diagnostic workup ■ Diagnosis ■ Communicating diagnosis to family/friends/coworkers/employer ■ Initiation of cancer treatment ■ Completion of cancer treatment ■ Cancer follow-up appointments ■ Anniversaries of cancer diagnosis ■ Recurrence (personal) ■ Recurrence (friends/acquaintances) ■ Transfer of care from oncologist to primary care

The ASCO guidelines recommend assessment of depression with the PHQ-9 measure and the assessment of anxiety with the Generalized Anxiety Disorder 7-item (GAD-7) scale (see"Assessment Measures Specifically Designed for Cancer Survivors" that follows) and a problem checklist to explore social, occupational, and other sources of stress. Assessment should include signs and symptoms of depression and anxiety, cancer-related symptoms, stressors, risk factors, use of prescribed and non-prescribed substances (including alcohol and other drugs) that may affect mood, and target "times of vulnerability." Finally, screening and assessment outcomes should be shared with the clinical team and appropriate referrals made.

Assessment for Quality of Life in Cancer Survivors

In addition to depression or anxiety, cancer survivors may have individualized experiences with cancer-related side effects that impact their quality of life. In 1996 Betty Ferrell and her colleagues published a "Quality of Life Conceptual Model Applied to Cancer Survivors" (Ferrell et al., 1996). This model still stands as a comprehensive summary of the components of quality of life for cancer survivors and is useful for conceptualizing a comprehensive assessment of the cancer survivor in the primary care setting. The model posits that quality of life is dependent on four components: physical well-being, psychological well-being, social well-being, and spiritual well-being. We have added some specific factors to the original model including a sense of personal control under psychological well-being and satisfaction with sexual functioning under physical well-being since recent research indicates that these are important components of quality of life for cancer survivors (Burg et al., 2014).

Assessment Measures Specifically Designed for Cancer Survivors

There are many measures designed specifically for use with cancer patients and survivors. The Functional Assessment of Chronic Illness Therapy (FACIT) measurement system is a compilation of health-related quality-of-life questionnaires for use in clinical trials, patient outcomes studies, and individual patient care management (Cella et al., 1993). The FACIT system includes a core measure, the Functional Assessment of Cancer Therapy-General (FACT-G), which provides a comprehensive evaluation of cancer patients including their physical well-being, social/family well-being, emotional well-being, and functional well-being, appropriate for use with patients with any form of cancer. The FACIT system includes measures for use with patients with specific types of cancer including breast, bladder, brain, colorectal, cervical, esophageal, endometrial, head and neck, lung, leukemia, liver, lymphoma, melanoma, nasal-pharyngeal, multiple myeloma, ovarian, prostate, and vulvar cancer (FACIT, 2014). There are also symptom-specific measures for cancer-related problems such as fatigue and lymphedema. The FACIT organization has over 50 scales that are free to the public and are translated into many languages and used around the world.

The Cancer Survivors' Unmet Needs (CaSUN) is an instrument designed specifically for cancer survivors that can be used for screening and assessment purposes and focuses on "unmet needs" of cancer survivors including (a) information needs and medical care issues, (b) quality of life, (c) emotional and relationship issues, (d) life perspective, (e) positive changes, and (f) an open-ended question permitting identification of additional needs (Hodgkinson et al., 2007a).

Many other cancer survivor measures exist, ranging in focus (somatic and psychological symptoms, unmet needs, distress, quality of life, concerns, body image, health and functioning, social/family well-being, stressors, relationship with providers, behavioral symptoms, spirituality well-being and positive benefits of cancer). Some of the most commonly used are reviewed in an article by Chopra and Kamal (2012). Determining which of the available screening and assessment measures are appropriate for use in the primary care setting may depend on the focus, cost, length, type of administration (self-administered vs. clinical interview), and cultural appropriateness and sensitivity.

In recent years researchers have utilized the concept of the "Distress Continuum" and the measure of "distress" as a marker for the need for psychological support in cancer patients. The term "distress" was suggested as a label for psychosocial and psychological/psychiatric concerns by the National Comprehensive Cancer Network working group, which developed initial clinical practice guidelines for psychosocial care of cancer patients. This global term serves to normalize the experience of psychosocial distress during the cancer period in efforts to reduce stigma relative to psychosocial and psychiatric concerns associated with the cancer experience and to develop a common language for use among cancer teams. "Distress" is a fairly common experience that varies in intensity for patients throughout the cancer continuum. A common method of measuring distress is a visual analog scale, the "Distress Thermometer" (Hoffman, Zevon, D'Arrigo, & Cecchini, 2004). The Distress Thermometer has been used primarily with cancer patients during their treatment but it is also a useful measure to screen for distress in cancer survivors and any patient in the outpatient setting. Research utilizing the Distress Thermometer finds that persons at highest risk for post-treatment cancer-related distress are women, those with comorbid conditions and functional limitations, and those with significant concerns with basic needs and family dysfunction (Jacobsen et al., 2005). Rates of psychological distress are also found higher for persons with terminal cancers and those with cancers of highest risk of mortality including pancreatic cancer and lung cancer (Brintzenhofe-Szoc, Levin, Li, Kissane, & Zabora, 2009). The Distress Thermometer is a simple, brief, culturally sensitive, and free initial screening instrument that has been shown to be as good as other well-studied instruments, for example, the Hospital Anxiety and Depression Scale (HADS; Zigmond & Snaith, 1983) and the Brief Symptom Inventory (BSI-18; Derogatis & Savitz, 2000) in discriminating between patients with or without clinically significant distress (Rohan, 2012). When combined with a cancer-relevant problem checklist, the Distress Thermometer can be a quickly administered, patient-friendly method of screening, which can be followed by more specific and precise diagnostic assessment tools if indicated. The National Comprehensive Cancer Network's Distress Thermometer and problem checklist are an excellent example of an easy to utilize screen for use in the primary care setting.

Behavioral Factors in Disease Management and Adherence

Newly diagnosed and pre treatment cancer patients are typically engaged—and often overwhelmed—with absorbing new clinical information about their cancer diagnosis, submitting to diagnostic tests, working on treatment decisions with their oncologist, and making preparations for treatment. In this period they may be advised by their oncologist to visit their primary care provider if they have chronic conditions such as diabetes, heart disease, or pulmonary conditions, all of which need close management throughout the process of cancer treatment, particularly since some chronic disease medications can be contraindicated when cancer therapies are being administered and since some cancer therapies can be toxic to the organs affected by chronic diseases.

In collaboration with the primary care provider, the BHS can help support the newly diagnosed cancer patient by helping them work through the information and options being presented to them by oncology providers. Due to the acute, stressful nature of this initial period on the cancer continuum, the BHS can help the cancer patient to identify and mobilize existing strengths and resources for the weeks and months ahead during cancer treatment. For some cancer patients this may also be a time to initiate cognitive behavioral stress management strategies, which are useful through the ups and downs of the cancer treatment period.

New, treatment-complete survivors can be surprisingly vulnerable. Depending on the type of cancer therapies they had they may experience some disabling side effects from the treatment and these problems can interfere with their ability to manage other premorbid chronic conditions. Because newly treatment-complete survivors often experience a kind of "dropping off" of both medical and social support, leaving them feeling scared and isolated, they are likely to be referred to the BHS for problems with anxiety or depressed mood, or with difficulty managing non-cancer-related chronic disease.

The experience of cancer survivors at this stage presents a unique window of opportunity for engagement in beneficial and life-affirming behavioral interventions (Demark-Wahnefried, Aziz, Rowland, & Pinto, 2005). If the patient has been referred for chronic disease management, the BHS will make that a focus of interventions. It is important to realize that the patient's recent experience with transitioning from active cancer treatment to cancer survivor can be used in discussion as a critical time for the patient to reinvest in healthy behaviors and chronic disease management. The cancer survivor's willingness to engage in self-management with respect to health and well-being is integral for coping and adapting to having had cancer and cancer treatment. Depending on their physical and emotional condition, patients at this stage may be especially motivated (sometimes for the first time in their lives) to be interested in improved nutrition and exercise spurred by the hope that their healthy behaviors might help reduce the risk for recurrence or the development of new cancers.

Cancer patients completing primary treatment may struggle to manage their self-care and confidence may be low in this regard especially if support is limited (Foster & Fenlon, 2011). Physical and psychological recovery from having had cancer involves adjusting to a changed sense of self while simultaneously reentering daily life. In addition to developing a plan of action for chronic disease control, by helping patients explore their level of motivation and self-efficacy for achieving healthy livings the BHS can assist patients in regaining a sense of control over their lives and perhaps move them into a positive "new normal" where their overall health becomes a priority and a source of hope for the future. Cancer survivors can be encouraged to regain a sense of control by engaging in actions that lower their risk of recurrence including smoking cessation, increased physical activity, and better nutrition to reduce obesity (Morey et al., 2009; Siegel et al., 2012). The American Cancer Society has published guidelines for nutrition and physical activity for cancer survivors and the research evidence on how these activities can reduce recurrence in specific types of cancer (Kushi et al., 2006).

Cancer survivors may also welcome information and resources to supplement their personal treatment plan. For example, web-based interventions for patient empowerment and physical activity have demonstrated utility in helping cancer survivors manage chronic illness (Kuijpers, Groen, Aaronson, & van Harten, 2013).

Long-term survivors without recurrence may have few specific needs related to having had cancer and its treatment, but many still experience negative effects of their cancer experience and may continue to suffer from a sense of lost control over their lives, even years after being treatment-complete and cancer free (Burg et al., 2014). A small but substantial number of long-term survivors do suffer from various effects of cancer and its treatment such as reduced psychological well-being, neuropsychological deficits, and cancer-related fatigue. The research indicates that the number of needs expressed by the cancer survivor is associated with the level of anxiety (Hodgkinson et al., 2007b). Similar to cancer survivors who have recently completed treatment, long-term survivors can be responsive to encouragement in engaging in health behaviors that are associated with reducing the risk of cancer recurrence or the development of new cancers.

They may also need assistance with long-term and late effects of cancer and its treatment. For example, cancer survivors treated with anthracyclines (e.g., breast cancer) or mediastinal radiation (e.g., Hodgkin's disease) are particularly at risk for cardiovascular abnormalities and cardiac morbidity associated with these cancer treatments (Ho et al., 2010; Tukenova et al., 2010). Sexuality, sexual function, and body image are sometimes a significant problem for long-term survivors, especially survivors of testicular or prostate cancer or survivors of gynecological cancers (Greenwald & McCorkle, 2008; Rossen, Pedersen, Zachariae, & von der Maase, 2012). Women under age 40 diagnosed with invasive cervical cancer, breast cancer, Hodgkin's disease, or non-Hodgkin's lymphoma report distress even 10 years post-treatment with respect to unresolved grief with cancer-related infertility (Canada & Schover, 2012).

Chronic cancer survivors: Cancer survivorship as a broad descriptor align this line at the left encompasses persons with incurable cancer; yet, chronic cancer is not well-defined, nor does it fit precisely into chronic illness models (Harely, Pini, Bartlett, & Velikova, 2012). A description of chronic cancer includes the following: (a) a diagnosis of active advanced or metastatic cancer is made; (b) cancer-directed treatments are available to control symptoms, slow progression, or prolong life; (c) the patient is not considered to be at the end-of-life; and (d) chronic cancer ends when cancer-directed therapies are no longer effective or no further treatment options exist, and the patient's prognosis is only a few months (Harely et al., 2012). Chronic cancer patients may be receiving episodic cancer treatment including systemic and targeted therapies interspersed with periods of no treatment. Between treatments, they may report fewer symptoms and feel relatively well; thus, a challenge during this phase is maintaining quality of life during periods of cyclical side effects and symptoms. Over time these therapies can create multiple toxicities and become debilitating for the chronic cancer survivor.

When the patient's cancer has recurred or the initial diagnosis involves advanced disease, survivors have a different set of experiences with which to cope. The experience of chronic cancer is frequently marked by uncertainty and the anxiety that accompanies an unknown future. Chronic cancer patients may report psychological distress associated with burdening others (Harley et al., 2012). They may be more prone to existential distress, hopelessness, and a sense of isolation from others (Boerger-Knowles & Ridley, 2014). They also have practical needs such as work-related concerns, financial planning, and applying for disability benefits. Chronic cancer survivors are generally involved with multiple treatment decisions and lengthy medical appointments and may have varying involvement with a primary care provider. The behavioral health referral may likely to be focused on assisting the patient with the emotional aspects of the cancer; however, self-management continues to be an important component of care. The focus of care in the behavioral health visit will be to work with the chronic cancer patient on ways to improve quality of life and learn a "new normal" during good days or periods of time when the patient feels well. Some chronic cancer patients report reluctance to disclose symptoms or side effects for fear that their oncologist will stop treatment or the belief that side effects must be endured as a cost of continuing to fight the disease. Working with the chronic cancer survivor at this stage may involve strategies to manage sleep disturbance, poor appetite, fatigue, and emotional difficulty (Harley et al., 2012).

Patients at the end-of-life from recurrent or newly diagnosed advanced, metastatic cancer require different types of support from the BHS. Frequently, advanced, metastatic cancer patients with refractory disease are abruptly discharged from cancer care in the oncology setting, which can result in feelings of abandonment depending on how that transition is managed. A relationship with primary care providers can bridge that transition through supportive care services such as palliative care and emotional support. Depending on the role and structure of behavioral health services in the primary care setting, the BHS may focus on helping the patient and caregiver with advanced planning (e.g., advance directives, caregiving needs), and anticipatory guidance with respect to planning further care whether through hospice services or other palliative model of care. Managing pain and symptoms and focusing on remaining quality of life are important goals of care during this phase of the cancer trajectory.

Basic Needs and Social Service Referrals

While a patient is in active cancer treatment, the patient hopefully has access to an oncology social worker or a patient navigator at the treatment site to assist with supportive services and health insurance coverage for the cancer treatment. However, when the patient transitions out of treatment the patient typically loses access to this source of support.

Basic needs of cancer survivors are varied and often depend on the patient's stage of survivorship. They often include the following:

- Health insurance coverage
- Medication costs
- Legal assistance
- Transportation to treatment
- Financial assistance for housing costs, food, utilities
- Child care
- Employment-related concerns

Costs of Care

A large proportion of cancer patients have difficulty paying for their cancer care, especially for the high costs of certain oral chemotherapies and medications. For many patients the direct and indirect costs of cancer treatment result in lost wages, financial devastation, bankruptcy, and inability to pay for health insurance (Banegas & Yobroff, 2013; Kaiser Family Foundation, 2006). A study conducted by the Cancer Support Community (2013) found that cancer patients have many unexpected expenses, such as out-of-pocket costs, unexpected deductibles, office visits and prescription co-pays, childcare costs, parking fees, and home health costs (www.cancersupportcommunity.org/MainMenu/ResearchTraining/Research-Projects-2/Copy-of-Access-Study.html). Over a third of the patients in this study reported that no one (including physicians, nurses, and social workers) discussed costs of cancer care with them.

Even when survivors complete active cancer treatment they continue to have larger health care costs than most people without cancer histories. In addition to continuing primary care and chronic care costs, many survivors must continue on a course of adjuvant cancer treatments for a number of years. For example, some women treated for breast cancer (estrogen- or progesterone-positive tumor) receive tamoxifen, an oral hormone therapy medication for 5 years or more. Men with prostate cancer recurrence will often be treated with a hormone therapy called androgen deprivation therapy (ADT), an injection which slows the progression of recurrent prostate cancer. Uninsured or underinsured patients can find it impossible to pay for the care they need. One study of breast cancer patients reported that uninsured women were significantly less likely to have surgery for breast cancer or breast reconstruction after breast cancer surgery than those who were insured (Coburn et al., 2008). To complicate this problem, uninsured patients are more likely to present with later-stage cancers than insured patients—so their rates of survival are compromised at the outset.

Additionally, the time required for treatment and recovery may result in reduced work and wage loss for patients and caregivers and thereby delayed care. These direct and indirect costs of cancer can have significant and long-term financial, social, and emotional impacts on patients and their families.

Legal Issues

The fallout from costly cancer care often leaves cancer survivors with the need for legal assistance to help recover from bankruptcy and other financial liabilities as well as employment disputes. The National Cancer Legal Services Network (NCLSN) assists cancer survivors and their families with insurance disputes, public benefits, housing, employment issues, future care and custody planning, immigration, and advance directives (NCLSN, 2014). Survivors can also be directed to inquire into the services of local legal aid associations. The National Coalition for Cancer Survivorship (NCCS, 2014) is another useful resource for information on the legal rights of cancer patients.

There are many cancer-specific sources for patient support and assistance for basic needs. The Leukemia and Lymphoma Society helps persons with blood cancers across the cancer continuum. The Society has chapter organizations located throughout the United States. Another organization, Cancer Care, Inc., based in New York provides support throughout the United States with education, financial support, online and telephone support groups, and counseling. The Cancer Financial Assistance Coalition (CFAC) is a 14-member organization consisting of various cancer support organizations in the United States and functions as a clearinghouse for individual financial requests as well as a database of organizations known to assist cancer patients with financial needs.

Brief Counseling Methods

After the initial consultation, assessment, and identification of the patient's behavioral health targets, the BHS might engage the patient in a discussion of how his or her particular situation may be helped through a process of merging the goals of chronic health management with the patient's goals to reduce cancer-related anxiety. This discussion can be organized in the following way:

- *Normalize* the patient's experience by discussing how research shows that many cancer survivors have more difficulty with diabetes management.
- *Encourage* the patient to consider that change is attainable and how working on both problems will result in better overall health and quality of life.
- *Review personal strengths* the patient utilized throughout the cancer treatment journey. Inquire what personal strengths were helpful through that difficult process and how they might be utilized at this stage in the patient's life to work toward goals of reducing anxiety and improving diabetes management.
- *Develop a plan of action* for helping the patient organize his or her life to make positive change. The patient should be asked for ideas of what he or she might be willing to do and how he or she might overcome barriers to engaging in and succeeding in goal setting. Remember that cancer survivors often express a general feeling of lack of personal control in their lives; this theme is one you can identify with the patient as a target for the treatment plan and discuss how becoming behaviorally active and working toward realistic goals may result in a renewed sense of personal control.
- *Review and summarize* what has been discussed in options put forth for creating change. Ask the patient to suggest any other options he or she might have for regaining a sense of empowerment and control. Attempt to gain agreement for an action plan that incorporates the patient's goals and strengths.

Behavioral activation has been shown to be a key step in patients moving toward improvement in both mood and control over chronic disease. Help the patient identify any processes that might inhibit activation and trigger the loss of self-control such as escape and avoidance behaviors, ruminative thinking, and cognitive distortions. Review the common types of cognitive distortions and teach the patient to challenge these thoughts and to choose to think and react differently. Develop a plan for how the patient can avoid triggers to cognitive distortions.

In helping the patient develop a plan, have planning tools available that you can help the patient complete. Specify the activities that the patient has agreed to engage in that promote health and build physiological reserve such as exercise, proper nutrition, social activation, and sleep. Explain other potential additional approaches to successful goal achievement including complementary and alternative therapies, such as relaxation therapy, meditation, and movement therapies. Provide the patient with a tool for monitoring mood and blood sugar to help the patient identify the intersection of the two over a period of time. Plan to review these regularly at follow-up visits.

Finally, if your setting allows for the scheduling of follow-up behavioral consultations, make a recommendation for a series of follow-up visits. These visits would focus on reviewing the patients' progress in working on their personal action plans and reviewing their changes in mood. Some cancer survivors, especially those with high recurrence anxiety or those with significant problems in certain areas of functioning, may need a course of focused cognitive behavioral therapy or possibly referral to other specialists.

Integrated Team Feedback and Response

Communicate with health care providers in your primary care setting about the patient's experience with cancer survival, and confirm the providers' knowledge of the patient's personal action plan in order to include the provider team in helping the patient with adherence to goals. Evidence suggests that active and sustained coordinated follow-up that is reliable, occurs at regular intervals, and is initiated by the provider team in the primary care setting leads to better outcomes (Sharpe et al., 2014).

You may want to advocate for provider training in your setting on the potential needs of cancer survivors including psychosocial support needs, so that those survivors who are less inclined to discuss their needs are routinely screened for undetected psychosocial distress and provided the opportunity for referral to behavioral health follow-up.

BEHAVIORAL HEALTH ASSESSMENT AND TREATMENT SUMMARY TO REFERRING PRIMARY CARE PROVIDER

Date:
From: Behavioral Health Specialist
To: Dr. Jones
Regarding: Behavioral Health Consultation With Ruby Smith

Presenting Problem

Mrs. Ruby Smith is a 59-year-old married woman who was referred for help with illness worry, insomnia, and diabetes management (diet, weight management, exercise). She is a small statured, obese, well-groomed woman who presents with a pleasant and humorous affect. She acknowledges that her diabetes management has not been optimal. She says that she has a hard time motivating herself to do a better job with nutrition and physical exercise because of her recent feelings of anxiety about the possibility of recurrence of her breast cancer. The onset of this heightened anxiety was her 5-year anniversary of being cancer-free and the termination of her tamoxifen therapy. She had expected to feel relief, but instead she has had increasing anxiety, sleep disturbance, and little to no motivation to work on self-care. She describes feelings of isolation because her family and friends expect her to act like she is now back to "normal" and don't understand her concern about recurrence or her fear that her two daughters might get breast cancer. She also describes frustration with trying to manage her lymphedema in her right arm (secondary to lumpectomy and removal of lymph nodes) and says it interferes with her ability to work out in the ways she used to for weight control.

Background and Current Functioning

Ms. Smith was diagnosed with Type 2 diabetes in 2006 and had good control of her blood sugar with combined physical therapy, increased physical activity with gym classes, and regular walking for 3 years. In 2009 she was diagnosed with Stage 2 breast cancer and underwent a lumpectomy and 11-week course of chemotherapy followed by 6 weeks of external radiation and 5 years of tamoxifen therapy. Although there has been no cancer recurrence, she developed lymphedema in her right arm and has a fitted sleeve for compression and undergoes lymphatic massage for swelling control with some success. She was post menopausal when she started tamoxifen therapy and says that she did not experience any significant hot flashes or other hormonal side effects with tamoxifen. She does not complain of any other cancer-related side effects. She describes herself as very healthy, apart from her weight gain following her cancer diagnosis, and other than the history of cancer and current diabetes, has no other chronic conditions. Her sleep disturbance began after her 5-year follow-up visit with her oncologist, and she describes it as waking up and not being able to get back to sleep because of her anxious thoughts.

Psychiatric/Medical/Substance Abuse/Interpersonal Violence History

She has no history of diagnosed mental illness; she has never had psychological treatment. She denies any prior history of depression or anxiety other than a period of sadness after the death of her mother from breast cancer in 2000. She drinks a glass of red wine each evening prior to dinner and denies any use of prescribed or recreational drugs. She denies any history of Intimate Partner Violence.

Social History

Ms. Smith has lived in her current residence for 30 years. She completed an AA degree in 1990 and has worked as an independent copy editor for 20 years. She describes her marriage of 30 years as very happy. Her husband, Mike, is a recently retired electrician. She has two daughters (26 and 32 years old) who both live locally. Both are married and have children. She has extended family in the area and two very close female friends whom she sees at least once per week. She is an active member of her church.

She has health insurance through her husband's union. There are no current financial or legal problems.

Overall Assessment

Ms. Smith is a gregarious and insightful woman. Her current mood problems and sleep disturbance appear to be related to her fear of recurrence and fear of her daughters' risk for breast cancer. Her understanding of the association among Type 2 diabetes mellitus (T2DM), obesity, and cancer recurrence is limited and she was quite surprised to learn about the evidence for such an association.

Ms. Smith has many positive behaviors that should be particularly helpful in her treatment plan. She said she took on her cancer treatment as a personal challenge and worked hard to maintain physical activity and good nutrition during the first 2 years after her surgery and chemotherapy. She continued to work throughout her cancer treatment and derives personal satisfaction from her work. She has been married for 30 years and feels her husband will do anything he can to support her. She has a close relationship with her two daughters, has good friends who she can rely on, and derives comfort from her religious beliefs and church activities. She appears to be highly motivated to work on ways to reduce her anxiety and improve her motivation for her diabetes control and weight management with an overall goal to reduce her risk of cancer recurrence. She says she would prefer to work on self-management strategies for anxiety reduction before trying pharmacological approaches.

Treatment Plan

I explained to Ms. Smith how recurrent anxiety was very common for cancer survivors and especially at certain stages such as the 5-year anniversary. We worked on reframing her thoughts about recurrence and her concerns about her daughters getting cancer into more positive and proactive actions. She plans to also utilize her spiritual beliefs in supporting herself through anxiety. She indicates a renewed sense of motivation for weight loss based on the new information provided to her today regarding her increased risk for cancer recurrence with respect to her diagnoses of T2DM and obesity. We also discussed how the anxiety, sleep disorder, and low motivation for exercise were connected and she agreed to start a steady and realistic behavioral activation plan to improve her current problems and improve her diabetes management.

We identified the following goals for the patient:

1. **Increased physical activity**: Prior to her cancer diagnosis she was in a neighborhood walking group. She agreed to resume walking approximately 2 miles, three nights/week with two friends in the neighborhood.
2. **Improved nutrition and weight management**: She agreed she could start being more conscious of carbohydrates in her daily meals. She is motivated to begin with monitoring her carbohydrate intake with a food diary and attempt to keep her daily carb intake at the level of ____.
3. **Improved sleep hygiene**: She will not eat in the 2 hours prior to going to bed. She will not have the TV on in her bedroom, but will read a book prior to going to sleep.
4. **Brief counseling and monitoring**: She will return to the clinic for two more sessions for monitoring of her progress on her behavioral activation goals and for motivational therapy for sustained maintenance.

REFERENCES

Adorno, G. (2015). Between two worlds liminality and late-stage cancer-directed therapy. *OMEGA-Journal of Death and Dying*, *71*(2), 99–125.

Alfano, C. M., & Rowland, J. H. (2006). Recovery issues in cancer survivorship: A new challenge for supportive care. *Cancer Journal*, *12*(5), 432–443.

Anderson, B. L., DeRubeis, R. J., Berman, B. S., Gruman, J, Champion, V. L., Massie, M. J., ... Rowland, J. H. (2014). Screening, assessment, and care of anxiety and depressive symptoms in adults with cancer: An American Society of Clinical Oncology guideline adaptation. *Journal of Clinical Oncology*, 32, 1605–1619.

Arroll, B., Goodyear-Smith, F., Crengle, S., Gunn, J., Kerse, N., Fishman, T., ... Hatcher, S. (2010). Validation of PHQ-2 and PHQ-9 to screen for major depression in the primary care population. *Annals of Family Medicine, 8*(4), 348–353. doi:10.1370/afm.1139

Banegas, M. P., & Yabroff, K. R. (2013). Out of pocket, out of sight? An unmeasured component of the burden of cancer. *Journal of the National Cancer Institute, 105*(4), 252–255.

Boerger-Knowles, K., & Ridley, T. (2014). Chronic cancer: Counseling the individual. *Social Work in Health Care, 53*, 11–30. doi:10.1080/00981389.2013.840355

Brintzenhofe-Szoc, K. M., Levin, T. T., Li, Y., Kissane, D. W., Zabora, J. R. (2009). Mixed anxiety/depression symptoms in a large cancer cohort: Prevalence by cancer type. *Psychosomatics, 50*, 383–391.

Broder, H., Gottlieb, R. A., & Leport, N. E. (2008). Chemotherapy and cardiotoxicity. *Reviews in Cardiovascular Medicine, 9*, 75–83.

Burg, M. A., Adorno, G., Lopes, E. D. S., Loerzel, V., Stein, K., Wallace, C., Sharma, D. K. (2014). Current unmet needs of cancer survivors: Analysis of open-ended responses to the American Cancer Society Study of Cancer Survivors II. *Cancer*. 2015, *121*(4), 623–630.

Canada, A. L., & Schover, L. R. (2012). The psychosocial impact of interrupted childbearing in long-term female cancer survivors. *Psycho-Oncology, 21*(2), 134–143.

Cancer Support Community. (2013). Retrieved June 19, 2014, from www.cancersupportcommunity.org/General-Documents-Category/Research-and-Training-Institute/Posters-and-Presentations/2013-American-Public-Health-Association-Annual-Meeting-A-Four-Year-Review-of-the-Financial-Burden-o.pdf

Cella, D. F., Tulsky, D. S., Gray, G., Sarafian, B., Linn, E., Bonomi, A., ... Brannon, J. (1993). The functional assessment of cancer therapy scale: Development and validation of the general measure. *Journal of Clinical Oncology, 11*(3), 570–579.

Chopra, I., & Kamal, K. M. (2012). A systematic review of quality of life instruments in long-term breast cancer survivors. *Health and Quality of Life Outcomes, 10*(1), 14.

Coburn, N., Fulton, J., Pearlman, D. N., Law, C., DiPaolo, B., & Cady, B. (2008). Treatment variation by insurance status for breast cancer patients. *Breast Journal, 14*(2), 128–134.

Demark-Wahnefried, W., Aziz, N. M., Rowland, J. H., & Pinto, B. M. (2005). Riding the crest of the teachable moment: Promoting long-term health after the diagnosis of cancer. *Journal of Clinical Oncology*, 23(24), 5814–5830.

Demark-Wahnefried, W., Platz, E. A., Ligibel, J. A., Blair, C. K., Courneya, K. S., Meyerhardt, J. A., ... Goodwin, P. J. (2012). The role of obesity in cancer survival and recurrence. *Cancer Epidemiological Biomarkers Prevention, 21*(8), 1244–1259. doi:10.1158/1055-9965.EPI-12-0485

Derogatis, L. R., Savitz, K. L. (2000). The SCL-90-R and brief symptom inventory (BSD in primary care. In M. E. Maruish, (Ed.), *Handbook of Psychological Assessment in Primary Care Settings* (pp. 297–334). Mahwah. NJ: Lawrence Erlbaum Associates.

Economou, D., Hurria, A., & Grant, M. (2012). Integrating a cancer-specific geriatric assessment into survivorship care. *Clinical Journal of Oncology Nursing, 16*(3), E78–E85.

Epstein R. M., & Street, R. L. (2007). *Patient-centered communication in cancer care: Promoting healing and reducing suffering—NIH Publication No. 07-6225*. Bethesda, MD: National Cancer Institute.

FACIT (2014). www.facit.org/FACITOrg

Ferrell, B. R., Grant, M., Funk, B., Garcia, N., Otis-Green, S., & Schaffner, M. L. (1996). Quality of life in breast cancer. *Cancer Practice, 4*, 331–340.

Forsythe, L. P., Alfano, C. M., Leach, C. R., Ganz, P. A., Stefanek, M. E., & Rowland, J. H. (2012). Who provides psychosocial follow-up care for post-treatment cancer survivors? A survey of medical oncologists and primary care physicians. *Journal of Clinical Oncology, 30*(23), 2897-2905.

Forsythe, L. P., Kent, E. E., Weaver, K. E., Buchanan, N., Hawkins, N. A., Rodriguez, J. L., ... Rowland, J. H. (2013). Receipt of psychosocial care among cancer survivors in the United States. *Journal of Clinical Oncology, 31*(16), 1961–1969.

Foster, C., & Fenlon, D. (2011). Recovery and self-management support following primary cancer treatment. *British Journal of Cancer, 105*, S21–S28.

Giovannucci, E., Harlan, D. M., Archer, M. C., Bergenstal, R. M., Gapstur, S. M., Habel, L. A., ... Yee, D. (2010). Diabetes and cancer: A consensus report. *Diabetes Care, 33*, 1674–1685.

Greenwald, H. P., & McCorkle, R. (2008). Sexuality and sexual function in long-term survivors of cervical cancer. *Journal of Women's Health, 17*(6), 955–963. doi:10.1089/jwh.2007.0613

Harely, C., Pini, S., Bartlett, Y. K., & Velikova, G. (2012). Defining chronic cancer: Patient experiences and self-management needs. *BMJ Supportive & Palliative Care*, 2(3), 248–255. doi:10.1136/bmjspcare-2012-000200

Hewitt, M. E., Greenfield, S., Stovall, E., National Cancer Policy Board, Committee on Cancer Survivorship: Improving Care and Quality of Life. (2005). *From cancer patient to cancer survivor: Lost in transition* (p. 506). Washington, DC: National Academies Press. Retrieved May 10, 2015, from www.loc.gov/catdir/toc/ecip 0518/2005024963.html

Ho, E., Brown, A., Barrett, P., Morgan, R. B., King, G., Kennedy, M. J., Murphy, R. T. (2010). Subclinical anthracyclines- and trastuzumab-induced cardiotoxicity in the long-term follow-up of asymptomatic breast cancer survivors: A speckle tracking echocardiographic study. *Heart, 96*, 701–707. doi:10.1136/hrt.2009.173997

Hodgkinson, K., Butow, P., Hunt, G. E., Pendlebury, S., Hobbs, K. M., & Wain, G. (2007a). Breast cancer survivors' supportive care needs 2–10 years after diagnosis. *Supportive Care in Cancer, 15*(5), 515–523.

Hodgkinson, K., Butow, P., Hunt, G. E., Pendlebury, S., Hobbs, K. M., Lo, S. K., & Wain, G. (2007b). The development and evaluation of a measure to assess cancer survivors unmet supportive care needs: The CaSUN (Cancer Survivors' Unmet Needs measure). *Psycho-oncology, 16*(9), 796–804.

Hoffman, B. M., Zevon, M. A., D'Arrigo, M. C., & Cecchini, T. B. (2004). Screening for distress in cancer patients: The NCCN rapid-screening measure. *Psycho-Oncology, 13*(11), 792–799. doi:10.1002/pon.796

Holland, J. C., & Reznik, I. (2005). Pathways for psychosocial care of cancer survivors. *Cancer, 104*(11 Suppl), 2624–2637. doi:10.1002/cncr.21252

Institute of Medicine. (2007). *Cancer care for the whole patient: Meeting psychosocial health needs*. A Consensus Report. Washington, DC: National Academies Press.

Institute of Medicine. (2013). *Committee on improving the quality of cancer care: Addressing the challenges of an aging population*. Washington, DC: National Academies Press.

Jacobsen, P. B., Donovan, K. A., Trask, P. C., Fleishman, S. B., Zabora, J., Baker, F., & Holland, J. C. (2005). Screening for psychologic distress in ambulatory cancer patients. *Cancer, 103*(7), 1494–1502.

Kaiser Family Foundation. (2006). *Spending to survive: Cancer patients confront holes in the health insurance system*. Retrieved June 19, 2014, from http://jnci.oxfordjournals.org/content/early/2013/01/12/jnci.djs641.full.pdf+html

Koch, L., Jansen, L., Brenner, H., & Arndt, V. (2013). Fear of recurrence and disease progression in long-term (≥5 years) cancer survivors—a systematic review of quantitative studies. *Psycho-Oncology*, 22(1), 1–11.

Kuijpers, W., Groen, W. G., Aaronson, N. K., & van Harten, W. H. (2013). A systematic review of web-based interventions for patient empowerment and physical activity in chronic diseases: Relevance for cancer survivors. *Journal of Medical Internet Research, 15*(2), e37. doi:10.2196/jmir.2281

Kushi, L. H., Byers, T., Doyle, C., Bandera, E. V., McCullough, J., Gansler, T., Andrews, K. S., Thun, M. J.; American Cancer Society 2006 Nutrition and Physical Activity Guidelines Advisory Committee. (2006). American Cancer Society guidelines on nutrition and physical activity for cancer prevention: Reducing the risk of cancer with health food choices and physical activity. *CA: A Cancer Journal for Clinicians, 56*, 254–281.

Kwak, M., Zebrack, B. J., Meeske, K. A., Embry, L., Augilar, C., Block, R., ... Cole, S. (2013). Prevalence and predictors of post-traumatic stress symptoms in adolescent and young adult cancer survivors: A 1-year follow-up study. *Psycho-Oncology*, 22, 1798–1806.

Morey, M. C., Snyder, D. C., Sloane, R., Cohen, H. J., Peterson, B., Hartman, T. J., ... Demark-Wahnefried, W. (2009). Effects of home-based diet and exercise on functional outcomes among older, overweight long-term cancer survivors: RENEW: A randomized controlled trial. *JAMA*, *301*(18), 1883–1891.

Mukherjee, S. (2010). *The emperor of all maladies: A biography of cancer*. New York, NY: Scribner.

National Cancer Legal Services Network. Retrieved June 19, 2014, from www.nclsn.org

National Coalition for Cancer Survivorship (NCCS). (2014). Defining cancer survivorship. Retrieved from www.canceradvocacy.org/news/defining-cancer-survivorship

Nekhlyudov, L., & Wenger, N. (2014). Institute of Medicine recommendations for improving the quality of cancer care: What do they mean for the general internist? *Journal of General Internal Medicine*, *29*, 1404–1409. doi:10.1007/s11606-014-2931-9

Oeffinger, K. C., Mertens, A. C., Sklar, C. A., Kawashima, T., Hudson, M. M., Meadows, A. T., ... & Robison, L. L. (2006). Chronic health conditions in adult survivors of childhood cancer. *New England Journal of Medicine*, *355*(15), 1572–1582.

Rohan, E. A. (2012). Removing the stress from selecting instruments: Arming social workers to take leadership in routine distress screening implementation. *Journal of Psychosocial Oncology*, *30*(6), 667–678.

Rossen, P., Pedersen, A. F., Zachariae, R., & von der Maase, H. (2012). Sexuality and body image in long-term survivors of testicular cancer. *European Journal of Cancer*, *48*(4), 571–578. doi:10.1016/j.ejca.2011.11.029

Scott, J. G., Suh, J. H., Elson, P., Barnett, G. H., Vogelbaum, M. A., Peereboom, D. M., ... Chao, S. T. (2011). Aggressive treatment is appropriate for glioblastoma multiforme patients 70 years old or older: A retrospective review of 206 cases. *Neuro-Oncology*, *13*(4), 428–436. doi:10.1093/neuonc/nor005

Sequist, L. V., & Lynch, T. J. (2003). Aggressive treatment for the fit elderly with non-small-cell lung cancer? Yes! *Journal of Clinical Oncology*, *21*(17), 3186–3188. doi:10.1200/JCO.2003.04.002

Sharpe, M., Walker, J., Hansen, C. H., Martin, P., Symeonides, S., Gourley, C., ... Murray, G. (2014). Integrated collaborative care for comorbid major depression in patients with cancer (SMaRT Oncology-2): A multicentre randomised controlled effectiveness trial. *The Lancet*, *384*(9948), 1099–1108

Shaw, M. G., & Ball, D. L. (2013). Treatment of brain metastases in lung cancer: Strategies to avoid/reduce late complications of whole brain irradiation. *Current Treatment Options in Oncology*, *14*, 553–567. doi:10.1007/s11864-013-0258-0

Siegel, R., DeSantis, C., Virgo, K., Stein, K., Mariotto, A., Smith, T., ... Ward, E. (2012). Cancer treatment and survivorship statistics, 2012. *CA: A Cancer Journal for Clinicians*, *62*(4), 220–241.

Sussman, J., & Baldwin, L. (2012). The interface of primary and oncology specialty care: From diagnosis through primary treatment. *Journal of the National Cancer Institute Monographs*, *40*, 18–24.

Tukenova, M., Guibout, C., Oberlin, O., Doyon, F., Mousannif, A., Haddy N., ... de Vathaire, F. (2010). Role of cancer treatment in long-term overall and cardiovascular mortality after childhood cancer. *Journal of Clinical Oncology*, *28*(8), 1308–1315.

Wikman, A., Johar, A., & Lagergren, P. (2014). Presence of symptom clusters in surgically treated patients with esophageal cancer: Implications for survival. *Cancer*, *120*(2), 286–293.

Zigmond, A. S., & Snaith, R. P. (1983). The hospital anxiety and depression scale. *Acta Psychiatrica Scandinavica*, *67*, 361–370.

TEN

ADDRESSING SUBSTANCE ABUSE IN PRIMARY CARE

THOMAS W. BISHOP, BETH A. BAILEY, TIMOTHY A. URBIN, JACK WOODSIDE, MICHAEL FLOYD, AND FRED TUDIVER

S.O.A.P. NOTE FROM REFERRING PRIMARY CARE PROVIDER

S: Mrs. Peters is a 58-year-old female with reports of elevated blood pressure. For the preceding 2 years, her blood pressure has been at the upper limits of normal (144/92). Prior to that, all of her blood pressure readings had been normal (below 135/85). She has never been diagnosed with hypertension, nor taken any medication for hypertension. She has additional complaints of frequent heartburn (for which she takes multiple OTC antacids) and stress. She denies chest pain, cough, shortness of breath, headache, or dizziness. She also denies exertional or paroxysmal nocturnal dyspnea, nocturia, hematuria, melena, or hematochezia. Bowels are regular, no recent changes.

She and her husband lead very busy lives as she works in real estate and her husband is an attorney. Her work has become increasingly stressful. Her real estate agency let her go and she is now starting her own business. They frequently "entertain" and her husband (who accompanied her today) expresses concerns regarding her drinking behavior. There is noticeable tension between them on the topic and she indicates minimal concern in her use of alcohol. She admits that she often drinks more than she intended while entertaining. She gets to talking and loses count. However, she never is drunk while entertaining despite having several drinks. She denies any other consequences to alcohol overuse/abuse. However, she is worried about her blood pressure and frequent heartburn. She also reports smoking cigarettes, approximately one pack a day for 40 years.

Her sleep is characterized by episodic difficulty falling asleep and she admits that she occasionally has a drink to help her fall asleep. Furthermore, on those "rare" occasions when she admits to drinking more than she should when entertaining she often has early morning awakening on those nights. She denies any other recreational drug use currently or historically. Family history is positive for hypertension (both parents), diabetes (mother), hyperlipidemia (both parents), and alcoholism (father).

O: BP 162/104, pulse 100, respirations 16, temperature 99, height 5′08″, weight 135 (BMI 20.5)

General: Alert and oriented to person, place, and time. Presents as somewhat depressed

HEENT: PERRLA. Fundoscopic exam reveals mild arteriolar narrowing. TMs intact bilaterally, throat and posterior pharynx without erythema, exudate, or masses

Neck: Without adenopathy or masses. No thyroid enlargement or asymmetry

Lungs: Clear to auscultation bilaterally without crackles or wheezes

Heart: RRR without murmur or gallop

Abdomen: Mild epigastric and right upper quadrant abdominal tenderness, with negative Murphy's sign (*a test for an inflamed gallbladder*), no guarding, normal bowel sounds, liver palpable on deep inspiration with normal span and percussion

Extremities: Strong pedal pulses. No edema

Neurologic: Motor and sensory intact. Patellar DTRs 2+ to 3+ bilaterally, gait normal, Babinski sign negative. PHQ-9 depression screening reveals a score of 8 consistent with mild depression. AUDIT screening reveals a score of 17 consistent with harmful alcohol use, while drug use was denied

Past Medical History: Bilateral tubal ligation after the birth of second child

Current Medications: Extra-strength TUMS® and Tylenol as needed

A:
1. Hypertension uncontrolled (401.1)
2. Alcohol use disorder, moderate (303.90)
3. Other Specified Depressive Disorder (311)
4. Tobacco use disorder (305.1)
5. Probable GERD/reflux esophagitis (530.81)

P:
1. Hypertension (uncontrolled): Run a complete metabolic panel, fasting lipid panel, and TSH. Discuss the negative effect of alcohol on blood pressure, discuss (and provide) a low sodium diet; begin lisinopril 20 mg/day. Follow-up BP readings in 1 month.
2. Alcohol use (ongoing): Engage in motivational interviewing and refer to behavioral health specialist for brief treatment.
3. Depression NOS (ongoing): Assess for potential suicidal/homicidal ideation or plans. Review stress management skills and refer to behavioral health specialist for further assessment and counseling. Also consider a trial of an SSRI antidepressant (e.g., citalopram 20 mg/day). Be wary of any suicidal ideation before prescribing.
4. Tobacco use disorder (ongoing): Discuss the need to quit smoking. Discuss and consider nicotine replacement therapy (e.g., nicotine patches). If deemed appropriate at the next appointment, discuss and consider referral to behavioral health specialist for additional motivational interviewing.
5. GERD (ongoing): Discuss the lifestyle issues that cause/aggravate the condition (smoking, alcohol use, stress). Start an H2 blocker (e.g., ranitidine 150 mg bid), or a PPI (e.g., omeprazole 20 mg daily).

INTRODUCTION

Substance use, including the abuse of alcohol, the use of illicit drugs, the misuse of prescription medications, and the use of tobacco, is common in the United States, and contributes significantly to morbidity and mortality. According to a report by the Robert Wood Johnson Foundation (RWJF), drug, alcohol, and tobacco abuse is the cause of more deaths, illnesses, and disabilities than any other preventable health condition (RWJF, 2001). Data from the most recent National Survey on Drug Use and Health reveal that over 21 million Americans are dependent on alcohol and/or illicit drugs, with the rate over 5% among adolescents (Substance Abuse and Mental Health Services Administration [SAMHSA], 2014). Unhealthy substance use, which includes the full spectrum of risky to dependent use of alcohol and other drugs, is substantially more common. Indeed, as many as one in three adults engage in at-risk drinking (National Institute on Alcohol Abuse and Alcoholism [NIAAA], 2005), including one in four who binge drink at least monthly (SAMHSA, 2014). Rates of illicit drug use remain high, with nearly one in ten Americans aged 12 and older reporting use in the last month (SAMHSA, 2014). Marijuana continues to be the most commonly used illicit drug (over 21 million report use in the past 30 days), followed by cocaine (1.6 million U.S. users in 2012), hallucinogens (1.1 million users), and heroin (700,000 users; SAMHSA, 2014). See Table 10.1 for current U.S. drug use rates.

Prescription drug misuse has also emerged as a challenge over the past decade, with one in six Americans reporting ever misusing prescription medication, and 4.6% reporting doing so in the last year (National Institute on Drug Abuse [NIDA], 2012, 2014a). Prescription drug misuse rates vary by region with 18 U.S. states seeing more than one in 20 adults misusing prescription drugs each year, with painkillers most commonly abused, followed by tranquilizers and stimulants (NIDA, 2012, 2014). Prescription drug misuse has been referred to by the Office of National Drug Control Policy as the "nation's fastest-growing drug problem" (Office of National Drug Control Policy [ONDCP], 2011), and as

TABLE 10.1 Current Substance Use Rates in the United States

Substance	Percentage of U.S. Population
Tobacco, current use[a]	18%
Alcohol, current risk drinking[b]	30%
Alcohol, current monthly + binge drinking[c]	23%
Any illicit drug use, past month[c]	9%
Marijuana use, past month[c]	7%
Prescription drug misuse, lifetime[d]	17%
Prescription drug misuse, past year[d]	5%
Alcohol or drug dependency, current[c]	9%

[a] Centers for Disease Control and Prevention (2012)
[b] National Institute on Alcohol Abuse and Alcoholism (2005)
[c] Substance Abuse and Mental Health Services Administration (2014)
[d] National Institute on Drug Abuse (2012, 2014)

an "epidemic" by the Centers for Disease Control and Prevention (CDC, 2013). Finally, more than one in five U.S. adults continue to smoke cigarettes, with rates exceeding 25% in several southern states and approaching 30% in nonmetropolitan counties nationwide (Agaku, King, & Dube, 2014; CDC, 2012).

The health consequences of substance use are significant. Alcohol and drug use are established risk factors for many common medical conditions including diabetes, hypertension, chronic obstructive pulmonary disease (COPD), osteoporosis, liver disease, and many types of cancer (Brick, 2008; Howard, Arnsten, & Gourevitch, 2004; McFadden, Brensinger, Berlin, & Townsend, 2005; Mehra, Moore, Crothers, Tetrault, & Fiellin, 2006; Rehm, Room, Graham, Monteiro, Gmel, & Sempos, 2003; U.S. Department of Health and Human Services [HHS], 2014). In addition, substance use is linked to many mental health conditions including anxiety and major depression (Grant et al., 2004; Sullivan, Fiellin, & O'Connor, 2005). Substance users have substantially reduced rates of use of preventive health care services, and reduced rates of compliance with prescribed medical treatment (Lasser et al., 2011). Alcohol and/or drug use intoxication is a leading risk factor for injury (Rivara et al., 1993; Soderstrom et al., 1997) and is implicated in more than two of every five automobile accidents (National Highway Traffic Safety Administration [NHTSA], 2006). Given the health consequences it is not surprising that substance use results in substantial costs and leads to a significant number of deaths. The annual cost of excessive alcohol consumption exceeds $225 billion per year in the United States (Bouchery, Harwood, Sacks, Simon, & Brewer, 2011) and results in approximately 76,000 deaths annually (CDC, 2004). The annual cost of illicit drug use and prescription drug misuse is estimated at $193 billion in the United States (NDIC, 2011), and 114 people die each day from accidental overdoses (SAMHSA, 2013).

Tobacco use also deserves attention when discussing substance abuse. Because it is not a "mood altering" substance such as alcohol and many other drugs, tobacco is not always initially considered when substance abuse is addressed. However, tobacco use is estimated to cost $289 billion annually in the United States (HHS, 2014), more than either alcohol or all other drug use combined. Additionally, tobacco use is the leading cause of preventable death, responsible for 443,000 deaths per year in the United States (HHS, 2014), not including fetal deaths due to maternal smoking, which are estimated at as many as 140,000 per year (DiFranza & Lew, 1995). Thus, while the challenges and most useful approaches may vary when the drug addressed is tobacco, efforts to identify and treat substance abuse should always include plans for identifying and intervening with tobacco users as well. As many as 80% of heavy alcohol users are also tobacco smokers (Hughes, 1996), while more than 70% of illicit drug users smoke (Richter, Ahluwalia, Mosier, Nazir, & Ahluwalia, 2002), making those who use "mood altering" substances four or more times as likely to be smokers as other patients. Indeed, several studies have demonstrated that alcohol abusers are more likely to die from smoking-related diseases than alcohol-related diseases (Hurt et al., 1996). In addition, patients who have agreed to treatment for alcohol and/or illicit drugs are more than twice as likely as other patients to also attempt to quit smoking

(Prochaska, Delucchi, & Hall, 2004). Given this finding, it certainly makes sense to identify and address all types of unhealthy substance use in order to ultimately improve patient health.

Substance users are significantly overrepresented in primary care populations (Cherpital & Ye, 2008), providing an opportunity for intervention. Primary care providers are frequently overwhelmed and may be reluctant to address substance-related problems given few resources. Settings that have integrated a behavioral health specialist (BHS) may increase the likelihood of early detection of potential substance abuse and assist the clinical team in treatment and intervention. Indeed, direct collaboration with a BHS co-located within the primary care clinic results in increased efficiency and better treatment outcomes (American Hospital Association [AHA], 2012; McDaniel & deGruy III, 2014). When this is not possible, referrals can be made to specialty behavioral health services. Every effort should be made to facilitate connecting patients to external behavioral health agencies given many patients fail to follow through on these referrals on their own (Cummings, Cummings, & Johnson, 1997).

IDENTIFICATION OF SUBSTANCE ABUSE

In order for substance abuse to be addressed in primary care settings, those using substances must first be identified. Unfortunately, most primary care physicians have little training in this area (Miller, Sheppard, Colenda, & Magen, 2001), lack confidence in their ability to identify substance use (Beich, Gannik, & Malterud, 2002), and report discomfort with discussing substance use with patients (McCormick et al., 2006). Consequently, family physicians have been found to fail to identify more than 90% of patients with early alcohol abuse and as many as 40% of patients with classic drug abuse (D'Amico, Paddock, Burnam, & Kung, 2005). Despite the fact that both the Institute of Medicine (IOM, 2005) and the U.S. Preventive Services Task Force (USPSTF, 2004) recommend that primary care providers screen all patients for substance use, this clearly does not routinely occur in practice (Ernst, Miller, & Rollnick, 2007; National Center on Addiction and Substance Abuse [NCASA], 2000). Even in primary care settings that include a BHS, substance users are still frequently substantially underidentified because a high percentage of psychologists and counselors feel they lack sufficient training in this area (DeAngelis, 2001). This is despite the fact that substance abuse disorders collectively are the most frequently occurring mental health problems in the United States (DeAngelis, 2001).

Validated approaches and tools for substance use screening exist, and should be the first step in effectively addressing substance use in primary care settings. The most useful tools will identify both those likely to have substance use disorders or dependence, as well as those with earlier stage risky use that increases the likelihood of serious health problems or later dependence (American Public Health Association [APHA], 2008). Generally, anyone currently using tobacco at any level, or with any recent (last 90 days) use of an illicit drug or use of a prescription medication other than as prescribed, would be considered to be engaging in risky substance use (HHS, 2012). With respect to alcohol, risky use is gender and age specific. For adult males under the age of 65, consumption of more than 14 drinks per week, or more than four drinks per occasion, at any point in the past 12 months is considered outside of "safe consumption" guidelines (NIAAA, 2005). For women of all ages, and men over 65, consumption of more than seven drinks per week, or more than three drinks per occasion, is considered as risk drinking (NIAAA, 2005).

Both prescreening tools, those that consist of one or two initial questions followed by more comprehensive screening for those who are positive, and regular screening tools with anywhere from three to 20 or more questions, have been found to be highly sensitive in identifying both risky and dependent substance users (NIDA, 2013). These tools can be used as part of an overall validated screening and intervention process, such as SBIRT (Screening, Brief Intervention, and Referral to Treatment). SBIRT is an evidence-based practice used to identify, reduce, and prevent problematic use, abuse, and dependence on alcohol and illicit drugs (SAMHSA, 2008). The SBIRT model was developed in response to the IOM recommendation for universal substance use screening in primary care settings (IOM, 2005), and has been found to be effective in reducing substance use, as well as substance-related health and social consequences in dozens of different studies over the last several years (Gryczynski et al., 2011; InSight Project Research Group, 2009; Madras et al., 2009). The initial "screening" step most commonly involves both a prescreen given to all patients and then a follow-up, more detailed screen for those who are positive.

The most widely used and effective prescreen questions (Smith, Schmidt, Allensworth-Davies, & Saitz, 2009, 2010) are presented in Table 10.2. With a single question for alcohol use and a single question for drug use, these questions can be easily incorporated into a triage or vital sign assessment at the beginning of a primary care appointment. As part of the SBIRT model, SAMHSA recommends annual drug and alcohol screening for all patients. However, recent data have suggested that patient disclosure of substance use increases if prescreens are administered at every visit (Bailey, Urbin, Bishop, & Floyd, 2014). While these prescreen questions are highly sensitive in identifying those with potential substance use issues, false-positives do result. Thus, it is necessary to administer a more detailed screening with those who prescreen positive. Several well-validated tools exist for this purpose (Table 10.3), and the choice

TABLE 10.2 Common Drug and Alcohol Prescreen Questions for Use in Primary Care

How many times in the past year have you used an illegal drug or used a prescription medication for nonmedical reasons?[a]
How many times in the past year have you had five or more (four or more for women) drinks in a day?*

[a]A response of one or greater is considered positive.
Source: Smith et al. (2009, 2010).

TABLE 10.3 Commonly Used Validated Alcohol and Drug Screening Tools

Tool	Substance	Length	Reliability/Validity	Comment
AUDIT (Alcohol Use Disorders Test)[a]	Alcohol	10 items	High internal consistency (>.80) and test-retest reliability (>.80) For a cut-off score of 8, sensitivity ranges from 85% to 98%, specificity from 78% to 97%; cut-off score of 5 still highly sensitive and specific, especially for women and younger adults[g]	Self-administered Queries both amount of alcohol used and consequences of drinking
MAST (Michigan Alcohol Screening Test)[b]	Alcohol	25 items	High test-retest reliability (>.85) For a cut-off score of 12, sensitivity >90%, specificity >80%[h]	Self-administered Queries a multitude of drinking consequences; scores discriminate early from problem drinkers
SMAST (Short Michigan Alcohol Screening Test)[c]	Alcohol	13 items	Minimal info available	Self-administered Shorter version of MAST; scores correlate highly with scores on longer MAST
CAGE[d]	Alcohol	4 items	High test-retest reliability (.80–.95) For a cut-off score of 2, sensitivity >70%, specificity >90% Performs less well with women of child-bearing age and college students[i]	Clinician-administered Name is acronym for four markers of an alcohol problem: Criticism about drinking, Annoyed by others commenting on drinking, Guilty about drinking, need for *Eye-opener* (drink first thing in morning)

(*continued*)

TABLE 10.3 Commonly Used Validated Alcohol and Drug Screening Tools (*continued*)

Tool	Substance	Length	Reliability/Validity	Comment
DAST (Drug Abuse Screening Test)[e]	Drug Use	28 items	High internal consistency (>.90) and test-retest reliability (.85) Scores correlate with reports of specific substance use (>.50) For a cut-off score of 6, sensitivity ranges from 81% to 96%, specificity from 71% to 94%[j]	Self-administered Parallels the MAST; asks about consequences of drug use in the past 12 months, including prescription drug misuse
DAST-10 (Drug Abuse Screening Test – 10 Items)[e]	Drug Use	10 items	High internal consistency (.94) and test-retest reliability (.71); high correspondence (>.90) with full DAST[i]	Self-administered Shorter version of DAST; scores correlate highly with scores on longer DAST and still includes a total score indicating level of problem
CAGE-AID (CAGE Adapted to Include Drugs)[f]	Alcohol Drug Use	4 items	For a cut-off score of 1, sensitivity of 79%, specificity of 77%	Clinician-administered Each question asks about both alcohol and drug use consequences

[a]Babor et al. (2001).
[b]Selzner (1971).
[c]Selzner, Vinocker, and Van Rooijen (1975).
[d]Ewing (1984).
[e]Skinner (1982).
[f]Brown and Rounds (1995).
[g]Reinert and Allen (2007).
[h]Gibbs (1983).
[i]Dhalla and Kopec (2007).
[j]Yudko, Lozhkina, and Fouts (2007).

of which to use will depend upon practice/provider goals, including whether intervention will be offered inhouse, and also on patient characteristics. Generally, the most commonly used and recommended tools are the Alcohol Use Disorders Identification Test (AUDIT; Babor, Higgins-Biddle, Saunders, & Monteiro, 2001) for risky alcohol use screening, and the Drug Abuse Screening Test (DAST; Skinner, 1982) for drug abuse (Table 10.3).

The assessment and treatment of tobacco abuse is not discussed in depth in this chapter; however, there are excellent resources available for the BHS who will provide tobacco abuse interventions in the primary care setting (Agency for Healthcare Research and Quality, 2008; Patnode et al., 2013; HHS, 2008; World Health Organization [WHO], 2013). A commonly used assessment and intervention strategy for tobacco abuse is the 5 As approach: ASK every patient at every visit if they smoke; ADVISE smokers in a clear manner to quit smoking, providing personal benefits to quitting; ASSESS the smoker's willingness to quit smoking; ASSIST the smoker in quitting using counseling and pharmacotherapy; and ARRANGE for follow-up contact (see www.etsu.edu/tips/participating/intervention.aspx for a comprehensive resource on the 5 As approach for pregnant smokers that can be used with any tobacco user). The 5 As approach can be used with alcohol and drug abusers but other interventions are more commonly used for these patient populations and have more empirical support as already discussed.

For those patients who are positive for either alcohol or drugs as part of a screening process, further evaluation is needed before a substance use diagnosis can be made. The *Diagnostic and Statistical Manual of Mental Disorders*, Fifth Edition (*DSM-5*) provides the most widely accepted criteria for classifying substance use problems (American Psychiatric Association [APA], 2013). Diagnosis of a substance-related problem hinges on an individual's continued use of any substance despite significant problems as exhibited in poor cognitive, behavioral, and physiological functioning. In general, a diagnosis of a substance use disorder is a maladaptive use of a substance resulting in a pathological pattern of behaviors in four areas: impaired control, social impairment, risky use, and pharmacological criteria (Table 10.4). An individual's behavior is thought to be reflective of a substance use disorder if use and associated behaviors lead to clinically significant impairment or distress, manifesting at least two symptoms/behaviors over a 12-month period. Unlike previous editions of the *DSM*, the fifth edition does not make a distinction between abuse and dependence, but rather conceptualizes the extent of the problem along a continuum from mild to severe, where an individual demonstrates more symptoms with greater intensity.

Substance abuse often disguises itself as a medical or other psychiatric condition, hampering identification efforts, and symptoms may manifest themselves in marital, emotional, occupational, spiritual, financial, or legal struggles. Cummings and Cummings (2000) have suggested that the identification of substance-related problems should include close attention to one or more "signposts" suggesting a substance use problem (Table 10.5). Collins and his colleagues (Collins, McAllister, & Adury, 2010), in providing an overview of drug abuse and addiction, have identified several physical factors that patients may exhibit (Table 10.6).

TABLE 10.4 *Diagnostic and Statistical Manual of Mental Disorders*—Fifth Edition Criteria for Substance Abuse (Modified to Reflect Overview of Criteria for Any Substance Use)

1. Substance is taken in larger amounts or for a longer period than is intended
2. There is a persistent desire or unsuccessful efforts to cut down or control use
3. A great deal of time is spent in activities necessary to obtain a substance or recover from its effects
4. Craving, or a strong desire or urge to use a substance
5. Recurrent substance use resulting in a failure to fulfill major role obligations at work, school, or home
6. Continued use despite having persistent or recurrent social or interpersonal problems caused or exacerbated by the effect of the substance
7. Important social, occupational, or recreational activities are given up or reduced because of substance use
8. Recurrent substance use in situations in which it is physically hazardous
9. Substance use is continued despite knowledge of having a persistent or recurrent physical or psychological problem that is likely to have been caused or exacerbated by the substance
10. Tolerance, as defined by either of the following:
    - A need for markedly increased amounts of the substance to achieve intoxication or desired effect
    - A markedly diminished effect with continued use of the same amount of the substance
11. Withdrawal, as manifested by either of the following:
    - The characteristic withdrawal syndrome expected for a particular substance
    - A substance or similar substance is taken to relieve or avoid withdrawal symptoms

Based on: American Psychiatric Association (2013).

TABLE 10.5 Signposts of Potential Substance Abuse

Frequent auto accidents

Two or more bone fractures in a 3- to 5-year period

Spousal battery, physical abuse of children, or both

Tweaking (picking the face or the skin on the forearm)

Unusual physique

Paranoia

Stains on clothing, red eyes or nose, sores around the mouth, poor muscle control, and loss of appetite

Missed adolescence—having to function early as an adult

Source: Cummings and Cummings (2000).

TABLE 10.6 Physical Findings and Complications of Chronic Drug Addiction

Skin	Needle marks, injection "tracks" over veins, scars, ulcerations, cellulitis, necrotic tissue, jaundice
Eyes	Pupillary constriction (opiates) or dilation (stimulant, opiate, or benzodiazepine withdrawal), sclera icterus
Respiratory	Nasal mucosal inflammation or septal perforation, coarsened voice, or chronic bronchitis from cocaine freebasing or marijuana smoking
Cardiovascular	"No veins" limiting intravenous access and blood for laboratory sampling, bacterial endocarditis
Autonomic nervous system	Elevated blood pressure, abnormal heart rate (bradycardia or tachycardia), tremor, diaphoresis, brisk reflexes
Liver	Tenderness or enlargement
Neuromuscular	Seizures, aseptic necrosis of large muscle masses causing scarring, fibrosis, and board-like rigidity of affected muscles

Source: Collins et al. (2010).

BEHAVIORAL FACTORS IN MANAGING THE PATIENT WITH SUBSTANCE ABUSE

A number of behavioral factors should be considered in effectively addressing substance use and abuse in the primary care setting. Intervention begins with first appreciating a patient's "readiness to change" and "stage matching" interventions according to the level of a patient's contemplated change (DiClemente, Schlundt, & Gemmell, 2004). Very brief exposure to treatment may result in gains for patients possessing a high level of readiness to change, while others with little motivation toward change may have minimal improvement even with more intensive interventions. The level or type of intervention provided by a primary care provider should match a patient's readiness for change (as described in the following). However, a patient's desire, ability, or motivation for change is dependent on the level of the patient's commitment (Amrhein, Miller, Yahne, Palmer, & Fulcher, 2003). A patient may have a high level of readiness to change, but in fact lack a firm commitment to doing things differently, resulting in little improvement. In spite of a patient's readiness or commitment to change, it has been demonstrated that change is possible through provider's initiation of brief interventions. Brief interventions can reduce substance use, may facilitate adherence with medical treatment as it relates to substance abuse problems, and assist in bridging patients to more intensive treatment (Fleming, 2002; Fleming, Barry, Manwell, Johnson, & London, 1997).

The ability to effectively address substance abuse also requires the recognition that substance abuse is frequently comorbid with mental health struggles, such as depression, anxiety, posttraumatic stress disorder, trauma, and other mood disorders. Adequately screening for these conditions and addressing them more fully may lead to better gains and improvement in managing substance use problems as well. Primary care providers should also be alert to unexplained vague symptoms, somatic complaints, difficulty with sleep, anxiousness, frequent life disruptions or chaotic lifestyle, and a family history of mental health problems or substance abuse. Screening tools such as the Patient Health Questionnaire 9 (PHQ-9; Kroenke, Spitzer, & Williams, 2001) and Generalized Anxiety Disorder 7 (GAD-7; Spitzer, Kroenke, Williams, & Löwe, 2006) could be utilized in assessing current mental health problems. Finally, risk factors such as peers, family history and dynamics, temperament or personality style, and genetics may also contribute to vulnerability for substance abuse. These factors should be explored in addressing substance abuse as they could lead to insight into potential challenges, treatment approaches, and the effectiveness of interventions. Thus, they should be included in a thorough history taking.

Additional consideration should be given when dealing with substance use problems in special populations including geriatrics, adolescents, and different ethnic groups. Older adults (age 65 and older) are less likely to abuse illicit drugs and are more vulnerable to the effects of alcohol than their younger cohorts. However, there is a growing trend in the number of older adults who are abusing substances. With an increased risk of comorbid diseases, use of prescription and over-the-counter medications, and increased vulnerability to poor or negative lifestyle behaviors, older adults may present with health problems that do not immediately suggest substance abuse. Older adults experience slowed absorption rates, decreased availability of plasma proteins, declining liver functioning, and decreased kidney functioning (Cummings, 2005), which can lead them to be more sensitive and reactive to medications and other substances. Treatment of older adult substance abuse is most effective and reduces relapse if it addresses specific concerns and is personalized by the primary care provider (Blow, Brockmann, & Barry, 2007; Fink, Elliot, Tsai, & Beck, 2005).

The first use of substances can occur as early as in elementary school, but is more common in adolescence. Substance use in adolescence has been understood for some time to be associated with peers, although first experimentation is often a means of coping with family stress and conflict. Substance abuse is more often seen in young people who feel alienated and are disenfranchised with authority figures, have negative peer influences, experience family conflict, and perceive substance use as being condoned by parents. Substance use by some young people may be a means of obtaining negative attention when little other is given or to draw attention away from family conflict (Gomez, Nunes, & Ragnauth, 2012). Young people are often unwilling to seek treatment independently, but do tend to be open to discussion when approached within a primary care setting (Stern, Meredith, Gholson, Gore, & D'Amico, 2007). The top five abused substances for eighth graders, in order, are marijuana, alcohol, inhalants, synthetic marijuana, and cough medicine. This trend is a little different for high school seniors, who use, in order, alcohol, marijuana, Adderall, synthetic marijuana, and Vicodin (NIDA, 2014b).

In terms of ethnic differences related to substance abuse, the diagnostic criteria of the *DSM-IV* do not vary between African Americans and Caucasians (Horton, Compton, & Cottler, 2000). However, it has been suggested that there are cultural considerations in terms of the language used to describe the criteria of substance abuse and dependence in the *DSM-5* in that it may be more appropriate to exclude criteria emphasizing hazardous behavior, such as drinking and driving, and give more attention to pathological behaviors and poor psychological functioning (Caetano, 2011). Specifically, differences in rates of alcohol abuse among different ethnic groups as determined by the *DSM-5* criteria may be more a factor of access to cars and alcohol rather than a true indication of abuse and preoccupation in obtaining alcohol. Differences tend to be most important in access to substance abuse treatment, the course of treatment, and treatment endurance. For example, there may be fewer treatment options in communities that are largely Hispanic (Archibald, 2007), and Native Americans are less likely to seek treatment while African Americans are more likely to leave treatment early (Campbell, Weisner, & Sterling, 2006).

BASIC NEEDS AND SOCIAL SERVICE REFERRALS (ALCOHOL AND ILLICIT SUBSTANCE ABUSE)

Social and economic factors are important to the selection of treatment and its effectiveness. The work of Walton and colleagues suggests that low income, being single, and having lower self-efficacy contribute to drug and alcohol use even after 2 years following treatment (Walton, Blow, Bingham, & Chermack, 2003). Ethnic differences in substance use and abuse are believed to be more a factor of socioeconomics, culture, and experiences of discrimination than other contributors (Buka, 2002). While addressing behavioral risk factors of substance use and abuse is necessary, behavior is only one component of substance abuse prevention. It is also necessary to address other social determinants such as socioeconomic status, homelessness, social support, residential considerations, and possibly incarceration (Galea & Vlahov, 2002). Most communities have social support agencies that could serve a role in substance abuse treatment plans. Self-help organizations and community support groups should be considered as well, as detailed further in the following.

BRIEF COUNSELING METHODS

Despite a common hesitancy to engage patients with a substance use disorder in nonaddiction services settings (Miller & Brown, 1997; Washton, 2001), most BHSs have the necessary basic skills that can be easily enhanced to address risky substance use with patients seen in the primary care environment. For example, all brief interventions for risky substance use emphasize the need for proficiency in client-centered counseling skills as these skills are important predictors of successful outcomes (Miller & Brown, 1997; Miller & Moyers, 2006). These basic skills are the foundation of most behavioral health training programs (Duncan, 2014; Egan, 2002.)

Adequate situational awareness (Singh et al., 2012) is important for the BHS to develop in order to address the challenges to both screening and responding to substance abuse problems in the primary care clinic. Despite the increased focus on integrated care, the majority of patients expect their primary care visit to be focused on what they perceive as their medical issues. As a result, risky substance use may not be reported even though the behaviors are currently occurring (Bailey et al., 2014). If the risky substance use is affecting the patient's ability to benefit from medical interventions, inaccurate reporting can hide a significant barrier to effective medical treatments. Assisting patients in understanding the need to identify contributors to their medical problems and barriers to effective treatment can be a very important role for the BHS during screenings or during follow-up on screenings that have been completed.

In addition, challenges are frequently multidimensional. For patients, the potential stigma associated with acknowledging substance use when seeking medical care can be a major barrier to sharing that information with the primary care provider (Corrigan, 2014). One attempt to reduce stigma is the recommended implementation of universal screening guidelines (SAMHSA, 2011) to normalize the screening process.

At the same time, a medical provider's negative personal reactions to substance use may reinforce the stigma, or the medical provider's response to multiple new demands on them can be a major challenge to appropriately addressing substance use issues at all. McDaniel (2014) points out: "In the emerging health care culture of physician accountability for patient outcomes, physicians are even more tempted to 'double down' on ineffective methods of behavior change such as reciting the information, using scare tactics that haven't worked before, or even antagonizing the patient enough so that he or she leaves the practice. Unprocessed provider frustration is a hidden threat to good health care" (McDaniel, 2014, p. 148).

The BHS working in an integrated care setting can enhance the environment/context for addressing these important substance use issues. McDaniel (2014) notes that the BHS is in a unique position of bringing a systems approach to intervention that includes all team members as well as the patient and his or her family. She points out that the core skill of accurate empathy should be used when the behavioral health provider is interacting with patients and with medical providers. In particular, avoiding a lecturing approach in giving feedback to a medical provider about his or her approach to addressing substance use issues with a patient (e.g., "being critical of the doctor for being critical of the patient") is important.

The best known comprehensive model of brief interventions used in the primary care setting is motivational interviewing (MI) (Miller & Rollnick, 2013; Rollnick, Miller, & Butler, 2008). MI-based interventions are appropriate for a wide variety of health-related problems that benefit from behavior change (Rollnick, Mason, & Butler, 1999). For substance use behaviors, SAMHSA has integrated MI into the SBIRT model that has been implemented in many primary care practices (O'Donnell, et al., 2014; SAMHSA, 2011). In the SBIRT model, following the initial "screening" discussed earlier in this chapter, further assessment and verification of risky substance use behaviors are completed and the identification of the current Stage of Change is made. The type of intervention that may be most beneficial in modifying substance use behavior is selected based on the extent of substance use (e.g., risky use vs. dependency) as well as the patient's current readiness to change.

The Stage of Change model (Connors, DiClemente, Velasquez, & Donovan, 2013; DiClemente, 2003; Prochaska & DiClemente, 1992; Prochaska, DiClemente, & Norcross, 1992) focuses on the patient's resistance to change and interventions that may help move the patient toward an active commitment to change behaviors. The Stages include Precontemplation, Contemplation, Preparation, Action, Maintenance, and Recurrence (Center for Substance Abuse Treatment, 2006). Research on activities that help patients move toward a commitment to change has led to approaches such as MI (Miller & Rollnick, 2002). To help move toward a commitment to change, the primary focus is on the patient's level of ambivalence regarding the change. By exploring the pros and cons of the behavior with the patient, the BHS facilitates the patient's own identification of reasons to change. The "decisional balance" is used to guide the process and when the cons for not changing the behavior outweigh the pros, movement toward a change plan will typically occur (Connors et al., 2013; Prochaska, 1994).

SAMHSA (2011) suggests the following goals for each Stage of Change as a guideline:

Precontemplation: Raising awareness of the problem
Contemplation: Resolving ambivalence and choosing positive change
Preparation: Identifying appropriate change strategies
Action: Implementing change strategies, learning to avoid/limit relapse
Maintenance: Developing new skills for maintaining recovery
Recurrence: Recovering quickly and resuming the change process

To achieve these goals, the two broad categories of brief counseling interventions are Brief Intervention (BI) and Brief Treatment (BT). Most BIs in primary care incorporate skills from MI (Miller & Rollnick, 2013) as a foundation but also expand into skills from cognitive behavioral therapy (CBT) models depending on the complexity of the identified problems. It should be noted that MI is not based on the "transtheoretical model" of the Stages of Change but "are, in essence, kissing cousins" (Miller & Rollnick, 2009, p. 130). MI is a directive, client-centered approach for eliciting behavior change by helping clients explore and resolve ambivalence (Miller & Rollnick, 2002). In the MI approach to behavior change, "It is the patient who should be voicing the arguments for change" (Rollnick et al., 2008, p. 8). In fact, one of the self-assessment questions suggested by the Center for Evidence-Based Practices for determining "Am I doing this right?" is "Do I listen more than I talk?" (www.centerforebp.case.edu/resources/tools/mi-reminder-card; retrieved January 22, 2015). This method of facilitating behavior change has been well supported by research over the past several decades (Miller & Rollnick, 2013).

Skills in MI include both basic and advanced components. A study of fidelity with the MI model conducted by Dunn and colleagues (Dunn et al., 2015) indicated that skills using the basic components ("beginning proficiency in MI") were demonstrated by both medical professionals and BHSs up to 40 months posttraining, but more advanced skills in MI ("competency in MI") were more likely to be demonstrated by BHSs. This study indirectly supports the idea that behavioral health providers have foundational skills that enhance the development of competency in using more advanced skills such as MI for effectively addressing substance use issues in the primary care setting.

Miller and Moyers (2006) summarize the learning process in developing skills in MI: "Based on our research and experience in providing training on MI, practitioners acquire expertise in this method through a sequence of eight stages: (a) openness to collaboration with clients' own expertise, (b) proficiency in client-centered counseling, including accurate empathy, (c) recognition of key aspects of client speech that guide the practice of MI, (d) eliciting and strengthening client change talk, (e) rolling with resistance, (f) negotiating change plans, (g) consolidating client commitment, and (h) switching flexibly between MI and other intervention styles." Training programs for implementing an SBIRT program in health care settings incorporate these skills (Center for Substance Abuse Treatment, 2006).

BI is defined as "a time-limited, patient-centered strategy that focuses on changing a patient's behavior by increasing insight and awareness regarding substance use" (SAMHSA, 2014). The goal of BI is primarily to educate patients about the behavior and to enhance their motivation to reduce risky behavior. BI is considered most appropriate if (a) the initial screening indicates mild-to-moderate substance use that may place them at future risk but is not currently risky or dependent, (b) the patient appears to be at risk for experiencing negative consequences as a result of current patterns but isn't ready to change or modify the behavior, (c) the patient has coexisting illness or medical conditions that may be worsened by continued drinking or may interfere with medications that are being used to treat those conditions, or (d) the patient refuses referral for further assessment or treatment of probable addiction. Typically, BI involves one to five sessions lasting anywhere from 5 to 60 minutes each, with a minimum of 15 minutes required for billing for the service (SAMHSA, 2011). For those in the early stages of a substance use problem, BI in the context of an SBIRT model can be highly effective and has been shown to save $4.30 in primary care costs for every $1.00 spent (Fleming et al., 2002). In the case of probable addiction, facilitating referral for treatment is the primary goal for the BHS. Recent studies have indicated that BI is inadequate for achieving behavior change if dependency is likely (Saitz, 2010).

The focus of BT as defined in the SBIRT model is on more in-depth issues such as addressing long-term problems with risky substance use or comorbid issues such as depression. Advanced techniques beyond basic MI skills may be needed including the use of CBT techniques discussed by Sanchez and Burg in Chapter 3 of this volume. Depending on the nature of these additional issues, CBT techniques such as motivational enhancement, behavioral activation, and problem-solving therapy may be used. BI may be used initially to increase the motivation of patients to engage in BT. While BI may be provided by medical providers as well as BHSs, BT is usually provided by the BHS. BT may involve five to 12 sessions with each session usually being of greater length than BI sessions. In some cases, BT may be focused on helping the patient accept referral for treatment in a specialized program when either addiction or complexity, beyond what can be addressed in the primary care setting, is present.

The typical scenario for BHSs varies depending on their immediate availability in the clinic. If the BHS is available at the time the patient agrees with the plan, a "warm handoff" while the patient is still in the clinic may occur (the patient is introduced to the BHS by the primary care provider). In this instance, the BHS may complete a full assessment, clarifying the focus of subsequent interventions, or may schedule a follow-up time that is more convenient for the patient. In the latter instance, assessment of the Stage of Change should be accomplished and initial use of MI to facilitate the follow-up contact is recommended. When the BHS is unavailable for a "warm handoff," the primary care provider should provide the initial use of MI focused on facilitating the patient's acceptance of the referral. Frequently, this is a critical initial step that increases the likelihood the referral process will be completed.

When the BHS makes contact with the patient, a typical encounter involves the following seven steps. Examples of possible responses at each step are provided:

1. Asking permission to discuss with them the primary care provider's assessment and agreed upon plan:
   "I appreciate your agreement to meet with me. Could we take a minute or so to discuss the plan you made with your primary care provider?"
2. After receiving permission to proceed, discussion of the plan described in the referral is followed by conducting a full screen of current substance use (e.g., AUDIT, DAST):
   "To help us provide the best services we can for you, would you mind if I asked you a few more questions that can help identify what may be the best plan for your care?"
3. Providing feedback on the results of the screening such as risk level indicated by the score on the AUDIT/DAST:
   If scores fall in the "At Risk" or "Harmful/High Risk" levels: "I appreciate you answering these questions. Your answers indicate that your current level of substance use can be harmful to your health and possibly be responsible for some of your current medical problems."
   The patient's reaction to this statement should guide the subsequent steps. A focus on their current Stage of Change is necessary in facilitating motivation to change.
4. Eliciting change talk and enhancing motivation to consider and possibly make changes:
   "What are the good things about your substance use?"/"What are the not so good things about it?"
   "On a scale of 1 to 10 with 10 being the most important, how important would it be for you to cut back or quit?" (For any response other than 1, "That's great. Why did you choose that number and not a lower one?")
   "Have you ever previously considered cutting back or quitting?" If so, "why did you consider it?" If not, "what would have to happen for you to consider it?"
5. When the patient desires more information, providing advice on possible steps to take or identifying additional information that may help the patient decide about the need to change.

6. Identifying the next steps that the patient is willing to take:
   "If you were to make a change, what would be your first step?"
7. Closing on good terms by summarizing the conversation, emphasizing the patient's strengths, reinforcing the patient's change talk through positive affirmation, and arranging any necessary follow-up:
   "I really appreciate your time today discussing issues that may be uncomfortable. We really want to provide you the best care possible and these are important issues to address for your future well-being."

CASE VIGNETTE (SUBSTANCE USE FOCUS)

In the case described at the beginning of this chapter, the primary care provider's plan that initiated the referral to the BHS includes two important components to be considered: (a) alcohol use—engage in MI and refer to BHS for brief treatment, and (b) Other specified depressive disorder—review stress management skills and refer to BHS for further assessment and counseling.

A "warm handoff" did occur and the BHS followed the MI model by asking for permission to discuss the primary care provider's assessment and plan. The patient was initially defensive when the alcohol issue was brought up. Though initially appearing to be in the Precontemplation stage of change relative to alcohol consumption (i.e., "I don't have a problem"; "I'm not an alcoholic"), an initial brief intervention using MI techniques was provided. Permission to conduct a full screening using the AUDIT to help clarify whether or not risky behavior was present was obtained. Her responses were consistent with a "Harmful/High Risk" level of use.

Her initial reaction to the risk level was surprise that her drinking behavior could be causing her medical problems. As the MI-based conversation progressed, she was able to identify her history of an alcohol-related "blackout" and her increasing medical issues potentially caused or exacerbated by alcohol use as her motivating factors to at least explore possible changes. She also identified a 2-week vacation last summer when she did not consume any alcohol at all, which was positively affirmed as an important indicator of past coping behavior. At the end of the session, the patient was identified as being in the Contemplation stage of behavior change.

Discussion of the possible next steps to take indicated she was not ready to quit/abstain from alcohol, but would be willing to cut down on the amount of alcohol consumed per day. She also agreed to further exploration of her emotional distress at the follow-up session and declined initiation of antidepressant medication at this time.

Training Materials

Many resources for developing skills in this approach are available on the Internet including demonstration videos for different risk levels and for different substances. YouTube as well as SBIRT-specific sites contain useful training materials. For example, see www.sbirtoregon.org/videos.php (retrieved January 22, 2015) to view intervention skills specifically related to primary care and how this approach can be implemented in the least disruptive manner possible. In addition, the website contains tools for use including screening forms and visual prompts to guide the discussion with a patient. Other websites containing useful information and tools for implementing this approach include improvinghealthcolorado.org and www.samhsa.gov/sbirt/resources.

Addiction and Withdrawal

The BHS will frequently be involved in facilitating a referral to treatment for patients with signs of addiction. MI skills are important to help the patient identify reasons to engage in specialized treatment. Familiarity with local resources, including the personnel working in those programs, will make this process easier. Many patients will become frustrated with a complicated referral process and have an increased likelihood of reversing their decision to engage in outside treatment. Support and information from the BHS can be very helpful in maintaining the motivation to change. It is even more critical for there to be collaboration between the BHS and medical providers when there is suspicion of withdrawal, which may require more urgent intervention. This would include instances when patients present with anxiety, hyperactivity, shakiness, sweating, nausea and vomiting, insomnia, uncharacteristic irritability, fatigue, or loss of appetite. The BHS can serve an integral role in bridging between outpatient services and more intensive medical or inpatient treatment programs.

Community and Treatment Resources

Community resources beyond specialized treatment programs are usually available and the BHS should be familiar with these additional options. The importance of patient engagement in these opportunities cannot be underestimated. For example, Alcoholics Anonymous (AA) and Narcotics Anonymous (NA) can be valuable resources for clients struggling with addictions, and offer an additional referral avenue. Outcome studies for 12-step groups are difficult due to the groups' anonymity. However, Project MATCH conducted a randomized, prospective comparison of motivational enhancement therapy (MET), CBT, and 12-step facilitation (TSF; Project MATCH Working Group, 1998). Outcomes at 36 months for over 1,700 patients were similar for the three approaches with approximately 30% abstinent. Subgroup analysis revealed that those high in anger responded somewhat better to MET, whereas those with social networks supporting drinking did better with TSF.

Twelve-step groups have the advantage of being free and easily accessed. These programs offer long-term support spanning months to years, whereas professional programs typically conclude after several weeks (AA, 2002). The groups also provide access to friends and social activities supporting sobriety. However, the groups do lack the safeguard of a professionally trained moderator. There may be members who are abusive or exploitive that the group neglects to deal with. Newcomers are advised to associate with members who are healthy and doing well but that distinction may be beyond the ability of those actively struggling with their addiction. Health professionals can assist the patient participating in a 12-step program by inquiring about the patient's experience with the group and offer guidance. In addition, the health professional may also cultivate a relationship with an AA member who is available to work with clients who may be initially reluctant to attend a meeting.

There are many other self-help programs similar to AA, such as NA and Alateen, and faith-based programs such as Celebrate Recovery or Teen Challenge. The following represents just a few other resources to consider:

www.samhsa.gov A great resource for general information regarding assessment, intervention, and treatment options. There is also information regarding faith-based initiatives.

www.ncbi.nlm.nih.gov/books/NBK64827 This site provides a guide for substance abuse for primary care clinicians.

www.integration.samhsa.gov/clinical-practice/SBIRT This site has information regarding SBIRT and how this approach can be implemented for more effective substance abuse assessment and intervention.

https://findtreatment.samhsa.gov This site provides assistance in locating treatment options.

https://findtreatment.samhsa.gov/TreatmentLocator/faces/quickSearch.jspx This site is an extension of SAMHSA and provides assistance in locating treatment facilities.

www.helpguide.org/articles/addiction/choosing-a-drug-treatment-program.htm Providers and patients can find resources in selecting treatment programs and in overcoming drug addiction.

BEHAVIORAL HEALTH ASSESSMENT AND TREATMENT SUMMARY TO REFERRING PRIMARY CARE PROVIDER

Chief Complaint: Mrs. Peters is new to the clinic and was referred by her gynecologist. She is a married, 58-year-old Caucasian female with an elevated blood pressure of 162/104. She has additional complaints of frequent heartburn and stress.

Subjective/Objective

Behavioral observations: Mrs. Peters was on time for her appointment accompanied by her husband of 32 years. She was neatly dressed and groomed, and alert and oriented X4. Mrs. Peters presented with a moderately bright affect and an unrestricted range of emotion, although there did appear to be tension between her and her husband. While she expressed concerns about her current symptoms, her husband frequently broke into the discussion to express his concerns, particularly in regard to Mrs. Peters' use of alcohol, which he initially described as her "poor diet." Mrs. Peters initially appeared to be cooperative but became increasingly anxious as her husband asked questions about her substance use behavior. Defensiveness was exhibited as the substance use was explored including a strong verbal statement of "I am not an alcoholic" in response to being asked about the quantity of alcohol consumed in a typical day. She presented as being above average intellectual functioning. Her speech fluency was within normal limits. There was no tangentiality, circumstantiality, pressured speech, or indications of a thought disorder. Mrs. Peters denied any history of suicidal or homicidal ideation. She willingly signed and engaged in informed consent for treatment and expressed understanding of confidentiality and the limits of confidentiality.

Overview of psychological history: Mrs. Peters denied any history of previous inpatient or outpatient treatment. She did acknowledge periods of both depressed mood and anxiety, stating she drinks wine primarily to "relax." After further exploration of alcohol use, Mr. Peters expressed a concern over his wife having had a "blackout" after a Christmas party over 1 year ago. He described the "blackout" as having no recall of the party the next day. Mrs. Peters acknowledged the event had occurred and it was a matter of concern. No subsequent similar events were reported. No description of seizure-like activity was elicited.

She described her early years as positive. Mrs. Peters denied any history of trauma or abuse. There is a family history of alcoholism and depression, as well as heart disease.

Social situation: Mrs. Peters resides with her husband of 32 years in a geographic location close to the clinic. She and her husband have three adult children and she characterized her family as being "normal," although her husband expressed concerns that Mrs. Peters is minimizing the tension that exists between her and her children. One son has moved back into the family home after completing college, which they mutually agreed was stressful. Both of Mrs. Peters' parents are deceased, as well as her in-laws. She acknowledged that there have been some significant periods of hostility in her family relationships and in her marriage. She is very active with her business and with her husband's work as an attorney, both requiring frequent entertainment resulting in stress. Mrs. Peters belongs to several community organizations and is involved in many monthly social events. She reported that they had belonged to a church, but finds it difficult to consistently attend. There are no current financial or legal stressors.

Medical problems/health behaviors

Hypertension
Probable gastritis with frequent heartburn
Laparoscopic cholecystectomy 9 months ago

Alcohol use (AUDIT=17): Mrs. Peter's responses to the AUDIT produced a total score of 17, which falls in the "Harmful/At Risk" zone.

Dysphoric mood (PHQ-9=8): Mrs. Peter's responses to the PHQ-9 produced a total score of 8, which falls in the "Mild" category.

Assessment

Hypertension (401.1), alcohol use disorder, moderate (303.90), other specified depressive disorder (311), tobacco use disorder (305.1), GERD (530.81)

Assessment of Stage of Change: Though initially appearing to be in the Precontemplation stage of change relative to alcohol consumption, an initial brief intervention using MI techniques was provided. She identified her history of an alcohol-related "blackout" and her increasing medical issues potentially caused or exacerbated by alcohol use as her motivating factors to at least explore possible changes. She also identified a 2-week vacation last summer when she did not consume any alcohol at all, which was positively affirmed as important indicator of past coping behavior. Mrs. Peters was ultimately assessed to be in the Contemplation stage of behavior change.

Plan

Mrs. Peters participated in establishing the following goals:

1. She will reduce the number of drinks per day to the current recommendation of no more than one per day.
2. She will not attempt to adhere to the recommendation of no more than seven drinks per week due to the number of social events she and her husband engage in. However, she agrees to revisit the total number of drinks per week at a future visit.
3. She will continue brief treatment sessions focused on assisting in the achievement of the above goals, addressing the mild emotional distress indicated by her responses to the PHQ-9, and facilitating any additional goals that are identified. At this time, she declines initiation of medication for depression but will revisit this recommendation if symptoms of depression are not alleviated by brief treatment.
4. To reduce potential stress associated with increased frequency of being away from her office for multiple clinic appointments, we agree to schedule follow-up sessions in coordination with her medical appointments whenever possible.
5. To continue working with the primary care provider in addressing her tobacco use disorder. While the primary care provider is considering the use of nicotine replacement options and possible pharmacological intervention, the BHS is available for collaborative care. There is discussion of the challenge in addressing more than one significant behavior change at a time and how this would impact the achievement of a positive outcome.

Mrs. Peters verbally agreed with this assessment and plan.

REFERENCES

Agaku, I. T., King, B. A., & Dube, S. R. (2014). Current cigarette smoking among adults—United States, 2005–2012. *Morbidity and Mortality Weekly Report, 63*(2), 29–34.

Agency for Healthcare Research and Quality (2008). *Treating Tobacco Use and Dependence: 2008 Update,* Washington, DC: Department of Health & Human Services. Retrieved from http://www.ahrq.gov/professionals/clinicians-providers/guidelines-recommendations/tobacco/clinicians/update/treating_tobacco_use08.pdf

Alcoholics Anonymous. (2002). *Alcoholics Anonymous big book.* New York, NY: AA World Services.

American Hospital Association. (2012). *Bringing behavioral health into the care continuum: Opportunities to improve quality, costs, and outcomes.* Retrieved from www.aha.org/research/reports/tw/12jan-tw-behavhealth.pdf

American Psychiatric Association. (2013). *Diagnostic and statistical manual of mental disorders* (5th ed.). Washington, DC: Author.

American Public Health Association (APHA). (2008). *Alcohol screening and brief intervention: A guide for public health practitioners.* Washington, DC: NHTSA, U.S. Department of Transportation. Retrieved from http://integration.samhsa.gov

Amrhein, P. C., Miller, W. R., Yahne, C. E., Palmer, M., & Fulcher, L. (2003). Client commitment language during motivational interviewing predicts drug use outcomes. *Journal of Consulting and Clinical Psychology, 71,* 862–878.

Archibald, M. E. (2007). Socioeconomics and racial/ethnic disparities in substance abuse treatment provision, treatment needs and utilization. *Research in the Sociology of Health Care, 25,* 171–200.

Babor, T. F., Higgins-Biddle, J. C., Saunders, J. B., & Monteiro, M. G. (2001). *AUDIT: The Alcohol Use Disorders Identification Test: Guidelines for use in primary care* (2nd ed.). Geneva, Switzerland: Department of Mental Health and Substance Dependence, World Health Organization.

Bailey, B. A., Urbin, T. A., Bishop, T., & Floyd, M. (2014, November). *More often may be better: Annual vs repeated substance use screening in primary care.* Paper presented at the annual meeting of the American Public Health Association, New Orleans, LA.

Beich A., Gannik, D., & Malterud, K. (2002). Screening and brief intervention for excessive alcohol use: Qualitative interview study of experiences of general practitioners. *British Medical Journal, 325,* 870–876.

Blow, F. C., Brockmann, L. M., & Barry, K. L. (2007). Relapse prevention with older adults. In K. Witkiewitz & G. A. Marlatt (Eds.), *Therapist's guide to evidence-based relapse prevention* (pp. 313–337). Burlington, MA: Elsevier.

Bouchery, E. E., Harwood, H. J., Sacks, J. J., Simon, C. J., & Brewer, R. D. (2011). Economic costs of excessive alcohol consumption in the U.S., 2006. *American Journal of Preventive Medicine, 41*(5), 516–524.

Brick, J. (2008). *Handbook of the medical consequences of alcohol and drug abuse* (2nd ed.). New York, NY: Haworth Press.

Brown, R. L., & Rounds, L. A. (1995). Conjoint screening questionnaires for alcohol and other drug abuse: Criterion validity in a primary care practice. *Wisconsin Medical Journal, 94*(3), 135–141.

Buka, S. L. (2002). Disparities in health status and substance use: Ethnicity and socioeconomic factors. *Public Health Report, 117*(Suppl 1), s118–s125.

Caetano, R. (2011). Commentary on O'Brien's "Addiction and Dependence in *DSM-V*": There is potential for cultural and social bias in *DSM-V. Addiction, 106*(5), 885–887.

Campbell, C. I., Weisner, C., & Sterling, S. (2006). Adolescents entering chemical dependency treatment in private managed care: Ethnic differences in treatment initiation and retention. *Journal of Adolescent Health, 38,* 343–350.

Centers for Disease Control and Prevention (CDC). (2004). Alcohol-attributable deaths and years of potential life lost—United States, 2001. *Morbidity and Mortality Weekly Report, 57*(45), 1226–1228.

Centers for Disease Control and Prevention (CDC). (2012). *Prevalence and trends data: Tobacco 2012*. Retrieved from http://apps.nccd.cdc.gov/brfss/list.asp?cat=TU&yr=2012&qkey=8161&state=All

Centers for Disease Control and Prevention (CDC). (2013). *Addressing prescription drug abuse in the United States*. Retrieved from www.cdc.gov/HomeandRecreationalSafety/pdf/HHS_Prescription_Drug_Abuse_Report_09.2013.pdf

Center for Substance Abuse Treatment. (2006). *Enhancing motivation for change inservice training*. DHHS Publication No. (SMA) 06-4190. Rockville, MD: Substance Abuse and Mental Health Services Administration.

Cherpital, C. J., & Ye, Y. (2008). Drug use and problem drinking associated with primary care and emergency room utilization in the U.S. general population: Data from the 2005 national alcohol survey. *Drug and Alcohol Dependence*, *97*(3), 226–230.

Collins, G. B., McAllister, M. S., & Adury, K. (2010). *Drug abuse and addiction*. Cleveland Center for Continuing Education. Retrieved from www.clevelandclinicmeded.com/medicalpubs/diseasemanagement/psychiatry-psychology/drug-abuse-and-addiction/#prevalence

Connors, G. J., DiClemente, C. C., Velasquez, M. M., & Donovan, D. M. (2013). *Substance abuse treatment and the stages of change*. New York, NY: Guilford Press.

Corrigan, P. W. (2014). *The stigma of disease and disability: Understanding causes and overcoming injustices*. Washington, DC: American Psychological Association.

Cummings, J. L. (2005). Identification and treatment of substance abuse in primary care settings. In W. T. O'Donohue, M. R. Byrd, N. A. Cummings, & D. A. Henderson (Eds.), *Behavioral integrative care: Treatments that work in the primary care setting* (pp. 143–160). New York, NY: Brunner-Routledge.

Cummings, N. A., & Cummings, J. L. (2000). *The first session with substance abusers: A step-by-step guide*. San Francisco, CA: Jossey-Bass.

Cummings, N. A., Cummings, J. L., & Johnson, J. N. (Eds.). (1997). *Behavioral health in primary care: A guide for clinical integration*. Madison, CT: Psychosocial Press.

D'Amico, E. J., Paddock, S. M., Burnam, A., & Kung, F. Y. (2005). Identification of and guidance for problem drinking by general medical providers: Results from a national survey. *Medical Care*, *43*, 229–236.

DeAngelis T. (2001). Substance abuse treatment: An untapped opportunity for practitioners. *Monitor on Psychology*, *32*(6). Retrieved from www.apa.org/monitor/jun01/treatopp.aspx

Dhalla, S., & Kopec, J. A. (2007). The CAGE Questionnaire for alcohol misuse: A review of reliability and validity studies. *Clinical and Investigative Medicine*, *30*(1), 33–41.

DiClemente, C. C. (2003). *Addiction and change: How addictions develop and addicted people recover*. New York, NY: Guilford Press.

DiClemente, C. C., Schlundt, D., & Gemmell. L. (2004). Readiness and stages of change in addiction treatment. *American Journal of Addiction*, *13*, 103–119.

DiFranza, J. R., & Lew, R. A. (1995). Effect of maternal cigarette smoking on pregnancy complications and sudden infant death syndrome. *Journal of Family Practice*, *40*(4), 385–394.

Duncan, B. L. (2014). *On becoming a better therapist: Evidence-based practice one client at a time* (2nd ed.). Washington, DC: American Psychological Association.

Dunn, C., Darnel, D., Carmel, A., Atkins, D. C., Bumgardner, K., & Roy-Byrne, P. (2015). Comparing the motivational interviewing integrity in two prevalent models of brief intervention service delivery for primary care settings. *Journal of Substance Abuse Treatment*, *51*, 47–52.

Egan, G. (2002). *The skilled helper: A problem-management and opportunity-development approach to helping* (7th ed.). New York, NY: Wadsworth.

Ernst, D., Miller, W. R., & Rollnick, S. (2007). Treating substance abuse in primary care: A demonstration project. *International Journal of Integrated Care*, *7*, e36.

Ewing, J. A. (1984). Detecting alcoholism: The CAGE Questionnaire. *Journal of the American Medical Association*, *252*, 1905–1907.

Fink, A., Elliot, M. N., Tsai, M., & Beck, J. C. (2005). An evaluation of an intervention to assist primary care physicians in screening and educating older patients who use alcohol. *Journal of the American Geriatrics Society*, *53*, 1937–1943.

Fleming, M. F. (2002). Screening, assessment, and intervention for substance use disorders in general health care settings. In M. R. Haack & H. A. Adger (Eds.), *Strategic plan for interdisciplinary faculty development: Arming the nation's health professional workforce for a new approach to substance use disorders* (pp. 47–65). Providence, RI: Association for Medical Education and Research in Substance Abuse.

Fleming, M. F., Barry, K. L., Manwell, L. B., Johnson, K., & London, R. (1997). Brief physician advice for problem alcohol drinkers: A randomized controlled trial in community-based primary care practice. *Journal of American Medical Association*, *277*(13), 1039–1045.

Fleming, M. F., Mundt, M. P., French, M. T., Manwell, L. B., Stauffacher, E. A., Barry, K. L. (2002). Brief physician advice for problem drinkers: Long-term efficacy and benefit–cost analysis. *Alcoholism: Clinical and Experimental Research*, *26*, 36–43.

Galea, S., & Vlahov, D. (2002). Social determinants and the health of drug users: Socioeconomic status, homelessness, and incarceration. *Public Health Reports*, *117*(Suppl 1), s135–s145.

Gibbs, L. E. (1983). Validity and reliability of the Michigan Alcoholism Screening Test: A review. *Drug and Alcohol Dependence*, *12*(3), 279–285.

Gomez, M. F., Nunes, J. V., & Ragnauth, A. K. (2012). Substance abuse. In O. J. Z. Sahler & J. E. Carr (Eds.), *The behavioral sciences and health care* (3rd ed.) (pp. 206–211). Cambridge, MA: Hogrefe Publishing.

Grant, B. F., Stinson, F. S., Dawson, D. A., Chou, S. P., Dufour, M. C., Compton, W., & Kaplan, K. (2004). Prevalence and co-occurrence of substance use disorders and independent mood and anxiety disorders: Results from the National Epidemiological Survey on Alcohol and Related Conditions. *Archives of General Psychiatry*, *61*, 807–816.

Gryczynski, J., Mitchell, S. G., Peterson, T. R., Gonzales, A., Moseley, A., & Schwartz, R. P. (2011). The relationship between services delivered and substance use outcomes in New Mexico's Screening, Brief Intervention, Referral and Treatment (SBIRT) initiative. *Drug and Alcohol Dependence*, *118*(2–3), 152–157.

Horton, J., Compton, W., & Cottler, L. B. (2000). Reliability of substance use disorder diagnosis among African-Americans and Caucasians. *Drug and Alcohol Dependence*, *57*, 203–209.

Howard, A. A., Arnsten, J. H., Gourevitch, M. N. (2004). Effect of alcohol consumption on diabetes mellitus: A systematic review. *Annals of Internal Medicine*, *140*, 211–219.

Hughes, J. R. (1996). Treating smokers with current or past alcohol dependence. *American Journal of Health Behavior*, *20*, 286–290.

Hurt, R. D., Offord, K. P., Croghan, I. T., Gomez-Dahl, L., Kottke, T. E., Morse, R. M., & Melton, L. J. (1996). Mortality following inpatient addictions treatment. *Journal of the American Medical Association*, *275*, 1097–1103.

InSight Project Research Group. (2009). SBIRT outcomes in Houston: Final report on InSight, a hospital district-based program for patients at risk for alcohol and drug use problems. *Alcoholism: Clinical and Experimental Research*, *33*(8), 1374–1381.

Institute of Medicine (IOM) (2005). *Improving the quality of health care for mental and substance-use conditions: Quality chasm series*. Washington, DC: National Academies Press.

Kroenke, K., Spitzer, R., & Williams, W. (2001). The PHQ-9: Validity of a brief depression severity measure. *Journal of General Internal Medicine*, *16*, 606–616.

Lasser, K. E., Kim, T. W., Alford, D. P., Cabral, H., Saitz, R., & Samet, J. H. (2011). Is unhealthy substance use associated with failure to receive cancer screening and flu vaccination? *BMJ Open*, *1*(1), e000046.

Madras, B. K., Compton, W. M., Avula, D., Stegbauer, T., Stein, J. B., & Clark, H. W. (2009). Screening, brief interventions, referral to treatment (SBIRT) for illicit drug and alcohol use at multiple healthcare sites: Comparison at intake and six months. *Drug and Alcohol Dependence*, *99*(1–3), 280–295.

McCormick, K. A., Cochran, N. E., Back, A. L., Merrill, J. O., Williams, E. C., & Bradely, K. A. (2006). How primary care providers talk to patients about alcohol: A qualitative study. *Journal of General Internal Medicine*, *21*, 966–972.

McDaniel, S. (2014). *Medical family therapy and integrated care* (2nd ed.). Washington, DC: American Psychological Association.

McDaniel, S. H., & deGruy III, F. V. (2014). An introduction to primary care and psychology. *American Psychologist*, *69*(4), 325–331.

McFadden, C. B., Brensinger, C. M., Berlin, J. A., & Townsend, R. R. (2005). Systematic review of the effect of daily alcohol intake on blood pressure. *American Journal of Hypertension*, *18*, 276–286.

Mehra, R., Moore, B. A., Crothers, K., Tetrault, J., & Fiellin, D. A. (2006). The association between marijuana smoking and lung cancer: A systematic review. *Archives of Internal Medicine, 166*, 1359–1367.

Miller, N. S., Sheppard, L. M., Colenda C. C., & Magen, J. (2001). Why physicians are unprepared to treat patients who have alcohol- and drug-related disorders. *Academic Medicine, 76*, 410–418.

Miller, W., & Moyers, T. (2006). Eight stages in learning motivational interviewing. *Journal of Teaching in the Addictions*, *5*(1), 3–17.

Miller, W. R., & Brown, S. A. (1997). Why psychologists should treat alcohol and drug problems. *American Psychologist, 52*, 1267–1279.

Miller, W. R., & Rollnick, S. (2002). *Motivational interviewing: Preparing people for change* (2nd ed.). New York, NY: Guilford Press.

Miller, W. R., & Rollnick, S. (2009). Ten things that motivational interviewing is not. *Behavioural and Cognitive Psychotherapy, 37*, 129–140.

Miller, W. R., & Rollnick, S. (2013). *Motivational interviewing: Helping people change* (3rd ed.). New York, NY: Guilford Press.

National Center on Addiction and Substance Abuse (NCASA). (2000). *Missed opportunity: National Survey of Primary Care Physicians and Patients on Substance Abuse.* Retrieved from www.casacolumbia.org/templates/publications_reports.aspx

National Drug Intelligence Center (NDIC). (2011). *The economic impact of illicit drug use on American society*. Washington, DC: United States Department of Justice.

National Highway Traffic Safety Administration (NHTSA). (2006). *Traffic safety facts 2005: Alcohol*. DOT HS 810 616. Washington, DC: U.S. Department of Transportation.

National Institute on Alcohol Abuse and Alcoholism (NIAAA.) (2005). *Helping patients who drink too much: A clinicians' guide*. Bethesda, MD: National Institutes of Health.

National Institutes on Drug Abuse (NIDA). (2012). *2010–2011 National Survey on Drug Use and Health: Model-based prevalence estimates*. Retrieved from http://archive.samhsa.gov/data/NSDUH/2k11State/NSDUHsae2011/ExcelTabs/NSDUHsaeTables2011.pdf

National Institutes on Drug Abuse (NIDA). (2013). *Chart of evidence based screening tools of adults and adolescents*. Retrieved from www.drugabuse.gov/nidamed-medical-health-professionals/tool-resources-your-practice/screening-assessment-drug-testing-resources/chart-evidence-based-screening-tools-adults

National Institute on Drug Abuse (NIDA). (2014a). *High school and youth trends*. Retrieved from www.drugabuse.gov/publications/drugfacts/high-school-youth-trends

National Institutes on Drug Abuse (NIDA). (2014b). *Popping pills: Prescription drug abuse in America*. Retrieved from www.drugabuse.gov/related-topics/trends-statistics/infographics/popping-pills-prescription-drug-abuse-in-america

O'Donnell, A., Anderson, P., Newbury-Birch, D., Schulte, B., Schmidt, C., Reimer, J., & Kaner, E. (2014). The impact of brief alcohol interventions in primary healthcare: A systematic review of reviews. *Alcohol and Alcoholism, 49*, 66–78.

Office of National Drug Control Policy (ONDCP). (2011). *A response to the epidemic of prescription drug misuse*. Retrieved from https://www.whitehouse.gov/sites/default/files/ondcp/Fact_Sheets/prescription_drug_abuse_fact_sheet_4-25-11.pdf

Patnode, C. D., O'Conner, E., Whitlock, E. P., Perdue, L. A., Soh, C., & Hollis, J. (2013). Primary-care—relevant interventions for tobacco use prevention and cessation in children and adolescents: A systematic evidence review for the U.S. Preventive Services Task Force. *Annals of Internal Medicine, 158*(4), 253–260. Retrieved from http://annals.org/article.aspx?articleid=1476724

Prochaska, J., Delucchi, K., & Hall, S. M. (2004). A meta-analysis of smoking cessation interventions with individuals in substance abuse treatment or recovery. *Journal of Consulting and Clinical Psychology*, 72, 1144–1156.

Prochaska, J. O. (1994). Strong and weak principles for progressing from precontemplation to action on the basis of twelve problem behaviors. *Health Psychology, 13*(1), 47–51.

Prochaska, J. O., & DiClemente, C. C. (1992). Stages of change in the modification of problem behaviors. In M. Hersen, R. M. Eisler, & P. M. Miller (Eds.), *Progress in behavior modification* (pp. 184–218). Newbury Park, CA: Sage.

Prochaska, J. O., DiClemente, C. C., & Norcross, J. C. (1992). In search of how people change: Applications to addictive behaviors. *American Psychologist*, *47*(9), 1102–1114.

Project MATCH Working Group. (1998). Matching alcohol treatments to client heterogeneity: Project MATCH three-year drinking outcomes. *Alcoholism: Clinical and Experimental Research*, *22*(6), 1300–1307.

Rehm, J., Room, R., Graham, K., Monteiro, M., Gmel, G., & Sempos, C. T. (2003). The relationship of average volume of alcohol consumption and patterns of drinking to burden of disease: An overview. *Addiction*, *98*, 1209–1228.

Reinert, D. F., & Allen, J. P. (2007). The Alcohol Use Disorders Identification Test: An update of research findings. *Alcoholism: Clinical and Experimental Research*, *31*(2), 185–199.

Richter, K. P., Ahluwalia, H. K., Mosier, M. C., Nazir, N., & Ahluwalia, J. S. (2002). A population-based study of cigarettes smoking among illicit drug users in the United States. *Addiction*, *97*(7), 861–869.

Rivara, F. P., Jurkovich, G. J., Gurney, J. G., Seguin, D., Fligner, C. L., Ries, R., ... Copass, M. (1993). The magnitude of acute and chronic alcohol abuse in trauma patients. *Archives of Surgery*, *128*, 907–912.

Robert Wood Johnson Foundation (RWJF). (2001). *Substance abuse: The nation's number one health problem*. Retrieved from www.rwjf.org/content/dam/farm/reports/reports/2001/rwjf13550

Rollnick, S., Mason, P., & Butler, C. (1999). *Health behavior change*. New York, NY: Churchill Livingstone.

Rollnick, S., Miller, W. R., & Butler, C. C. (2008). *Motivational interviewing in health care: Helping patients change behavior*. New York, NY: Guilford Press.

Saitz, R. (2010). Alcohol screening and brief intervention in primary care: Absence of evidence for efficacy in people with dependence or very heavy drinking. *Drug and Alcohol Review*, *29*(6), 631–640.

Selzner, M. L. (1971). The Michigan Alcoholism Screening Test (MAST): The quest for a new diagnostic instrument. *American Journal of Psychiatry*, *127*, 1653–1658.

Selzner, M. L., Vinocker, A., & Van Rooijen, L. (1975). A self-administered short version of the Michigan Alcoholism Screening Test (SMAST). *Journal of Studies on Alcoholism*, *36*, 117–126.

Singh, H., Giardina, T. D., Petersen, L. A., Smith, M., Wilson, L., Dismukes, K., ... Thomas, E. J. (2012). Exploring situational awareness in diagnostic errors in primary care. *BMJ Quality & Safety*, *21*, 30–38.

Skinner, H. A. (1982). The Drug Abuse Screening Test. *Addictive Behavior*, *7*(4), 363–371.

Smith, P. C., Schmidt, S. M., Allensworth-Davies, D., & Saitz, R. (2009). Primary care validation of a single-question alcohol screening test. *Journal of General Internal Medicine*, *24*(7), 783–788.

Smith, P. C., Schmidt, S. M., Allensworth-Davies, D., & Saitz, R. (2010). A single-question screening test for drug use in primary care. *Archives of Internal Medicine*, *170*(13), 1155–1160.

Soderstrom, C. A., Dischinger, P. C., Smith, G. S., Hebel, J. R., McDuff, D. R., Gorelick, D. A., ... Read, K. M. (1997). Alcoholism at the time of injury among trauma center patients: Vehicular crash victims compared with other patients. *Accident Analysis and Prevention*, *29*, 715–721.

Spitzer, R. L., Kroenke, K., Williams, J. B., & Löwe, B. (2006). A brief measure for assessing generalized anxiety disorder: The GAD-7. *Archives of Internal Medicine*, *166*(10), 1092–1097.

Stern, S. A., Meredith, L. S., Gholson, J., Gore, P., & D'Amico, E. J. (2007). Project CHAT: A brief motivational substance abuse intervention for teens in primary care. *Journal of Substance Abuse Treatment*, *32*, 153–165.

Substance Abuse and Mental Health Services Administration (SAMHSA). (2008). *SBIRT: Screening, brief intervention, and referral to treatment*. Retrieved from www.integration.samhsa.gov/clinical-practice/SBIRT

Substance Abuse and Mental Health Services Administration (SAMHSA). (2011). *White paper: Screening, brief intervention and referral to treatment (SBIRT) in behavioral healthcare*. Retrieved from www.samhsa.gov/sites/default/files/sbirtwhitepaper_0.pdf

Substance Abuse and Mental Health Services Administration (SAMHSA). (2013). *Highlights of the 2011 Drug Abuse Warning Network (DAWN) findings on drug-related emergency department visits. The DAWN report*. Rockville, MD: U.S. Department of Health and Human Services. Retrieved from www.samhsa.gov/data/2k13/DAWN127/sr127-DAWN-highlights

Substance Abuse and Mental Health Services Administration (SAMHSA). (2014, September 4). Substance use and mental health estimates from the 2013 National Survey on Drug Use and Health: Overview of findings. *The NSDUH Report*. Retrieved from http://store.samhsa.gov/shin/content/NSDUH14-0904/NSDUH14-0904.pdf

Sullivan, L. E., Fiellin, D. A., & O'Connor, P. G. (2005). The prevalence and impact of alcohol problems in major depression: A systematic review. *American Journal of Medicine, 118*, 330–341.

U.S. Department of Health and Human Services (HHS). (2012). *Screening for drug use in general medical settings: A resource guide*. Retrieved from www.drugabuse.gov/sites/default/files/resource_guide.pdf

U.S. Department of Health and Human Services (HHS). (2014). *The health consequences of smoking—50 years of progress: A report of the Surgeon General*. Atlanta, GA: Author.

U.S. Preventive Services Task Force (USPSTF). (2004). Screening and behavioral counseling interventions in primary care to reduce alcohol misuse: Recommendation statement. *Annals of Internal Medicine, 140*, 554–556.

Walton, M. A., Blow, F. C., Bingham, C. R., & Chermack, S. T. (2003). Individual and social/environmental predictors of alcohol and drug use two years following treatment. *Addictive Behaviors, 28*, 627–642.

Washton, A. M. (2001). Why psychologists should know how to treat substance use disorders. *New Jersey Psychologist, Spring*. Retrieved from http://uwf.edu/rrotunda/psych/WhyPsych.ShouldTreatAddiction.htm

World Health Organization (WHO). (2013). *Strengthening health systems for treating tobacco dependence in primary care. Part III: Training for primary care providers*. Retrieved from http://apps.who.int/iris/bitstream/10665/84388/4/9789241505413_eng_Part-III_service_providers.pdf

Yudko, E., Lozhkina, O., & Fouts, A. (2007). A comprehensive review of the psychometric properties of the Drug Abuse Screening Test. *Journal of Substance Abuse Treatment, 32*, 189–198.

ELEVEN

OBESITY IN PRIMARY CARE

SHAWN A. LAWRENCE AND EILEEN MAZUR ABEL

S.O.A.P. NOTE FROM REFERRING PRIMARY CARE PROVIDER

S: *CC*: Obesity. *History of present illness*: 69-year-old white male started on Qsymia 2 weeks ago secondary to obesity. He has been thoroughly pleased with the results. He notes his weight is down 18 pounds over the past 2 weeks. He states that he feels great. He denies any palpitations or increased anxiety. He denies any added difficulty sleeping. He notes his appetite is dramatically controlled. He has avoided bread, butter, junk food, sugar, and other high glycemic index foods. He has been reading the calorie counts on all of the foods that he consumes. He has reduced the amount of coffee he consumes.

Patient has still not been doing any exercise outside of the limited amount of exercise he gets at helping to care for his grandchildren. Patient asked about the possibility of reducing some of his medications as he continues to lose weight. He is currently on levothyroxine 100 mcg daily as well as a blood pressure medication. He is tolerating all of these medications well without cough or myalgias.

Current Medications

Rx: Lisinopril 40 mg 1 tab daily—days, 90, Ref: 3
Rx: Levothyroxine sodium 100 mcg 1tab daily—days, 90, Ref: 3
Rx: Qsymia 3.75 mg/23 mg 1 tab every other day—days, 14, Ref: 0

He does not smoke. Has not been consuming significant amounts of alcohol.
No signs or symptoms of depression, anhedonia, or hopelessness.
Review of systems is negative for chest pain, shortness of breath, change in sleep habits, anxiety, palpitations, etc., as noted above.

O: On physical examination: Well-nourished well-developed obese White male in no apparent distress. Speech, mentation, and affect are normal.

Weight: 230 pounds
Height: 5 feet 11 inches
BMI: 32.1
Blood pressure: 130/80

Respirations: 16 and unlabored
Temperature: 98.3
Pulse: Initially 88 on arrival, dropping to 78 later in the office visit
Pulse oxygen: 96% on room air
Lungs: Clear
Cardiac: S1 and S2 normal without murmurs

A/P:
1. **Obesity**: Responding nicely to Qsymia 3.75 mg/23 mg daily. Because he is losing weight too rapidly, will reduce the dose to every other day and see how he responds. I recommend that he not exceed weight loss of greater than 5 pounds per week. Ideal weight loss might be closer to 2 pounds per week. He is not currently having any appreciable adverse effects to this medication. A new prescription for 14 tablets is provided, which should last him 1 month. Discussed with him the value of working with our behavioral health specialist (BHS) in reaching his weight loss goals. He is willing to accept the referral.
2. **Hypertension**: Under improved control with weight loss. Continue current medications but consider possible reduction in antihypertensive medication if blood pressure declines further as he loses more weight.
3. **Hypothyroidism**: Adequately corrected on 100 mcg of levothyroxine daily. No change in therapy at present time.

Follow up in 1 month.

The Changing Definition of Obesity

Obesity is a serious health problem in the United States, with almost 41 million women and more than 37 million men over the age of 20 meeting the criteria for obesity (Ogden, Carroll, Kit, & Flegal, 2014). According to the Centers for Disease Control and Prevention (CDC), obesity rates have dramatically increased over the past 20 years and now over one third of U.S. adults and 17% of children and adolescents are clinically obese (CDC, 2014).

The definition of obesity has been a controversial topic in public health circles and it is valuable to consider how the diagnosis of obesity has developed over time (Heymsfield & Cefalu, 2013). Obesity is currently defined by the federal government by body mass index (BMI). The calculation of BMI has changed over time so that a larger proportion of the population is now considered within the parameters of obesity compared to previous decades. Under the 1988 guidelines issued by the National Heart, Lung, and Blood Institute (NHLBI), clinical intervention for obesity was recommended when BMI was 30 or higher and when the patient had two or more obesity-related conditions (NHLBI, 1998). The 2013 NHLBI guidelines were changed to recommend that obesity treatment be provided to individuals with BMI rates of 25 or more with one or more obesity-related conditions (including waistline of 40 inches or more for a man and 35 inches or greater for a woman; Jensen et al., 2014). In 2013 the American Medical Association (AMA) officially

TABLE 11.1 Classification of Obesity

	Obesity Class	BMI
Underweight		<18.5
Normal		18.5–24.9
Overweight		25.0–29.9
Obesity	I	30.0–34.9
	II	35.0–39.9
Extreme obesity	III	>40

Source: Adapted from World Health Organization (1997).

recognized obesity as a disease in an attempt to bring more clinical attention to obesity and to advocate for reimbursement for obesity-related interventions (AMA, 2013).

BMI is calculated by dividing weight (in kilograms) by height (in meters) squared. CDC guidelines now identify "overweight" adult individuals as those having a BMI of 25 to 29.9 kg/m^2 and "obese" individuals as having a BMI of 30 kg/m^2 and higher (CDC, 2008). Thus, an adult who is 5′9″, whose weight is between 169 and 202 pound with a BMI of 25.0 to 29.9 would be considered overweight; if the weight is 203 pound or more and BMI is 30 or higher, the individual is considered obese. The BMI is used to classify adults into five categories (Table 11.1). Class III is also referred to as clinically severe or morbid obesity; this level of obesity has the most serious consequences for patients and is the most challenging for the primary care provider (Sturm & Hattori, 2013).

Obesity in children is determined by the CDC height and weight charts: Overweight is defined as a BMI above the 85th percentile and lower than the 95th percentile for children of the same age and sex, and obesity is defined as a BMI at or above the 95th percentile for children of the same age and sex (CDC, 2015a). The CDC provides online BMI calculators for both adults and for children and teens (CDC, 2015b).

Obesity Trends

Adult Obesity

Mortality rates associated with being overweight and obese are 5.0% and 15.6% for Black and White men, and 26.8% and 21.7% for Black and White women, respectively (Masters et al., 2013). However, the association between obesity and mortality is not straightforward. Although obesity is associated with higher all-cause mortality, recent research shows that this association may be true only in the two highest classes of obesity (BMI of ≥35) compared to normal and overweight classes, and furthermore, in their review of obesity and mortality research, Flegal and her co-authors found that being overweight is actually associated with a lower all-cause mortality compared to normal weight (BMI of 18.5 to <25) (Flegal, Kit, Orpana, & Graubard, 2013). The use of the BMI as the measure of obesity in epidemiological research is somewhat problematic since the effects of obesity on health outcomes are not determined by BMI but by the distribution of adipose (fat) tissue in the body (e.g., waist size) and the accumulation of other metabolic risk factors (hypertension risk, lipid profile, systemic inflammation, diabetes, and physical activity), which the BMI does not account for (Hamer & Stamatakis, 2012). In fact it is possible that individuals considered "metabolically healthy obese" are no more at risk for higher mortality than individuals of normal weight (Hamer & Stamatakis, 2012).

The prevalence of obesity in the United States varies somewhat by region of the country (CDC, 2013). There are no states that have an obesity prevalence of less than 20% and 18 states have obesity prevalence rates of between 30% and 35%. West Virginia and Mississippi have obesity prevalence rates of over 35% (CDC, 2013). Regional differences in obesity are primarily due to social and demographic factors.

Obesity is not a uniquely American issue. Obesity has increased worldwide in both adults and children. In Europe, estimates for 2008 indicated that 50% of both men and women in the World Health Organization (WHO) European Region were overweight, and roughly 23% of women and 20% of men were obese (WHO, 2014). It is estimated that 16% to 22% of European children are overweight and 4% to 6% are obese (European Association for the Study of Obesity, 2013).

Many low- to middle-income countries are experiencing what is referred to as a "double burden" of disease (WHO, 2014). These countries continue to deal with infectious disease and undernutrition while at the same time experiencing a drastic increase in disease risk factors including overweight or obesity. In fact, overweight and undernutrition exist side by side in communities and even within the same household (WHO, 2014). Individuals in these areas are more vulnerable to improper nutrition while at the same time are being exposed to high sugar, high fat, high salt, and micronutrient-poor foods. This dietary pattern combined with a decrease in physical activity has resulted in an increase in obesity in both adults and children while at the same time leaving the issue of poor nutrition unsolved (WHO, 2014).

Childhood Obesity

Particularly alarming is the increase in childhood obesity. Prior to 1980, only 6.5% of children aged 6 to 11 and 5% of children aged 12 to 19 were overweight or obese (Eliadis, 2006). By 2008, the percentage of overweight children increased to 19.6% of children aged 6 to 11 and 18.1% of children aged 12 to 19 (Ogden, Carroll, Curtin, Lam, & Flegal, 2010). In 2009/2010, approximately 12.5 million children and adolescents in the United States were reported as obese (Ogden et al., 2014). If the trend of elevating rates of childhood obesity is not reversed, the current generation of children may be the first in history to die younger than their parents' generation (Trust for America's Health and the Robert Wood Johnson Foundation, 2012).

Many factors contribute to the rise in obesity among school-age children (CDC, 2008) including parental (sedentary) lifestyle, a child's lack of exercise, reliance on fast food, and increased sedentary activity such as gaming, watching

TV, and the use of smartphones and tablets. While there is a genetic predisposition to being overweight (Francis, Ventura, Marini, & Birch, 2007), environmental factors appear to be a stronger contributor to childhood obesity (CDC, 2008). In addition to the physical consequences of being overweight or obese, overweight and obese children suffer psychosocial consequences including stigma, bullying, and diminished self-esteem and self-worth (Lawrence, Hazlett, & Abel, 2011).

Racial and Cultural Trends in Obesity

Obesity disproportionately affects African American women; approximately 50% of African American women in the United States are obese compared to 33% of Caucasian women (Kirby, Liang, Chen, & Wang, 2012). More than 60% of African American adults do not meet the guidelines for physical activity of 150 minutes per week (CDC, 2014). The reasons for the lower rates of physical activity include issues with body size stemming from cruel comments from children and adults (Baruth, Sharpe, Parra-Medina, & Wilcox, 2014); competing priorities (Miller & Marolen, 2012); lack of time; cost; and lack of a safe place to exercise (Siddiqi, Tiro, & Shuval, 2011). In addition, social norms about body weight may differ across ethnic groups. Research indicates that African American women perceive their body image differently from their White counterparts (Schuler et al., 2008), and that African American women who had a larger body shape reported less dissatisfaction with their body size and perceived themselves as thinner than their actual size (Lynch & Kane, 2014; Schuler et al., 2008). These findings speak to the importance of assessment of perceived body size when implementing obesity interventions (Schuler et al., 2008).

Costs of Obesity

The economic impact of obesity is substantial: Obesity-related medical care accounts for approximately .7% to 2.8 % of a country's total health expenditures (Withrow & Alter, 2011). If current trends continue by 2030, projections indicate a 33% increase in obesity, a 130% increase in severe obesity in the population, and obesity-related costs could reach over $950 billion, accounting for up to 18% of U.S. health expenditures (Finkelstein, Khavjou, & Thompson, 2012).

Obese individuals incur 30% higher costs for medical care than normal-weight individuals: They have significantly higher inpatient hospital costs, attend more outpatient visits, and spend more on prescription drugs than average-weight individuals (Go et al., 2014). They also experience decreased educational opportunities and lower overall job earnings (Lawrence, Hazlett, & Hightower, 2010).

Causes of Obesity

The rising obesity rate in the United States and worldwide has multiple causes and is often referred to as an "epidemic of obesity" (Mitchell, Catenacci, Wyatt, & Hill, 2011). While individual behavioral factors (food consumption and physical activity) are considered the most important cause of the obesity epidemic, Wright and Aronne (2012) review the complexity of causal factors.

They discuss the overall "food environment" as a main contributor, including the availability of higher calorie and higher fat foods, increasing fast food options, and increasing portion sizes. They also review clinical and structural causes, including certain commonly prescribed medications that can lead to weight gain including certain psychotropic medications, antihypertensives, and antihistamines. Additionally, social network studies have demonstrated that individuals are more likely to be obese if persons close to them in their social network (friends and family) are obese. Finally, U.S. social policies contribute to the obesity epidemic such as via agricultural subsidies that have increased the volume of affordable food in the United States (Wright & Aronne, 2012).

Lifestyle Factors

Lack of physical activity is clearly associated with overweight and obesity. Exercise is known to play a critical role in both the prevention and treatment of obesity among children and adolescents. In addition to weight loss and improving mood and appearance, exercise lowers blood pressure, reduces risk of coronary artery disease and hypertension, and lowers depression and anxiety (Davis et al., 2011).

While it is most often assumed that eating too much is the cause of obesity, numerous studies suggest that the lack of exercise may be equally or more important to weight control than eating habits (Stanford University School of Medicine, 2014). Studies have shown that lifestyle changes are effective in weight loss in the short term. Conversely, regular exercise has been shown to be one of the best predictors of successful weight maintenance, particularly beginning in childhood (Laguna, Ruiz, Gallardo, Garcia-Pastor, & Aznar, 2013).

Emotional Factors

Obesity is associated with several mental health disorders including depression (Beydoun & Wang, 2010; Ul-Haq et al., 2014), anxiety (Petry, Barry, Pietrzak, & Wagner, 2008), and eating disorders (Villarejo et al., 2013).

While depression has been linked to obesity there are inconsistent findings about the direction of causality between depression and obesity (Chou & Yu, 2013). To examine the relationship between obesity and depression in adults, Ul-Haq et al. (2014) conducted a cross-sectional study examining several measures of adiposity (BMI, waist circumference, waist–hip ratio, and body fat percentage). Results indicated that being overweight or obese was significantly associated with major depression, regardless of the measurement utilized. The association of overall obesity to depression was stronger in women (Carpenter, Hasin, Allison, & Faith, 2000; Dragan & Akhtar-Danesh, 2007; Heo, Pietrobelli, Fontaine, Sirey, & Faith, 2006; Onyike, Crum, Lee, Lyketsos, & Eaton, 2003). Only men with Class III obesity were found to have a greater increased risk of depression than women. Heo et al. (2006) found higher rates of depressed mood among women who were obese or overweight as compared to those who were not overweight or obese, especially among Hispanic women. In a systematic review, Luppino et al. (2010) concluded that depression was predictive of developing obesity in males and females.

One possible explanation for some of the inconsistent findings surrounding the relationship between depression and obesity is that depression presents in many different ways. Some depressed individuals experience insomnia and loss of appetite, while others experience hypersomnia and increased appetite. The latter of these two presentations may put the individual at a higher risk of obesity (Chou & Yu, 2013). Rates of sleep deprivation are associated with obesity (Knutson, Spiegel, Penev, & Van Cauter, 2007).

Sjöberg, Nilsson, and Leppert (2005) found that among 15 to 17 year olds, obesity was significantly related to depression, shame, and depressive symptoms (Anderson, Cohen, Naumova, & Must, 2006; Goodman & Whitaker, 2002). Shame in adolescents has been found to increase the risk of depression (Sjöberg et al., 2005). Prospective studies show childhood obesity can lead to future low self-esteem (Hesketh, Wake, & Waters, 2004; Strauss, Rodzlisky, Burack, & Colin, 2001; Tiggeman, 2005). Weight-based teasing and criticism from parents mediate this relationship between obesity and self-esteem and may mediate the relationship between depression and obesity in adolescents (Davison, Markey, & Birch, 2003; Eisenberg, Neumark-Sztainer, & Story, 2003; Keery, Boutelle, van den Berg, & Thompson, 2005; Puhl & Latner, 2007). The same result was found regarding the relationship between body dissatisfaction and body weight; actual body weight does not affect one's body image but rather the effect is moderated by teasing. In other words, it is not necessarily body weight that leads to body dissatisfaction but the teasing that often accompanies it (Keery et al., 2005).

Environmental Factors

Poverty and Obesity

Economically disadvantaged adults and children are especially at risk for poor nutrition, obesity, and related physical diseases (Trust for America's Health and the Robert Wood Johnson Foundation, 2012). Socioeconomic disadvantage may lead to weight differences later on in life, particularly for women, and immigrant status may also increase vulnerability to overweight and obesity (McCullough & Marks, 2014). The term "immigrant paradox" refers to the phenomenon wherein obesity is less prevalent in residents of home countries and new first-generation immigrants compared to second- and third-generation immigrants (Glick & Yabiku, 2014).

Weight issues may also be influenced by culture among different ethnic groups. Approximately one third of Spanish-speaking Latinos, the largest minority group in the United States making up 16.7% of the total population, are obese (United States Census Bureau, 2011). What is particularly concerning is that 30.7% of Latino/Hispanic persons lack health insurance and many have difficulty accessing the health care system to receive treatment or preventive services related to obesity (Gerchow et al., 2014). Research indicates that tobacco use, alcohol intake, consumption of fruits and vegetables, lack of physical activity, and general poor nutrition are associated with obesity in the Latino population (CDC, 2010).

Consequences of Obesity

Medical Consequences

The greater the BMI, the greater the risk for developing chronic illnesses such as hypertension, diabetes, osteoarthritis, coronary heart disease (CHD), sleep apnea, gallbladder disease, and some cancers such as endometrial, breast, and colon (WHO, 2014). Obstructive sleep apnea, where the upper airway is restricted when lying down, is associated with obesity, and sleep apnea is associated with cardiovascular disease (CVD) and diabetes (Imes & Burke, 2014). As mentioned earlier, it is clear that obesity is a significant risk factor for diabetes; however, the relationship appears to be more complicated in terms of mortality among diabetics. Findings from a cross-sectional study using National Health Interview Survey data (Jackson et al., 2014) indicated that mortality decreased with increasing BMI among individuals with diabetes. However, prospective studies of the relationship between obesity and diabetes are needed to understand the causal pathways between them.

A study conducted by Borrell and Samuel (2014) found that compared with average-weight adults, adults who are obese had at least a 20% significantly higher rate of all-cause death and CVD. The risk of death was greatest among adults aged 45 to 64 for all-cause and CVD mortality and among women for all-cause mortality (Borrell & Samuel, 2014).

Stigma

Stigma and discrimination against overweight individuals have increased along with rising obesity rates. One study reported a 66% increase in weight-based discrimination in the United States between 1995 and 2005 (Andreyeva, Puhl, & Brownell, 2008). Individuals who are overweight or obese are often perceived as less active, less intelligent, lazy, unattractive, less popular, less successful, and less athletic than people of average weight (Harris, Harris, & Bochner, 1982; Hebl & Heatherton, 1997; Latner & Stunkard, 2003).

A classic study on obesity stigmatization (Richardson, Goodman, Hastorf, & Dornbusch, 1961) asked adolescent children to rank pictures of children (four with disabilities, one "average," and one overweight) based on who they would most like to befriend. Results indicated that the overweight child was ranked as the most "unlikeable." This study was replicated by Latner and Stunkard (2003) and the findings were very similar.

Approximately 50% of obese boys and 58% of obese girls report having experienced significant problems with their peers (Warschburger, 2005). The victimization experienced by overweight and obese children typically includes verbal teasing, physical bullying, and relational victimization (Puhl & Latner, 2007).

PRIMARY CARE RESPONSE TO OBESITY

The rise in chronic disorders and diseases such as diabetes, heart disease, stroke, and cancers, which are often linked to obesity as well as other factors (substance use, culture, genetics, environment), has resulted in the utilization of a wide range of medical interventions for obesity and behavioral approaches aimed at preventing and treating obesity. Weight loss programs are especially important for preventing or delaying the onset of Type 2 diabetes, and for lowering blood lipid levels, waist circumference, and the risk for cardiovascular disease. Behavioral interventions are considered the first-line treatment for obesity and have been shown to lead to 8- to 15-pound weight loss (Moyer, 2012). For more severe obesity and/or intractable obesity, behavioral interventions can be paired with medical interventions, either pharmacologic or surgical.

Clinical Assessment of Obesity

The primary care team is critical in screening for obesity and providing guidance and support to overweight or obese patients (Kushner & Ryan, 2014). The U.S. Preventative Services Taskforce (USPSTF) Guidelines for Screening for and Management of Obesity in Adults recommends screening all adults for obesity and those with a BMI greater than or equal to 30 kg/m^2 be assigned to "intensive, multicomponent behavioral interventions" including setting weight loss goals, improving diet and nutrition and physical activity, addressing barriers to change, self-monitoring, and strategizing how to maintain these lifestyles (Moyer, 2012). The USPSTF also recommends intensive obesity interventions, specifically 12 to 26 sessions in the first year. Despite the high rates of obesity in our country and the USPSTF recommendations, identification and treatment rates for obesity remain low. As few as one third of obese adults are diagnosed with obesity; male patients and older patients are less likely to be diagnosed, and patients in Class II and Class III obesity are more likely to be diagnosed. Furthermore, only one fifth of obese adults are provided with weight reduction counseling and fewer are provided dietary or exercise counseling (Bleich, Pickett-Blakely, & Cooper, 2011).

Behavioral Assessment

A dietary and weight history is needed for all patients, and patients should be shown how to complete dietary record forms with the date, time, type of food eaten, and amount of each food eaten so that their progress can be evaluated. Identifying behavioral and biopsychosocial determinants of weight gain is also important to developing individualized treatment plans. Stressful life events, smoking cessation, hormone fluctuations, and/or changes in eating and exercise habits are all common triggers for weight gain (Ogden, Stavrinaki, & Stubbs, 2009). It is also important to assess an individual's mental health status. This information should be routinely obtained at patient visits. Mood disorders are common among the general population as well as among people with obesity and may interfere with motivation to lose weight (Luppino et al., 2010). If a person is found to be suffering from depression, mental health counseling should be part of the treatment plan (Ryan & Heaner, 2013).

Treatment Approaches

There is strong evidence that behavioral interventions, especially when paired with pharmaceutical obesity treatments, improve patients' weight loss in primary care settings. Intensity of behavioral interventions is associated with more weight loss (LeBlanc, O'Connor, Whitlock, Patnode, & Kapka, 2011). Weekly sessions for 4 to 6 months are recommended and group interventions may be more effective than individual sessions (Butryn, Webb, & Wadden, 2011).

Brief Counseling Methods

The core principles of counseling (empathy, respect, warmth) are key elements in producing successful patient outcomes (Coady & Lehmann, 2008). Several brief treatment approaches are recommended for working with clients struggling with being overweight or obese. The approaches focus on helping the patient find the eating/exercise strategies that are best tailored to the patient's life situation. This section provides an overview of six counseling approaches: readiness-for-change, motivational interviewing (MI), cognitive behavioral interventions(CBT), technology-supported multicomponent coaching, family counseling, and adjunctive pharmacological interventions.

Readiness-for-Change

Despite the best efforts of health professionals, we have begun to understand that individuals tend to embrace change when they are motivated to do so. Readiness-for-change perspectives have been increasingly used to help understand differences in behavior change among patients dealing with obesity (Logue, Sutton, Jarjoura, & Smucker, 2000). The readiness-for-change perspective proposes that the timing and client readiness for change may be the most important predictor of actual behavior change (Prochaska & DiClemente, 1992). A patient's readiness for embarking on a weight loss/weight management program can be quickly evaluated by the primary care provider or the BHS with the use of a short set of questions in a brief encounter (Flocke et al., 2014).

Motivational Interviewing

MI is an approach that sprung from the readiness-for-change model. Originally developed by Miller for targeting addictive behaviors, MI has been shown to be effective in a variety of venues including weight management and obesity reduction (Armstrong et al., 2011). It is a client-centered approach that is characterized by a warm, empathetic, and supportive therapeutic alliance between the patient and BHS. It requires the BHS to be nonjudgmental and accepting of the patient. The underlying rationale of the approach is that without external resistance, the patient is able to develop his or her own arguments, motivation, and timetable for engaging in healthy behaviors.

Cognitive Behavioral Interventions

In behavioral theory, individual behavior is said to be learned in response to the interaction of person, environment, rewards, and sanctions (Bandura, 1986). Cognitive theory is often incorporated into the behavioral treatment of obesity, resulting in an overall approach known as CBT. The underlying assumption of

CBT is that the manner in which an individual thinks will directly affect feelings and behaviors (Thomilson & Thomilson, 2011). CBT relies on cognitive restructuring and behavior change reinforced by education, role-play, and client homework and logs. CBT for obesity focuses on helping patients to change both the manner in which they think about food, their behaviors related to eating, and their attitudes and behaviors about physical activity. Within the context of CBT, patients work with the BHS to set realistic goals for weight and behavior change (e.g., walk for 20 minutes twice a day).

There is good evidence that CBT is effective in treating eating disorders, including binge eating (Hofmann, Asnaani, Vonk, Sawyer, & Fang, 2012). The evidence for the effectiveness of CBT-based interventions with weight loss in obese patients are inconclusive, but specific components of CBT may be effective and important to incorporate in any obesity intervention, including behavioral self-monitoring, behavior goal setting, and identification of barriers to behavior change in eating and exercising (Booth, Prevost, Wright, & Gulliford, 2014).

Technology-Supported Multicomponent Coaching

Technology-supported multicomponent coaching, which is summarized in the Guide to Community Preventive Services (2013), employs personal media devices (i.e., phone calls, texts, e-mails, push notices) to supportive interactions/counseling sessions between a coach or counselor and an individual or group focused on weight loss or weight maintenance. Evaluations of this intervention suggest that the multimodal aspects may offer more ongoing and creative ways of reinforcing and monitoring healthy eating patterns and exercise. Given the rise in access to social media and personal cell phones and computers, the use of technology to support weight reduction may be an effective means of obesity prevention.

Family Counseling

Behavioral health specialists working with families of obese children can assist them in creating environments that support healthy eating and exercise. This must be done in a gentle manner because research also suggests that parents should be discouraged from trying to prescribe or enforce strict diets as restrictive behavior may only serve to create conflict between parent and child (Birch & Fisher, 2000). Strategies for reducing household intake of unhealthy foods, for parents as well as children, may also be a part of family counseling (Lawrence, Zittel-Palamara, Wodarski, & Wodarski, 2003). Given that individuals who are obese exercise less than individuals who are lean, families are encouraged to provide opportunities for their children to become more physically active.

Medical Interventions

Pharmacology

In the 1990s there was a surge of prescription medications for the treatment of obesity (Anthes, 2014). Two drugs, phentermine and fenfluramine, were the most popular and most widely used. Dexfenfluramine was introduced as an alternative to fenfluramine with fewer side effects. Many patients were prescribed the combination of phentermine with fenfluramine or dexfenfluramine with good weight loss success. However, in the late 1990s after evidence of heart valve abnormalities traced to this combination of drugs, fenfluramine and dexfenfluramine were taken off the U.S. market by the Food and Drug Administration (FDA) (Anthes, 2014). There are currently 11 weight loss drugs approved for use in the United States. Ten of these drugs require a prescription to obtain, one is an over-the-counter drug, and eight of the prescription drugs are considered controlled substances (i.e., have the potential of causing abuse or dependence) by the Drug Enforcement Agency (DEA). Research indicates that people who take weight loss medications lose more weight than those taking a placebo (Yanovski & Yanovski, 2014) and these medications are effective in initiating weight loss and are well tolerated, but that safety concerns remain (Anthes, 2014; Hainer & Aldhoon-Hainerová, 2014). However, these medications are to be used in conjunction with lifestyle change (diet and exercise). BHS can assist patients with adherence to these medications, educate them about recognizing any side effects, and more importantly support patients in their concomitant lifestyle changes.

Bariatric Surgery

The 1991 National Institutes of Health Consensus Conference Statement on bariatric surgery, which is still in use, recommends that bariatric surgery be advised for patients whose BMI is over 40 and for patients with BMI between 35 and 40 and who also have significant high-risk conditions including cardiopulmonary conditions, diabetes, and joint disease (NIH, 1991). Bariatric surgery aims to restrict the amount of food the stomach can hold and the amount of absorption of calories and nutrients. There are four common forms of bariatric surgery in use today including gastric bypass, laparoscopic banding, sleeve gastrectomy, and duodenal switch with biliopancreatic diversion, (Mayo Clinic, 2015). In gastric bypass surgery, sleeve gastrectomy, and duodenal switch with biliopancreatic diversion, the surgeon surgically reduces the size of the stomach to limit the volume of food and drink and to some degree absorption. Banding involves a small balloon attached to the upper part of the stomach creating a small pouch and a narrow opening to the rest of the stomach, so that food intake is restricted but absorption is not.

Bariatric surgery has become an appropriate option for obesity treatment and is now much more readily accepted among both health care professionals and patients. In fact, bariatric surgery is the most efficacious treatment for severe obesity (Kohn, Galanko, Overby, & Farrell, 2009). However, it is important to note that approximately 10% of patients who undergo bariatric surgery will gain back the weight lost (Adams et al., 2012).

The 1991 consensus statement advises that all bariatric surgical candidates should be assessed by a multidisciplinary team in order to make sure the patient is well-informed about the benefits and risks of surgery and be able to participate in a follow-up program. The BHS is often asked to assess a primary care patient's appropriateness for bariatric surgery and to participate in the post surgery program of follow-up and maintenance. Components of a psychosocial–behavioral evaluation of the bariatric surgery candidate's appropriateness for surgery should include a formal mental health evaluation including assessment of substance abuse or dependence, assessment of the patient's understanding of the surgical procedure and clinical goals of surgery, and assessment of the patient's ability to incorporate nutritional and behavioral changes both pre- and post surgery.

Resources for Obesity Treatment

New technology has had a positive impact on weight loss and prevention of weight gain. Electronic personal devices such as computers, smartphones, and wristbands now make it easier to count steps, monitor exercise, and keep track of calories. These devices are viewed as "trendy" relative to previous efforts to monitor weight such as calorie charts and activity logs. Similarly, popular television shows and DVD products have made weight monitoring and health more interesting and desirable activities. The CDC offers a variety of resources aimed at increasing physical activity and nutrition at the individual, family, and community levels. The resources can be found at the following websites:

Increasing physical activity: www.cdc.gov/physicalactivity/index.html
Healthy Nutrition (including information from the U.S. Department of Agriculture and the FDA): www.cdc.gov/nutrition/everyone/index.html

Evidence-Based Obesity Prevention/Reduction Approaches

In light of the rising economic, social, and psychological costs of obesity, there is an implicit recognition that preventive approaches are needed to reduce childhood obesity and, in turn, adult obesity. The move toward primary prevention is a significant change from the secondary or tertiary care intervention focus historically used for obesity. It seems clear that without primary prevention, obesity rates will continue to climb. To reduce the systemic cost of the obesity epidemic, proactive (interactive) strategies are needed at various levels to replace reactive interventions.

Family and School-Based Prevention Strategies

While personal beliefs about health certainly impact behaviors, families and parents play a larger role in influencing the health behaviors of their minor children (Birch & Fisher, 2000). In relation to prevention, it may be that the parents of overweight children may require education about the health and mental health risk that continued weight gain may cause for their children. Parents can be extremely instrumental in helping children to self-regulate their eating (Cozolino, 2014; Schwartz & Puhl, 2003).

School-based interventions have also shown utility for preventing and reducing childhood obesity. These types of programs are community-based and often involve aspects of family, school, and community partners. Interventions focus on educating children about healthy eating, providing in-school and after-school exercise, offering healthy meals in the school cafeteria, working with parents to support at-home eating/activities, and changing the school culture to support lifelong health. This typically includes removing high-fat snacks from school events and vending machines.

School-based interventions have been demonstrated to be effective with children from various races and ethnicities. The Child Health Initiative for Lifelong Eating and Exercise (CHILE) is an evidence-based intervention to prevent obesity in children enrolled in 16 Head Start (HS) centers in rural communities (Davis et al., 2013). CHILE utilizes a school-based approach to improve children's diets and increase physical activity. The intervention included a classroom curriculum, teacher and cafeteria-staff training, family engagement, grocery store participation, and health care provider support. This study included not only majority-race children, but also Native American and Hispanic children. Findings affirm the effectiveness of school-based interventions for reducing obesity/overweight.

Community-Based Prevention

Beyond families, schools and communities are also important in terms of preventing childhood obesity. The American Academy of Pediatrics Council on School Health provides recommendations for schools to form school Wellness Councils composed of doctors, nurses, dieticians, parents, and other community members (Spear et al., 2007). These councils would play a key role in the creation of school wellness policies surrounding physical activity and dietary requirements within the schools. Community centers such as Boys and Girls Clubs are settings in which primary prevention of obesity might occur. These centers often offer opportunities for physical activity by providing educational workshops for parents and children on making healthy food choices and developing family-based physical activities (DeMattia & Denney, 2008).

SUMMARY

In a 2015 review article by the Director of the CDC, William Dietz, discussed the arc of the public and federal response to the obesity epidemic, from the time the first alarm was raised in a sentinel 1999 article in the *Journal of the American Medical Association* (Mokdad et al., 1999) to the current time. The federal response has expanded from the original standardization of the BMI measure, the CDC's development of growth charts and standards that included the BMI for screening and monitoring of childhood obesity, the funding of state- and school-based nutrition and physical activity and obesity programs, and ongoing production of a variety of surveillance data for informing policy and evaluating the progress of obesity prevention efforts across the country (Dietz, 2015). The Robert Wood Johnson Foundation and Kaiser Permanente have poured dollars into media campaigns and community interventions to combat obesity and encourage obesity research. In 2010, Michelle Obama launched the "Learn the Facts, Let's Move" campaign for combatting childhood obesity (Let's Move, 2015). These and other efforts, such as the publishing of calories in fast food restaurants, have certainly raised the public awareness of the obesity epidemic, but how much progress has been made in turning the epidemic around? There appears to be a plateauing in the prevalence of obesity among children and a leveling off of the rapid increase in adult obesity in the United States; however, in certain population groups rates of obesity continue to climb, specifically among non-Hispanic Black males and females, and Mexican American males and females (Imes & Burke, 2014). Global obesity rates are climbing rapidly especially in developing countries where rates have tripled between 1980 and 2008 (Imes & Burke, 2014).

There is a need to accelerate the fight against the obesity epidemic on multiple levels, but the primary care setting is a critical venue for combating the epidemic through obesity screening and intervention. However, it must be acknowledged that overweight and obese patients may find health care settings to be one of the main sources of weight-based stigmatization (Sikorski, Luppa, Brahler, Konig, & Riedel-Heller, 2013). Even in facilities that specialize in obesity, resources for obese patients such as size-appropriate gowns, stretchers, and scales are not always available (Sikorski et al., 2013). Obese patients often receive shorter examinations and are more often ascribed negative attributes such as being lazy, of low intelligence, and overeating by health care professionals (Brown, 2006; Hebl, Xu, & Mason, 2003). Thus, people who are obese are often reluctant to obtain medical care (Adams, Smith, Wilbur, & Grady, 1993; Amy, Aalborg, Lyon, & Keranen, 2006; Fontaine, Faith, Allison, & Cheskin, 1998; Friedman et al., 2005; Olson, Schumaker, & Yawn, 1994). This reluctance is the result of humiliating experiences, receiving disrespectful treatment, negative attitudes from health care providers, unsolicited advice about weight loss, and equipment failures related to their weight (Amy et al., 2006; Rogge, Greenwald, & Golden, 2004; Thomas, Hyde, Karunaratne, Herbert, & Komessaroff, 2008).

The BHS has the opportunity to be an advocate for improving the quality of care provided to patients who are overweight and obese by helping the primary care team to understand the effects of stigmatizing behaviors with patients. The BHS can also be an advocate for increased obesity screening of children, teens, and adults in the primary care setting and assist providers in helping to identify patients who need extended behavioral health support in managing their weight-loss program.

BEHAVIORAL HEALTH ASSESSMENT AND TREATMENT SUMMARY TO REFERRING PRIMARY CARE PROVIDER

Background and Referral Information

Mr. Q is a 69-year-old, Caucasian, married patient referred for assistance in reaching his weight loss goals. The patient is currently responding to Qsymia 3.75 mg/23 mg daily and has lost 18 pounds in 2 weeks. Mr. Q's PCP determined he was losing weight too quickly and suggested that he work on the goal of 5 pounds per week. His weight loss goal is 50 pounds.

Education and Employment

Mr. Q has a high school education and worked on the city police force for over 40 years and retired 3 years ago. He says he enjoys his retirement but believes that his lack of regular exercise since retirement contributed to his weight gain.

Social History

Mr. Q has been married for 50 years to his wife Irene. They live in a single family home and they have two children, Susan and Samantha, who are both married and live locally. They have five grandchildren and are busy helping with the care of the grandchildren.

Mr. Q says his wife is supportive of his weight loss and has helped in changing the foods they purchase and eat. He is pleasantly surprised at his lack of hunger or urges for junk food. He reports having very few stressors in his life and denies any current symptoms of depression or other mood disorders.

Health Behaviors

Mr. Q is confident that he can maintain the new eating patterns and denies any side effects of the weight loss medications. His major goal beyond that is to work on reducing his blood pressure so that he can get off blood pressure medication.

Mr. Q does not engage in regular exercise and has never had a routine physical fitness program. He believes that he would be able to start and maintain an exercise program if it did not require going to a gym. He would like to begin with a walking program and weight lifting.

Psychiatric Functioning

Mr. Q was appropriately dressed, alert and oriented (×3), talkative, and humorous. No deficits in memory or focus were evident.

Mr. Q denies any psychiatric history, any history of psychiatric medication use, or any current problems with mood. He denies any family history of psychiatric problems. He does have occasional sleep problems due to waking up and thinking about the "problems of the world" and how he can help his children and grandchildren avoid violence and financial problems.

Summary and Recommendations

This evaluation confirmed that the patient is adhering well to his medication and to his dietary changes for weight loss and is satisfied with his success in weight loss to date. His mood is stable and does not warrant any further assessment or planned intervention.

We discussed how his rapid weight loss to date may start to slow down and how his weight loss goals could be supported by engaging in a regular physical fitness program. We also discussed how long-term weight loss maintenance is more likely with continued physical activity and that physical activity could lead to better blood pressure control, which is a goal for the patient. Mr. Q agreed to begin a measured physical activity program including walking and weight lifting.

Recommendations:

1. Mr. Q will download a phone GPS application that allows him to track how far he walks and the calories expended. He will start to walk for 30 minutes daily for the first week and gradually increase that time until

he can walk for 3 miles. He will also explore some online weight lifting routines on several websites that we viewed together in my office and pick a routine that he believed he could maintain.

2. I also gave Mr. Q an exercise and a food diary to maintain for the next 2 weeks for the purpose of self-management and to review with me on a follow-up visit.
3. Five follow-up visits are recommended to assist the patient in weight loss maintenance and support of accelerated physical conditioning and exercise.

REFERENCES

Adams, C. H., Smith, N. J., Wilbur, D. C., Grady, K. (1993). The relationship of obesity to the frequency of pelvic examinations: Do physician and patient attitudes make a difference? *Women & Health*, *20*(2), 45–57.

Adams, T. D., Davidson, L. E., Litwin, S. E., Kolotkin, R. L., LaMonte, M. J., Pendleton, R. C, . . . Sherman, C. (2012). Health benefits of gastric bypass surgery after 6 years. *JAMA*, *308*(11), 1122–1131.

American Medical Association. (2013). AMA News Room. Retrieved February 3, 2015, from www.ama-assn.org/ama/pub/news/news/2013/2013-06-18-new-ama-policies-annual-meeting.page

Amy, N. K., Aalborg, A., Lyon, P., Keranen, L. (2006). Barriers to routine gynaecological cancer screening for White and African American obese women. *International Journal of Obesity*, *30*, 147–155.

Anderson, S. E., Cohen, P., Naumova, E. N., & Must, A. (2006). Association of depression and anxiety disorders with eight changes in a prospective community-based study of children followed up into adulthood. *Archives of Pediatrics & Adolescent Medicine*, *160*, 285–291.

Andreyeva, T., Puhl, R. M., & Brownell, K. D. (2008). Changes in perceived weight discrimination among Americans 1995–1996 through 2004–2006. *Obesity*, *16*(5), 1129–1134.

Anthes, E. (2014). Marginal gains: Behavioral interventions work, but not for everyone, and weight regain is common. Are there better ways to treat obesity? *Nature*, *508*(7496), s54–s56.

Armstrong, M. J., Mottershead, T. A., Ronksley, P. E., Sigal, R. J., Campbell, T. S., & Hemmelgarn, B. R. (2011). Motivational interviewing to improve weight loss in overweight and/or obese patients: A systematic review and meta analysis of randomized controlled trials. *Obesity Reviews*, *12*(9), 709–723.

Bandura, A. (1986). *Social foundations of thought and action: A social cognitive theory*. Englewood Cliffs, NJ: Prentice Hall.

Baruth, M., Sharpe, P. A., Parra-Medina, D., & Wilcox, S. (2014). Perceived barriers to exercise and health eating among women from disadvantaged neighborhoods: Results from a focus group assessment. *Women & Health*, *54*(4), 336–353.

Beydoun, M. A., & Wang, Y. (2010). Pathways linking socioeconomic status to obesity through depression and lifestyle factors among young US Adults. *Journal of Affective Disorders*, *123* (1–3), 52–63.

Birch, L. L., & Fisher, J. O. (2000). Mothers' child-feeding practices influence daughters' eating and weight. *American Journal of Clinical Nutrition*, *71*(5), 1054–1061.

Bleich, S. N., Pickett-Blakely, O., & Cooper, L. A. (2011). Physician practice patterns of obesity diagnosis and weight-related counseling. *Patient education and counseling*, *82*(1), 123–129.

Booth, H. P., Prevost, T. A., Wright, A. J., & Gulliford, M. C. (2014). Effectiveness of behavioural weight loss interventions delivered in a primary care setting: A systematic review and meta-analysis. *Family Practice*. doi:10.1093/fampra/cmu064

Borrell, L. N., & Samuel, L. (2014). Body mass index categories and mortality risk in U.S. adults: The effect of overweight and obesity on advancing death. *American Journal of Public Health*, *104*(3), 512–519.

Brown, I. (2006). Nurses attitudes towards adult patients who are obese: Literature review. *Journal of advanced nursing, 52*(2), 221–232.

Butryn, M. L., Webb, V., & Wadden, T. A. (2011). Behavioral treatment of obesity. *Psychiatric Clinics of North America, 34*(4), 841–859.

Carpenter, K. M., Hasin, D. S., Allison, D. B., & Faith, M. S. (2000). Relationships between obesity and *DSM-IV* major depressive disorder, suicide ideation, and suicide attempts: Results from a general population study. *American Journal of Public Health, 90*, 251–257.

Centers for Disease Control and Prevention. (2008). *Overweight and obesity*. Retrieved February 3, 2015, from www.cdc.gov/nccdphp/dnpa/obesity/index.htm

Centers for Disease Control and Prevention. (2010). *Behavioral risk factor surveillance*.

Centers for Disease Control and Prevention. (2013). *Obesity prevalence maps*. Retrieved June 22, 2015, from http://www.cdc.gov/obesity/data/adult.html

Centers for Disease Control and Prevention. (2014). *Facts about physical activity*. Retrieved February 3, 2015, from www.cdc.gov/obesity/data/facts.html

Centers for Disease Control and Prevention. (2015a). *Childhood overweight and obesity*. Retrieved February 3, 2015, from www.cdc.gov/obesity/childhood/basics.html

Centers for Disease Control and Prevention. (2015b). *Healthy weight: It's not a diet; it's a lifestyle*. Retrieved February 3, 2015, from www.cdc.gov/healthyweight/assessing/bmi/adult_bmi/english_bmi_calculator/bmi_calculator.html

Chou, K. L., & Yu, K. M. (2013). Atypical depressive symptoms and obesity in a national sample of older adults with major depressive disorder. *Depression and Anxiety, 30*, 574–579.

Coady, N., & Lehmann, P. (2008). The problem-solving model: A framework for integrating the science and art of practice. In N. Coady & P. Lehmann (Eds.). *Theoretical perspectives for direct social work practice*. New York, NY: Springer.

Cozolino, L. J. (2014). The neuroscience of human relationships: Attachment and the developing social brain (2nd ed.). New York, NY: W. W. Norton.

Davis, C. L., Tomporowski, P. D., McDowell, J. E., Austin, B. P., Miller, P. H., Yanasak, N. E. J. D., & Naglieri, J. A. (2011). Exercise improves executive function and achievement and alters brain activation in overweight children: A randomized controlled trial. *Health Psychology, 30*(1), 91–98.

Davis, S. M., Sanders, S. G., Fitzgerald, C. A., Keane, P. C., Canaca, G. F., & Volker-Rector, R. (2013). CHILE: An evidence-based preschool intervention for obesity prevention in Head Start. *Journal of School Health, 83*(9), 668–677.

Davison, K. K., Markey, C. N., & Birch, L. L. (2003). A longitudinal examination of patterns in girls' weight concerns and body dissatisfaction from ages 5 to 9 years. *International Journal of Eating Disorders, 33*(3), 320–332.

DeMattia, L., & Denney, S. L. (2008). Childhood obesity prevention: Successful community-based efforts. *Annals of the American Academy of Political and Social Science, 615*, 83–99.

Dietz, W. H. (2015). The response of the U.S. Centers for Disease Control and Prevention to the obesity epidemic. *Annual Review of Public Health, 36*, 575–596.

Dragan, A., & Akhtar-Danesh, N. (2007). Relation between body mass index and depression: A structural equation modeling approach. *BMC Medical Research and Methodology, 7*, 17.

Eisenberg, M. E., Neumark-Sztainer, D., & Story, M. (2003). Associations of weight-based teasing and emotional well-being among adolescents. *Archives of Pediatric & Adolescent Medicine, 157*, 733–738.

Eliadis, E. E. (2006). The role of social work in the childhood obesity epidemic [Commentary]. *Social Work, 51*, 86–88.

European Association for the Study of Obesity. (2013). *Facts and statistics*. Retrieved August 29, 2014, from http://easo.org/task-forces/childhood-obesity-cotf/facts-statistics

Finkelstein, E. A., Khavjou, O. A., & Thompson, H. (2012). Obesity and severe obesity forecasts through 2030. *American Journal of Preventive Medicine, 42*(6), 563–570.

Flegal, K. M., Kit, B. K., Orpana, H., & Graubard, B. I. (2013). Association of all-cause mortality with overweight and obesity using standard body mass index categories: A systematic review and meta-analysis. *JAMA, 309*(1), 71–82.

Flocke, S. A., Clark, E., Antognoli, E., Mason, M. J., Lawson, P. J., Smith, S., & Cohen, D. J. (2014). Teachable moments for health behavior change and intermediate patient outcomes. *Patient Education and Counseling, 96*(1), 43–49.

Fontaine, K. R., Faith, M. S., Allison, D. B., & Cheskin, L. J. (1998). Body weight and health care among women in the general population. *Archives of Family Medicine, 7*(4), 381–384.

Francis, L. A., Ventura, A. K., Marini, M., & Birch, L. L. (2007). Parent overweight predicts daughters' increase in BMI and disinhibited overeating from 5–13 years. *Obesity, 15*, 1544–1553.

Friedman, K. E., Reichman, S. K., Costanzo, P. R., Zelli, A., Ashmore, J. A., &, Mustante, G. (2005). Weight stigmatization and ideological beliefs: Relation to psychological functioning in obese adults. *Obesity Research, 13*(5), 907–916.

Gerchow, L., Tagliaferro, B., Squires, A., Nicholson, J., Savarimuthu, S. M., Gutnick, D., & Jay, M. (2014). Latina food patterns in the United States. *Nursing Research, 63*(3), 182–193.

Glick, J. E., & Yabiku, S. T. (2014). A moving paradox: A binational view of obesity and residential mobility. *Journal of Immigrant and Minority Health, 17*(2), 489–497.

Go, R. E., Hwang, K. A., Kim, S. H., Lee, M. Y., Kim, C. W., Jeon, S. Y., . . . Choi, K. C. (2014). Effects of anti-obesity drugs, phentermine and mahuang, on the behavioral patterns in Sprague–Dawley rat model. *Laboratory Animal Research, 30*(2), 73–78.

Goodman, E., & Whitaker, R. C. (2002). A prospective study of the role of depression in the development and persistence of adolescent obesity. *Pediatrics, 110*, 497–504.

Guide to Community Preventive Services. (2013). Obesity prevention and control: Technology-supported multicomponent coaching or counseling interventions to reduce weight and maintain weight loss (abbreviated). Retrieved from www.thecommunityguide.org/obesity/TechnicalCoaching.html

Hainer, V., & Aldhoon-Hainerová, I. (2014). Tolerability and safety of the new anti-obesity medications. *Drug Safety, 37*(9), 693–702.

Hamer, M., & Stamatakis, E. (2012). Metabolically healthy obesity and risk of all-cause and cardiovascular disease mortality. *Journal of Clinical Endocrinology & Metabolism, 97*(7), 2482–2488.

Harris, M. B., Harris, R. J., & Bochner, S. (1982). Fat, four-eyed and female: Stereotypes of obesity, glasses and gender. *Journal of Applied Social Psychology, 12*, 503–516.

Hattori, A., & Strum, R. (2013). The obesity epidemic and changes in self-report biases in BMI. *Obesity, 21*, 856–860. doi:10.1002oby.20313

Hebl, M., & Heatherton, T. F. (1997). The stigma of obesity: The differences are black and white. *Personality and Social Psychology Bulletin, 24*, 417–426.

Hebl, M. R., Xu, J., & Mason, M. F. (2003). Weighing the care: Patients' perceptions of physician care as a function of gender and weight. *International Journal of Obesity & Related Metabolic Disorders, 27*(2), 269–275.

Heo, M., Pietrobelli, A., Fontaine, K. R., Sirey, J. A., & Faith, M. S. (2006). Depressive mood and obesity in U.S. adults: Comparison and moderation by sex, age, and race. *International Journal of Obesity, 30*, 513–519.

Hesketh, K., Wake, M., & Waters, E. (2004). Body mass index and parent-reported self-esteem in elementary school children: Evidence for a causal relationship. *International Journal of Obesity, 28*, 1233–1237.

Heymsfield, S. B., & Cefalu, W. T. (2013). Does body mass index adequately convey a patient's mortality risk?. *JAMA, 309*(1), 87–88.

Hofmann, S. G., Asnaani, A., Vonk, I. J., Sawyer, A. T., & Fang, A. (2012). The efficacy of cognitive behavioral therapy: A review of meta-analyses. *Cognitive Therapy and Research, 36*(5), 427–440.

Imes, C. C., & Burke, L. E. (2014). The obesity epidemic: The USA as a cautionary tale for the rest of the world. *Current Epidemiology Reports, 1*(2), 82–88.

Jackson, C., Yeh, H-C., Szlko, M., Hu, F., Wang, N-Y., Dray-Spira, R., & Brancati, F. (2014). Body-mass index and all-cause mortality in U.S. adults with and without diabetes. *Journal of General Internal Medicine, 29*(1), 25–33.

Jensen, M. D., Ryan, D. H., Apovian, C. M., Ard, J. D., Comuzzie, A. G., Donato, K. A., . . . Yanovski, S. Z. (2014). 2013 AHA/ACC/TOS guideline for the management of overweight and obesity in adults: A report of the American College of Cardiology/American Heart Association

Task Force on Practice Guidelines and the Obesity Society. *Journal of the American College of Cardiology*, *63*(25_PA), 2985–3023.

Keery, H., Boutelle, K., van den Berg, P., & Thompson, J. K. (2005). The impact of appearance-related teasing by family members. *Journal of Adolescent Health*, *37*, 120–127.

Kirby, J. B., Liang, L., Chen, H-J., & Wang, Y. (2012). Race, place, and obesity: The complex relationships among community racial/ethnic composition, individual race/ethnicity, and obesity in the United States. *American Journal of Public Health*, *102*(8), 1572–1578.

Kohn, G. P., Galanko, J. A., Overby, D. W., & Farrell, T. M. (2009). Recent trends in bariatric surgery case volume in the United States. *Surgery*, *146*, 375–380.

Knutson, K. L., Spiegel, K., Penev, P., & Van Cauter, E. (2007). The metabolic consequences of sleep deprivation. *Sleep Medicine Reviews*, *11*(3), 163–178.

Kushner, R. F., & Ryan, D. H. (2014). Assessment and lifestyle management of patients with obesity: Clinical recommendations from systematic reviews. *JAMA*, *312*(9), 943–952.

Laguna, M., Ruiz, J. R., Gallardo, C., Garcia-Pastor, T., & Aznar, S. (2013). Obesity and physical activity patterns in children and adolescents. *Journal of Paediatrics and Child Health*, *49*, 942–949.

Latner, J. D., & Stunkard, A. J. (2003). Getting worse: The stigmatization of obese children. *Obesity Research*, *11*, 452–456.

Lawrence, S. A., Hazlett, R., & Abel, E. M. (2011). Obesity related stigma as a form of oppression: Implications for social work education. *Social Work Education: An International Journal*, *31*(1), 63–74. doi:10.1080/02615479.2010.541236

Lawrence, S. A., Hazlett, R., & Hightower, P. (2010). Understanding and acting upon the growing childhood and adolescent weight crisis: A role for social work. *Health & Social Work*, *35*(2), 147–153.

Lawrence, S. A., Zittel-Palamara, K. M., Wodarski, L. A., & Wodarski, J. (2003). Behavioral health: Treatment and prevention of chronic disease and implications for social work practice. *Journal of Health and Social Policy*, *17*(2), 49–65.

Let's Move. (2015). Retrieved June 18, 2015, from http://www.letsmove.gov

LeBlanc, E. S., O'Connor, E., Whitlock, E. P., Patnode, C. D., & Kapka, T. (2011). Effectiveness of primary care–relevant treatments for obesity in adults: A systematic evidence review for the U.S. preventive services task force. *Annals of Internal Medicine*, *155*(7), 434–454.

Luppino, F., de Wit, L. M., Bouvy, P. F., Stijen, T., Cuijpers, P., Penninx, B. W. J. H., & Sitman, F. G. (2010). Overweight, obesity, and depression: A systematic review and meta-analysis of longitudinal studies. *Archives of General Psychiatry*, *67*(3), 220–229.

Lynch, E. B., & Kane, L. (2014). Body size perception among African American women. *Journal of Nutrition Education and Behavior*, *46*(5), 412–417.

Masters, R. K., Reither, E. N., Powers, D. A., Yang, Y. C., Burger, A. E., & Link, B. G. (2013). The impact of obesity on U.S. mortality levels: The importance of age and cohort factors in population estimates. *American Journal of Public Health*, *103*(10), 1895–1901.

Mayo Clinic. (2015). *Tests and procedures: Gastric bypass surgery*. Retrieved February 3, 2015, from www.mayoclinic.org/tests-procedures/bariatric-surgery/in-depth/weight-loss-surgery/ART-20045334

McCullough, M. B., & Marks, A. K. (2014). The immigrant paradox and adolescent obesity: Examining health behaviors as potential mediators. *Journal of Developmental and Behavioral Pediatrics*, *35*(2), 138–143.

Miller, S. T., & Marolen, K. (2012). Physical activity-related experiences, counseling expectations, personal responsibility, and altruism among urban African American women with type II diabetes. *Diabetes Educator*, *38*(20), 229–235.

Mitchell, N. S., Catenacci, V. A., Wyatt, H. R., & Hill, J. O. (2011). Obesity: Overview of an epidemic. *Psychiatric Clinics of North America*, *34*(4), 717–732.

Mokdad, A. H., Serdula, M. K., Dietz, W. H., Bowman, B. A., Marks, J. S., & Koplan, J. P. (1999). The spread of the obesity epidemic in the United States, 1991–1998. *Journal of the American Medical Association*, *282*, 1519–1522.

Moyer, V. A. (2012). Screening for and management of obesity in adults: U.S. Preventive Services Task Force recommendation statement. *Annals of Internal Medicine*, *157*(5), 373–378.

National Heart Lung Blood Institute (NHLBI). (1998). *Clinical guidelines on the identification, evaluation and treatment of overweight and obesity in adults*. Bethesda, MD: Author.

National Institutes of Health. (1991). Gastrointestinal surgery for severe obesity. *Consensus Statement, NIH Consensus Development Conference March 25-27, 9*(1), Retrieved June 18, 2015, from http://consensus.nih.gov/1991/1991GISurgeryObesity084PDF.pdf

Ogden, C. L., Carroll, M. D., Curtin, L. R., Lamb, M. M., & Flegal, K. M. (2010). Prevalence of high body mass index in U.S. children and adolescents, 2007–2008. *Journal of the American Medical Association, 303*(3), 242–249.

Ogden, C. L., Carroll, M. D., Kit, B. K., & Flegal, K. M. (2014). Prevalence of childhood and adult obesity in the United States, 2011–2012. *JAMA, 311*(8), 806–814.

Ogden, J., Stavrinaki, M., & Stubbs, J. (2009). Understanding the role of life events in weight loss and weight gain. *Psychological Health and Medicine, 14*(2), 239–249.

Olson, C. L., Schumaker, H. D., & Yawn, B. P. (1994). Overweight women delay medical care. *Archives of Family Medicine, 3*(10), 888–892.

Onyike, C. U., Crum, R. M., Lee, H. B., Lyketsos, C. G., & Eaton, W. W. (2003). Is obesity associated with major depression? Results from the Third National Health and Nutrition Examination Survey. *American Journal of Epidemiology, 158*, 1139–1147.

Petry, N. M., Barry, D., Pietrzak, R. H., & Wagner, J. A. (2008). Overweight and obesity are associated with psychiatric disorders: Results from the National Epidemiologic Survey on alcohol and related conditions. *Psychosomatic Medicine, 70*, 288–297.

Prochaska J. O., & DiClemente, C. C. (1992). Stages of change in the modification of problem behaviors. *Progress in Behavior Modification, 28*, 183–218.

Puhl, R. M., & Latner, J. D. (2007). Stigma, obesity and the health of the nation's children. *Psychological Bulletin, 13*(4), 557–580.

Richardson, S. A., Goodman, N., Hastorf, A. H., & Dornbusch, S. M. (1961). Cultural uniformity in reaction to physical disabilities. *American Sociological Review, 26*, 241–247.

Rogge, M. M., Greenwald, M., & Golden, A. (2004). Obesity, stigma, and civilized oppression. *Advances in Nursing Science, 27*(4), 301–315.

Ryan, D., & Heaner, M. (2014). Guidelines (2013) for managing overweight and obesity in adults: Preface to the full report. *Obesity*, 22(52 Suppl), s1–s3.

Schuler, P. B., Vinci, D., Isosaari, R. M., Philipp, S. F., Todorovich, J., Roy, J. L., & Evans, R. R. (2008). Body-shape perceptions and body mass index of older African American and European American women. *Journal of Cross-Cultural Gerontology*, 23(3), 255–264.

Schwartz, M. B., & Puhl, R. (2003). Childhood obesity: A societal problem to solve. *Obesity Reviews*, 4(1), 57–71.

Siddiqu, Z., Tiro, J. A., Shuval, K. (2011). Understanding impediments and enablers to physical activity among African American adults. *Health Education Research, 26*(6), 1010–1024.

Sikorski, C., Luppa, M., Brahler, E., Konig, H. H., & Riedel-Heller, S. G. (2013). Attitudes of health care professionals towards female obese patients. *Obesity Facts, 6*(6), 1662–4033.

Sjöberg, R. L., Nilsson, K. W., & Leppert, J. (2005). Obesity, shame, and depression in school-aged children: A population based study [Electronic version]. *Pediatrics, 116*, 389–392.

Spear, B. A., Barlow, S. E., Ervin, C., Ludwig, D. S., Saelens, B. E., Schetzina, K. E., & Taveras, E. M. (2007). Recommendations for the treatment of child and adolescent overweight and obesity. *Pediatrics, 120*(Suppl 4), S254–S288.

Strauss, R. S., Rodzlisky, D., Burack, G., & Colin, M. (2001). Psychosocial correlations of physical activity in healthy children. *Archives of Pediatrics and Adolescent Medicine, 155*, 897–902.

Strum, R., & Hattori, A. (2013). Morbid obesity rates continue to rise rapidly in the United States. *International Journal of Obesity*, 37(6), 889–891.

Thomas, S., Hyde, J., Karunaratne, A., Herbert, D., Komessaroff, P. A. (2008). Being 'fat' in today's world: A qualitative study of the lived experiences of people with obesity in Australia. *Health Expectations, 11*, 321–330.

Thomilson, R. J., & Thomilson, B. (2011). In F. J. Turner (Ed.), *Social work treatment: Interlocking theoretical approaches* (5th ed., pp. 77–102). New York, NY: Oxford University Press.

Tiggeman, M. (2005). Body dissatisfaction and adolescent self-esteem: Prospective findings. *Body Image*, 2, 129–135.

Trust for America's Health and the Robert Wood Johnson Foundation. (2012). *F as in fat: How obesity threatens America's future, 2012.* Retrieved September 25, 2012, from http://www.healthyamericans.org/assets/files/TFAH2012FasInFatFnlRv.pdf

Ul-Haq, Z., Smith, D. J., Nicholl, B. I., Cullen, B., Martin, D., Gill J., . . . Pell, J. P. (2014). Gender differences in the association between adiposity and probably major depression: A cross-sectional study of 140,564 U.K. Biobank participants. *BMC Psychiatry*, *14*, 153.

United States Census Bureau. (2011). *National characteristics: Vintage 2011*. Retrieved January 8, 2015, from www.ensus.gov/popest/data/national/asrh/2011/index.html

Villarejo, C., Jimenez-Murcia, S., Alvarez-Moya, E., Granero, R., Penelo, E., Treasure, J., . . . Fernandez-Aranda, F. (2013). Loss of control over eating: A description of the eating disorder/obesity spectrum in women. *European Eating Disorders Review*, 22, 25–31. doi:10.1002/erv.2267

Warschburger, P. (2005). The unhappy obese child. *International Journal of Obesity*, *29*, s127–s129.

Withrow, D., & Alter, D. A. (2011). The economic burden of obesity worldwide: A systematic review of the direct costs of obesity. *Obesity Reviews*, *12*(2), 131–141.

World Health Organization. (1997, June). *Preventing and managing the global epidemic of obesity. Report of the World Health Organization Consultation of Obesity*. WHO, Geneva.

World Health Organization. (2014). *Obesity and overweight fact sheet*. Retrieved August 29, 2014, from http://www.who.int/mediacentre/factsheets/fs311/en/

Wright, S. M., & Aronne, L. J. (2012). Causes of obesity. *Abdominal Imaging*, *37*(5), 730–732.

Yanovski, S. Z., & Yanovski, J. A. (2014). Long-term drug treatment for obesity: A systematic and clinical review. *JAMA*, *311*(1), 74–86. doi:10.1001/jama.2013.281361

TWELVE

A SYSTEMS MEDICINE APPROACH TO BEHAVIORAL HEALTH IN THE ERA OF CHRONIC DISEASE

RUTH DEBUSK AND CATHY SNAPP

Health care is in transition, from a focus on acute care medicine in which infection and trauma play major roles to a new focus addressing the increase in the prevalence of chronic disease, which can be caused and exacerbated by inappropriate lifestyle choices throughout the life span. Major advances in science, particularly in neuroscience, genomics, epigenetics, and nutrition, accompany this new era of health care. These advances are facilitating the discovery of underlying mechanisms of chronic disease, the molecular basis for these mechanisms, and their influence on neural and behavioral outcomes. This information is critical for understanding chronic disorders at their root causes and for identifying the primary system imbalances that lead to dysfunction and disease. From this knowledge, health care professionals can develop therapeutic interventions that can help to prevent chronic disease and restore health to those with existing disease. Behavioral health specialists (BHSs) will increasingly be incorporated into chronic care teams and play a valuable role in (a) educating patients on the key lifestyle factors that trigger chronic disease, and (b) assisting patients in making behavioral changes to prevent disease and improve health.

This chapter explores the challenges that chronic disease presents to health care; introduces systems medicine and the emerging disciplines of genomics, epigenetics, and neuroscience; highlights the importance of patient education and behavioral therapy with respect to key modifiable lifestyle domains; and describes the integration of mindfulness into chronic disease care.

HEALTH CARE AND THE CHALLENGES OF CHRONIC DISEASE

Chronic disease is a growing concern in the United States and globally. The prevalence of chronic behavioral, metabolic, and physiological disorders has been escalating steadily over the past several decades (www.weforum.org/reports/global-economic-burden-non-communicable-diseases).

Chronic disease is accompanied by significant costs in terms of decreased quality of life and economic burden for individuals and for societies. The economic burden was estimated in 2010 to be $315.4 billion for heart disease and stroke by Go et al. (2014), $157 billion in 2010 for cancer by the National Cancer Institute (2013), and $245 billion for diagnosed diabetes in 2012 by the American Diabetes Association (2013). These costs are becoming unsustainable to our health care system.

SYSTEMS MEDICINE

Systems medicine is an approach to viewing chronic disease as distinct from acute disease and recognizes the complex interconnectivity of the various systems of the body. The theory behind systems medicine is that chronic disease is a complex web of systemic *imbalances*. These imbalances are generated by the interaction of the individual's genetic material with messages received from the internal and external environments that in turn influence gene expression and, ultimately, the organism's functional ability. These imbalances move the body from its natural state of balance (homeostasis) to dysfunction and disease.

Furthermore, systems medicine views chronic disease as lifestyle triggered, influenced by nutrition, physical activity, thoughts and emotions, relationships, and even sleep and relaxation. Collectively, these factors are cues that convey messages to our genetic blueprint that then influence the expression of our genes, ultimately influencing how well we are able to function within the environment in which we live.

From a behavioral health focus, if we view health and illness from a systems medicine perspective the goal of our interventions would be to intervene along this chain of events that influence the development and exacerbation of chronic illness. Each step in the process to the development of chronic disease is theoretically modifiable and such modifications can be learned, practiced, and sustained through effective behavioral therapy.

THE BRAIN–MIND–BODY CONNECTION

Although it is common in health care today to think in terms of organ systems in isolation (e.g., heart disease and brain trauma), neuroscience research reminds us that the brain, mind, and body are components of a complex, interconnected system that work seamlessly together to produce health and well-being. Imbalances in one part of the system have consequences to other parts that may be quite distant and distinct from the originating event. The body's complex mechanisms are designed to maintain homeostasis, a physiological state characterized by balance and stability. Upon detecting system imbalances it attempts to restore homeostasis. The degree the body achieves homeostasis influences whether we find ourselves functioning as healthy or unhealthy.

A major source of imbalance involves the contributions of the brain. The brain receives signals and translates them into molecular, biochemical, physiological, and behavioral responses. However, the brain can interpret signals inappropriately, termed "deceptive brain messages" by neuroscientist Jeffrey Schwartz (1997), and generate inappropriate physiological and behavioral responses that create system imbalances that in turn decrease health and well-being. For example, anxiety, self-doubt, or perfectionism may lead to the physiological responses of overeating, physical inactivity, or substance use/abuse. These in turn may bring about or perpetuate certain chronic illnesses such as hypertension, diabetes, or depression. In the next section we review the basic characteristics of the brain–mind–body connection and how this knowledge can be useful for behavioral health with respect to chronic disease. We will also explore the basics of psychoneuroimmunology as an example of this interconnectivity and the consequences of system imbalances.

The Brain

For our purposes of understanding how the brain–mind–body connection works and the consequences of imbalances on behavior and overall health, we describe the brain as the physical organ that receives signals, real or perceived, and is responsible for regulating molecular, biochemical, physiological, and behavioral responses. The evolved human brain consists of three main segments, each having developed at different times in human evolution and each contributing to our behavior patterns in different ways. Neuroscientist Paul MacLean (1990) coined the term "the triune brain" to describe these three segments: the reptilian brain, the paleo-mammalian brain, and the neo-mammalian brain. Although today's advances in neuroscience suggest that this characterization of the complex mammalian brain is an oversimplification, it remains a useful way to conceptualize the workings of the brain and provides clues to the brain's relationship to behavior.

The "reptilian brain" is the oldest of the brain segments and is present in many types of organisms. This segment encompasses the brainstem and cerebellum and is focused on ensuring the survival of the organism so that it can perpetuate the species. It is responsive to environmental cues that elicit fear, particularly in relation to the organism's safety. The "paleo-mammalian brain" is the next oldest segment and is motivated by satisfaction and reward. This segment houses the limbic system, which is considered to be the emotional center of the brain and that part of the brain that is essential for bonding/attachment and for emotions (Nieuwenhuys, Voogd, & van Huijzen, 2007). The newest segment to evolve is the "neo-mammalian brain," which is responsible for the higher order functions that characterize humans, such as language, reasoning, abstract thinking, compassion, empathy, cooperation, and altruism. This brain segment is motivated by attachment to others.

From a behavioral standpoint, each of these segments has ancient adaptive purposes that served the organism well in the evolutionary past but are not always appropriate for 21st-century living. Understanding the adaptive purposes of these brain segments and the cues that elicit responses can be helpful in changing behaviors to ones that are more appropriate for today's world. Rick Hanson, neuropsychologist at the University of California at Berkeley, describes how each segment relates to behavior (Hanson, 2013). The reptilian brain is motivated by safety. Providing a safe environment helps calm individuals so that they can focus attention on other aspects of their lives. The paleo-mammalian brain is motivated by feelings of satisfaction and contentment. Within a safe environment, helping individuals feel a sense of contentment with themselves and their surroundings helps to quiet this segment of the brain so that attention can be focused elsewhere. The neo-mammalian brain is motivated by connections with others and a sense of belonging.

The HPA Axis

Psychosocial stress has long been known to affect physiological systems. Hans Selye, as cited by Neylan (1998), first described the "fight-or-flight" stress response and is further credited with the discovery that the nervous system responds to both actual threats and perceived threats with the same physiological responses. Investigations by various research teams into the underlying mechanisms of these physiological responses to perceived stress have provided insight into the cascade of events that occurs with stress (Bellavance & Rivest, 2014; Benson et al., 2013).

The stress response occurs within the limbic system, which is formed by components of the paleo-mammalian brain. The limbic system controls functions necessary for self-preservation and species preservation that relate to emotions, memory, arousal, and motivational and reinforcing behaviors. The limbic system connects the parts of the brain responsible for low and high function. It essentially connects the feeling or receiving regions with the reacting regions, bridging the reptilian brain that receives input from the nervous system to the thinking brain (neo-mammalian brain) that is responsible for higher-order reactions (executive functions).

Of particular importance to the stress response is the hypothalamus-pituitary-adrenal (HPA) axis, formed by the hypothalamus and pituitary regions within the paleo-mammalian brain and the adrenal cortex glands that sit on top of each kidney. Through hormones secreted by these glands, threats (real or perceived) are conveyed to the brain and to multiple regions of the body, which influence a number of physiological processes such as digestive, cardiovascular, immune, reproductive, and central nervous system functioning. Corticotropin-releasing hormone (CRH) is secreted by the hypothalamus, which then stimulates the pituitary gland to secrete adrenocorticotropic hormone (ACTH), which then stimulates the adrenal glands to secrete mineralocorticoid and glucocorticoid hormones. In humans the primary mineralocorticoid is aldosterone, which promotes water and sodium retention and influences blood pressure. In humans the primary glucocorticoid secreted is cortisol. Together these adrenal hormones help prepare the body for the "fight-or-flight" response through such actions as increasing adrenaline levels and nutrient supplies and conserving water.

Cortisol is a major stress hormone that affects many parts of the body, including the brain. Its purpose is to sound the alarm and then retreat, as sustained levels of high cortisol have multiple negative effects on physiology. The body has a feedback mechanism by which elevated cortisol levels are detected and signals are sent to the hypothalamus and pituitary to reduce the secretion of CRH and ACTH, respectively, ending the immediate stress response. However, cortisol remains in the body until it has been degraded and excreted, a process that may take hours to days. Untamed stress leads to prolonged exposure to excess cortisol, which has been linked to damage to various regions of the brain, development of excess body fat, poor sleep quality, low libido, anxiety, digestive upset, and depressed immune function, which can increase vulnerability to respiratory and other infections. The more frequent the triggering of the stress response and the greater the magnitude of the response, the more cortisol circulates throughout the body, the longer it takes for clearance, and the longer the body is exposed to this powerful hormone.

Historically the stress response served the organism well by alerting it to physical dangers that threatened survival. In today's environment, however, this process continues to respond to what the organism perceives as danger, but the threats tend to be more often mental rather than physical. The end result, however, is the same: a negative influence on health. In spite of living in a stress-filled world, neuroscience research offers considerable hope that we can control our stress response, minimize our vulnerability to chronic disease, and enjoy vibrant health and a high quality of life.

One such area of neuroscience research has been the concept of neuroplasticity—that the brain's neural circuits are "plastic" or modifiable and can be rewired. Further, neuroplasticity can be self-directed, which offers BHSs new approaches to addressing chronic disease.

The Brain and Self-Directed Neuroplasticity

In contrast to earlier thinking that the mature brain is not able to synthesize new neurons, we now know that neurons can be synthesized and that they adapt to their environment (Davidson, Jackson, & Kalin, 2000; FitzGerald & Folan-Curran, 2002). Old neural circuits can be dismantled and new ones developed. From Hebb's Law (Hebb, 1949), a main principle of neuropsychology, we know that neurons that "fire together, wire together." Hebb and colleagues correctly postulated that, as the synapses between neurons were strengthened through greater activation, new neural structures—actual networks of synaptic connectivity—were built out within key regions of the brain. Neural circuits are shaped by mental activity. Focused attention creates neural pathways in targeted and discrete ways and neural substrates form in response to conscious learning (Layous & Lyubomirsky, 2014; Schwartz & Gladding, 2012). Specific experiential and motivational interventions could then positively influence the development of neural circuits and, by extension, behaviors that support health and well-being (Layous & Lyubomirsky, 2014; Layous, Chancellor, & Lyubomirsky, 2014). This outcome is indeed what has been observed over the past decade. Davidson and McEwen (2012) review existing data from animal and human studies that document the relationship of plasticity to behavioral change.

Genetic inheritance is estimated to play a primary role in the formation of the neural correlates of emotions and cognitive and motivational processes in the brain (Lyubomirsky, Sheldon, & Schkade, 2005). However, the nervous system is the product of over 600 million years of evolutionary development evolving by monitoring for and adapting to danger and potential extinction (Hanson, 2009). The neuroscience of plasticity and neurogenesis reveals that the human organism is not subject solely to genetic inheritance (nature) or its early childhood environment (nurture). The brain, like the rest of the body, is a complex, interconnected system that is modified by mental activity. We have the capacity to choose how and where we place our attention and this focused attention has a profound impact on each of the major domains of our lifestyle behaviors: diet, physical activity, thoughts and emotions, relationships, and sleep and relaxation. This self-directed neuroplasticity provides the basis for modifying our behaviors and thereby our neural circuits and consequently our health. Through self-directed neuroplasticity these behaviors become hard-wired as new neural circuits and structures that are critical for physical and mental well-being (Kabat-Zinn, 2003; Schwartz & Gladding, 2012).

In fact, mindfulness (training in focused awareness—to be discussed in the following section) offers such an approach. Neural circuit changes, accomplished through mindfulness-based interventions that train the brain to direct, focus, and maintain attention, appear to be an important tool in making sustainable behavior changes (Hanson, 2013).

MINDFULNESS

Mindfulness is defined as a state of focused attention, where one pays attention "on purpose, moment to moment and nonjudgmentally" (Kabat-Zinn et al., 1992). It is reported to have been a part of Eastern cultures for at least 26 centuries, with positive effects on quality of life, such as strengthened immune system; improved social relationships; reduced stress, anxiety, and depression; and increased well-being and happiness (Cayoun, 2005; Layous & Lyubomirsky, 2014). Mindfulness was successfully introduced into clinical practice in the United States in the 1980s by John Kabat-Zinn for stress reduction (Kabat-Zinn, 1982). Mindfulness training has subsequently been adapted by a number of researchers and clinicians to a variety of clinical applications, such as mindfulness-based cognitive therapy, mindfulness-based eating, and mindfulness-based positive psychology. See the works of Kabat-Zinn et al. (1992); Kristeller and Hallett (1999); Miller, Kristeller, Headings, Nagaraja, & Miser (2012); Segal, Williams, and Teasdale (2002); Schwartz (1997); Schwartz and Gladding (2012); Siegel (2007; 2012); and Ben-Shahar (2014) for an introduction to these adaptations. A recent review by Paulson, Davidson, Jha, and Kabat-Zinn (2013) provides an overview of the science of mindfulness.

Mindfulness training enhances our ability to focus our attention, which is reflected in changes throughout the body. Research has shown mindfulness training to improve immune function, strengthen equanimity and clarity, reduce pain, and potentially increase empathy and relational satisfaction (Baer, Smith, Hopkins, Krietemeyer, & Toney, 2006; Davidson et al., 2003; Gard et al., 2012; Siegel, 2007). Baer, Carmody, and Hunsinger (2012) found in 87 adults with chronic stress due to lifestyle-associated disorders that skills developed through mindfulness training preceded changes in perceived stress and led to greater emotional well-being and lesser degrees of emotional reactivity. Creswell et al. (2012) showed that mindfulness-based stress reduction reduced loneliness in mature adults and was correlated with changes in gene expression, particularly in the reduction in pro-inflammatory cytokines.

The changes in focused attention resulting from mindfulness training have been correlated with changes within the neo-mammalian brain. Davidson et al. (2003) were among the first to map the effects of mindfulness to specific regions of the brain. They found that subjects trained in mindfulness demonstrated increased activation of their left prefrontal cortex compared to a control group. Further, the effects of mindfulness training were still evident upon rescreening at 4 months. Hölzel et al. (2011) reported that mindfulness interventions targeting stress reduction correlated with decreased gray-matter density in the amygdala, which plays an important role in anxiety and stress. These and similar studies have solidified the concept of neuroplasticity as well as the value of mindfulness in promoting changes in neural circuits (Davidson & McEwan, 2012; Hölzel et al., 2011; Marchand, 2014).

Psychoneuroimmunology

It has long been known that biological, behavioral, and social factors influence health and disease. However, how this occurs has only been coming to light over the past 25 years. The interdisciplinary field of psychoneuroimmunology (PNI) is providing answers by using a systems approach to understand the interactions among the nervous system, endocrine system, and immune system; how stress influences these interactions; and the resultant implications for health (Vedhara, Fox, & Wang, 2013; see Irwin [2008] for an overview of the historical development of PNI). Key disciplines represented in this field include neuroscience, psychology, immunology, endocrinology, genetics, and behavioral health. Researchers have sought to identify these interactions, define their health outcomes, and elucidate the mechanisms by which stress can influence not only the immune system but many other physiological systems, such as the cardiovascular, respiratory, and digestive systems.

Before considering how stress-induced suppression of the immune system might occur, it is helpful to review a few immune system basics. The role of the immune system is to protect the body against invasion from foreign cells and organisms that are potentially harmful, which is essentially any type of cell that is different from the host's cells (e.g., bacteria, fungi, virus, parasites, and cancer cells). The immune system produces an innate/nonspecific (early phase) and an adaptive/highly specific (later phase) response to the threat of invasion. The innate response happens right away in direct response to the threat, real or perceived, of the presence of foreign cells in the body. The adaptive response happens more slowly (days) because it requires immune cells to be synthesized with specific surface antibodies and in sufficient numbers to attack the foreign cells.

In terms of how psychosocial stressors influence immune function, there are two systems that are primarily involved: (a) the central nervous system and its triggering of the HPA axis, and (b) the sympathetic nervous system, which elicits the arousal response and increases heart rate, constricts blood vessels, and raises blood pressure (Irwin, 2015). Together these systems prepare the body to fight the threat. The HPA axis elicits the classic stress response and the sympathetic nervous system orchestrates the release of neurotransmitters and hormones. The early, nonspecific immune response (also called the "sickness" response) has been mobilized, which includes the mobilization of macrophages (first-on-the-scene immune cells) and their secretion of pro-inflammatory cytokines, such as interleukin-1 (IL-1), interleukin-6 (IL-6), and tumor necrosis factor alpha (TNFalpha). These cytokines are small proteins that communicate the threat to the nervous system and promote inflammation, which is a normal part of the immune response to infection. This response enables the body to focus its resources on fighting infection and is characterized by both physiological and behavioral changes, such as fever, alterations in liver metabolism, suppression of appetite and libido, and activation of the stress response with its release of cortisol and other stress hormones.

Both real and perceived threats of infection can trigger the nonspecific immune response. When this response is chronically triggered, critical energy and nutrient resources are shifted away from the immune system, which can impair immune system function and leave the body with increased vulnerability to infection.

Behavioral professionals are familiar with the behavioral abnormalities characteristic of stressed patients, such as depression, anxiety, and disturbed sleep patterns. Depressed patients typically have elevated CRH, which leads to activation of the HPA axis. CRH triggers the pituitary to release ACTH, which triggers the adrenal cortex to secrete cortisol. Elevated CRH, ACTH, and glucocorticoid levels are correlated with decreased immune cell activity in animals and humans, which sets the stage for a suppressed immune response and increased risk of inflammatory and infectious disease (Irwin, 2015). A recent meta-analysis of studies on mind–body therapies on the immune system can be found in Morgan, Irwin, Chung, and Wang (2014).

Genomics and Epigenetics

Advances in genomics and epigenetics resulting from the Human Genome Project (www.genome.gov) have provided the foundation for examining chronic disease through the perspective of systems medicine. Although genetic material is relatively stable throughout an individual's life span, the environment can be highly variable. Changing the environment can change gene expression (explained in detail in the next section), which in turn can influence physiological function and ultimately one's personal health. Further, several categories of modifiable lifestyle factors have been identified that affect gene expression and influence the development or prevention of chronic disease. This section provides a brief overview of how genomics, epigenetics, and modifiable lifestyle factors provide the foundation for an effective approach to changing the trajectory of chronic disease.

Genomics is the study of an organism's DNA, its genetic material, which contains the blueprint for the operation of the organism—in other words, its operating system. The information for this operating system resides in the linear sequence of nucleotide building blocks that comprises the DNA. To be useful to the organism, the information encoded in the nucleotide sequence must first be translated into the proteins that do the work of the trillions of cells that collectively make up the organism. Examples of these proteins include enzymes, receptors, transport systems, hormones and other types of communication molecules, and structural and contractile components. Proteins are synthesized from genes, which are sequences of nucleotides whose encoded information ultimately generates the amino acid sequence of a protein. Just as words must be appropriate and in the right order to form a sentence that conveys meaning, the nucleotides within a gene are arranged such that their information can be used to order the amino acid building blocks of a protein that, when synthesized, is able to carry out its role in cellular health.

Changes to the DNA sequence occur and make each of us unique in our physical appearance and our functional abilities. These changes typically occur slowly over evolution, with little change during the lifetime of an individual. For humans, the DNA sequence is estimated to have evolved only slightly over the past 40,000 to 50,000 years (Konner & Eaton, 2010). The changes ("mutations" in genetic parlance) in the nucleotide sequence can cause changes in the proteins that result when genes are expressed. These changes within the genome may result in positive, negative, or neutral effects on how well an individual functions in his or her environment. In terms of clinical applications, genetics to date has typically focused on the negative effects on function, those changes that provide our genetic susceptibilities to disease.

In contrast, epigenetics is a process that does not affect the nucleotide sequence of the DNA, but instead alters the expression of the information encoded in the sequence (i.e., whether a gene is expressed and its protein is synthesized). As an example, by attaching chemical groups such as a methyl group to nucleotides, gene expression can be turned on or off. The sum total of all these changes throughout the genome is referred to as an individual's epigenome, which is unique to each person, even to siblings with an identical DNA nucleotide sequence, such as identical twins. Tammen, Friso, and Choi (2013) offer a comprehensive overview of how epigenetics is a key link between nature and nurture. As an interesting aside, the uniqueness of our epigenome is responsible for the fact that, over time, genetically identical siblings begin to look different and have different traits (Fraga et al., 2005).

Both an individual's genome (DNA sequence) and its epigenome (set of molecular tags) are of critical importance in chronic disease. We now know that, like the genome, the epigenome can be inherited. The genome contributes genetic susceptibilities through the structure and, thus, function of the proteins it encodes and the epigenome contributes control over gene expression, whether those proteins are expressed at all and at appropriate times during development and throughout the ensuing life span of an individual. Although many of the details remain to be elucidated, ancestors back at least two generations contribute to our epigenome. More detailed exploration of epigenetics and its influence on functional outcomes is available elsewhere (Cooney, 2006; Waterland & Jirtle, 2003; Waterland et al., 2006; Wolff, Kodell, Moore, & Cooney, 1998). Research on the role of epigenetics in behavioral health is also available elsewhere (Guintivano & Kaminsky, 2014; Hing, Gardner, & Potash,

2014; McEwen & Getz, 2013; Reul, 2014; Stankiewicz, Swiergiel, & Lisowski, 2013; Tammen et al., 2013; Zannas & West, 2014).

The disciplines of genomics and epigenetics are particularly relevant to the development of chronic disease because they provide the foundation for how internal and external messages communicate with the body, brain, and mind and influence outcomes throughout the organism. Think of genomics as "loading the gun" by endowing us with genetic susceptibilities and epigenetics as "pulling the trigger" by controlling the expression of our genes in response to messages received from the internal and external environment. These messages can turn genes on and off, appropriately or not, depending on the messages received and their timing. When the timing of the genes' expression is appropriate for the organism's needs, the influence on function is positive; when inappropriate, the influence is negative. These environmental messages appear to fall into only a few discrete domains that directly relate to our lifestyle choices: nutrition (the foods we eat and toxins we ingest), physical activity (whether we choose to exercise), thoughts and emotions (how we handle our positive and negative thoughts and emotions), sleep and relaxation (the quality and quantity of our sleep and rejuvenation), relationships with ourselves and others (our system of meaning and whether our relationships support or detract from our ability to thrive and flourish).

What is emerging is an understanding that each of the major lifestyle domains has an epigenetic influence on gene expression. It is through epigenetics that each of us becomes the product of the interaction between our individual genetic capabilities and limitations and our lifestyle choices. Fortunately, lifestyle choices within each of the lifestyle domains are modifiable and provide practitioners with targets for education and behavioral therapy to help patients live healthier.

MODIFIABLE LIFESTYLE FACTORS AND CHRONIC DISEASE

Over the past three decades, numerous studies have demonstrated the health benefits of lifestyle intervention. Among the earliest pioneering work was that of Dean Ornish and colleagues working with men who had cardiovascular disease (Aldana et al., 2003; Dod et al., 2010; Ornish et al., 1983; Silberman et al., 2010). These researchers were able to show that diet and lifestyle modifications—nutrition, physical activity, thoughts and emotions, relationships, and sleep—were powerful promoters of health, even in the face of existing cardiovascular disease. In 2010 the Centers for Medicare & Medicaid (CMS) began including the Ornish lifestyle program as an approved program for reversing heart disease (CMS memo available at www.cms.gov). In a cohort from the Look AHEAD trial of 5,000 overweight or obese adults with Type 2 diabetes, researchers found significant reductions in hospitalizations, medication use, and health care costs in subjects participating in the Ornish lifestyle program (Espeland et al., 2014). At the 10-year follow-up there was a 10% reduction in hospitalizations, 7% reduction in medication use, and a cost-savings of $5,280 per patient over the 10-year period.

More recently, lifestyle interventions for chronic disorders have been demonstrated to have positive effects on gene expression. Ornish and colleagues elegantly demonstrated the influence of lifestyle on gene expression in men with prostate cancer (Ornish et al., 2008a). The Prostate Cancer Lifestyle Trial was a 1-year randomized controlled clinical trial of 92 men with early-stage prostate cancer. The experimental arm opted not to undergo surgery or radiation therapy but instead to adopt a plant-based diet, exercise regularly, practice stress management techniques, and attend group support sessions. At the 2-year follow-up, only 5% (2 of 43) of the experimental subjects had undergone conventional prostate cancer therapy compared with 27% (13 of 49) of the control patients (Frattaroli et al., 2008). Ornish et al. (2008b) further demonstrated that diet and lifestyle therapy was effective in increasing telomerase activity, measured in peripheral blood mononuclear cells (immune system cells) from men with prostate cancer. Telomeres are the protective DNA-protein "caps" at the end of chromosomes that enhance chromosome stability, similar in concept to the cap at the end of a shoelace that prevents the shoelace from unraveling. The length of telomeres in human beings is becoming a prognostic indicator of longevity. Long telomeres are associated with increased longevity and short telomeres are associated with increase in disease risk and progression in several types of cancer. In a 5-year follow-up to this initial study, Ornish and colleagues found that both telomerase activity and telomere length increased in the experimental subjects but decreased in the controls (Ornish et al., 2013).

The following sections have a brief discussion of each of the major lifestyle domains and our current understanding of how they influence disease (see also Figure 12.1).

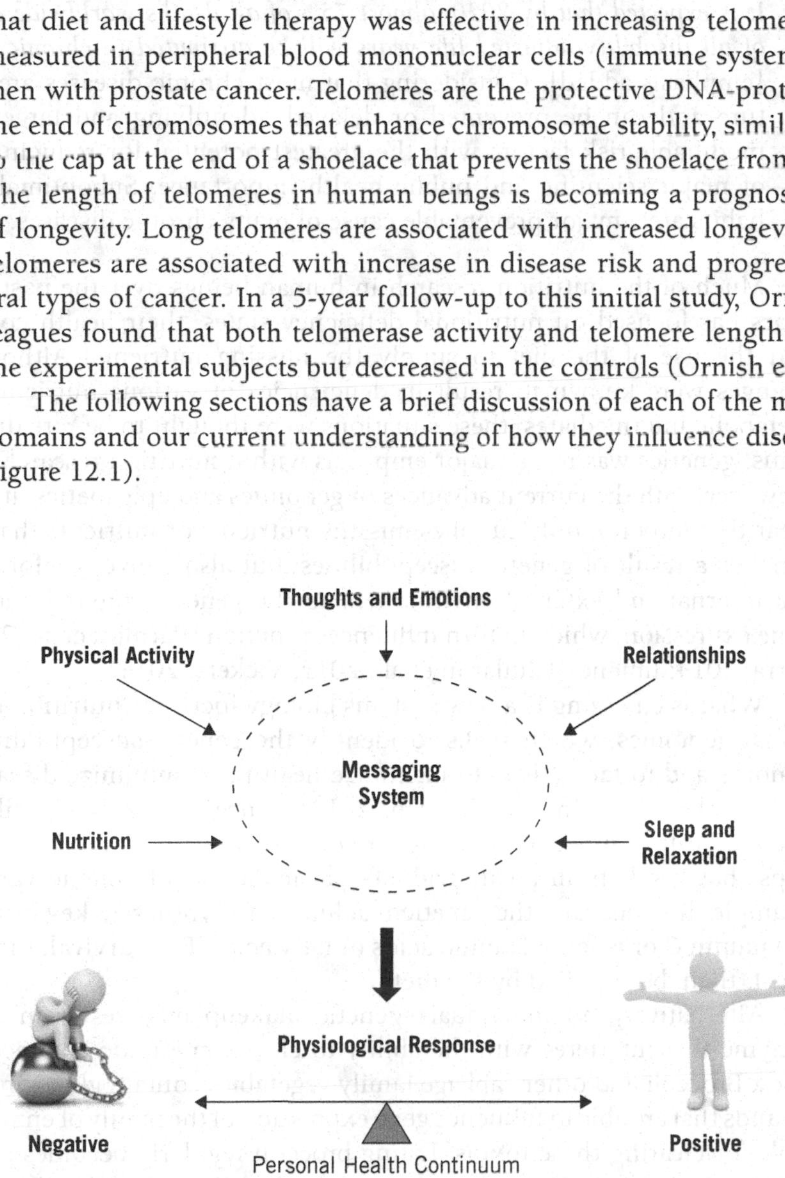

Figure 12.1 Key modifiable lifestyle domains that influence health outcomes. © Mindfulness-Based Therapeutic Lifestyle Change Program; used by permission.

LIFESTYLE DOMAIN: *NUTRITION*

The Academy of Nutrition and Dietetics, the largest organization of nutrition professionals in the world, addresses the role of nutrition in health promotion and chronic disease prevention in its official position and practice statements (Rosenbloom, Lacey, & Stang, 2013; Slawson, Fitzgerald, & Morgan, 2013). These publications summarize the strong association found between dietary choices and chronic diseases and the economic and quality of life costs of these disorders. Micha et al. (2012) succinctly summarize the central role of nutrition in health promotion and chronic disease prevention:

> *It is expected that by 2020, almost 75% of all deaths worldwide and 60% of all disability-adjusted life years will be attributed to chronic diseases* [emphasis added]. Considering that most chronic diseases are premature and can be prevented or delayed, identifying and targeting the modifiable risk factors with the greatest potential for reducing risk is of major scientific and public health importance. Suboptimal dietary habits are a major preventable cause of many chronic diseases. (p. 119)

Much of the nutrition research in human beings over the past 60 or more years has focused on nutritional deficiency states, their health consequences, and the use of the diet to supply the missing nutrients. Although genetic changes were known to result in deficiencies of various nutrients or critical metabolic intermediates, these situations were thought to be rare disease states. Thus, genetics was not a major emphasis within nutrition research or practice. However, with the current advances in genomics and epigenetics, it has become clear that food not only supplies missing nutrients or nutrients that are suboptimal as a result of genetic susceptibilities, but also conveys information from the internal and external environment to the genetic material and influences gene expression, which in turn influences function (Bacalini et al., 2014; Jang & Serra, 2014; Jiménez-Chillarón et al., 2012; Vickers, 2014).

What is emerging is a new systems biology focus for nutrition called nutritional genomics, which seeks to identify the genetic susceptibilities in one's genome and to tailor diets to maximize health and minimize disease (Fenech, 2014; Sales, Pelegrini, & Goersch, 2014). Once genetic susceptibilities have been identified, it becomes possible to develop a diet that can fill the metabolic gaps that result from an individual's particular set of genetic variations. For example, humans lack the genetic machinery to synthesize key nutrients, such as vitamin C or essential amino acids or fatty acids. For survival, these nutrients must, then, be supplied by the diet.

Alternatively, an individual's genetic makeup may result in an impaired enzyme that interferes with the ability to clear some toxic chemicals from the body. Broccoli and other cabbage family vegetables contain glucosinolates, compounds that are able to influence gene expression of the family of enzymes responsible for clearing these toxins. Eating broccoli regularly becomes a therapeutic strategy for these individuals and increases their protection against certain toxic chemicals they are exposed to in their food or environment. See Remely et al.

(2014); Henning, Wang, Carpenter, and Heber (2013); Joven et al. (2014); Miceli, Bontempo, Nebbioso, and Altucci (2014), and Milenkovic et al. (2014) for examples of the types of gene, diet, epigenome interactions that are being investigated, and the anticipated applications to chronic disease management and prevention.

Considering food in this way is part of the systems medicine approach that uses therapeutic interventions targeted to a chronic condition's underlying mechanisms. The technology is in place for this approach but a deeper understanding of nutrition through research must be achieved so that it is clear which gene alteration is associated with which dysfunction and what the appropriate nutritional intervention options are for restoring homeostasis. In the meantime, clinicians familiar with a systems approach and well-versed in metabolic pathways and their associations with various food components are increasingly targeting nutrition as one way to improve health and prevent chronic disease.

Of more immediate application are the many ways that food components influence the complex structures and reactions of the brain (Hing et al., 2014; McEwen & Getz, 2013; Stankiewicz et al., 2013; Virmani, Pinto, Binienda, & Ali, 2013). As with molecular nutrition, neuroscience is a young field and much research lies ahead before the mechanisms by which food influences brain activity and behavior are well understood. However, it is clear that nutrition plays an important role in brain health. For example, food supplies the building blocks needed to make neurotransmitters. The precursors for the synthesis of the complex neural circuits that transmit information and respond to neurotransmitters, hormones, and other chemical messengers through gene-encoded protein receptors also originate from what we eat. At a minimum a diet built on a healthy base of overall nutrient sufficiency and generous levels of omega-3 fatty acids and protein is needed.

LIFESTYLE DOMAIN: *PHYSICAL ACTIVITY*

Regular physical activity is recommended for health promotion for all age groups. The benefits are well documented in the prevention, management, and rehabilitation of chronic conditions, particularly for cardiovascular-related outcomes (Barlow et al., 2012; Gupta et al., 2011). Further, low levels of activity are associated with increased risk for all-cause mortality as well as for chronic disorders, such as heart disease and stroke, high blood pressure, insulin resistance and diabetes, and behavioral health conditions such as anxiety, depression, impaired cognition, and overall diminished quality of life (Park, Han, & Kang, 2014). Research with animals and humans suggests that physical activity results in greater neuroplasticity through multiple avenues, which in turn improves cognitive function and the capacity to respond to potential stressors with positive behavioral adaptations (Gary & Brunn, 2014; Hötting & Röder, 2013). Improving and sustaining neuroplasticity require cardiovascular fitness, further supporting the idea that physical activity needs to be regular and lifelong.

In addition to the conventional recommendations for aerobic, resistance, and stretching activities, the ancient practice of yoga has become a popular movement modality in the United States. In a meta-analysis of 18 studies, Patel, Newstead, and Ferrer (2012) found that for elderly participants a regular yoga practice was at least equal to other forms of exercise in terms of overall health benefits, aerobic fitness, and muscular strength. Additional benefits of improved executive function and other aspects of cognition have also been reported for those engaging in a regular gentle yoga practice (Gothe, Kramer, & McAuley, 2014). Bikram yoga ("hot yoga") has become popular for younger individuals, particularly for weight loss and weight maintenance, and appears to be a beneficial physical activity option (Pate & Buono, 2014). Research correlating yoga with changes in gene expression is in its infancy but promising, particularly with respect to the reduction in pro-inflammatory signaling (Black et al., 2013; Bower et al., 2014).

Research into the molecular basis for the various health benefits of regular physical activity focuses on the identification of gene variants together with physical activity and their roles in various chronic diseases as well as on the epigenetic influences on gene expression. Using insulin resistance-related conditions as just one chronic disease example, studies have found that the muscle contractions that occur during physical activity result in translocation of the GLUT4 receptor from the interior of cells to the cell membrane where it assists in blood glucose entry and facilitates energy production (Richter & Hargreaves, 2013; Strasser & Pesta, 2013). Further, exercise lowers the number of methyl groups attached to the region of DNA that controls the synthesis of the GLUT4 receptor, which increases the production of this receptor protein and further enhances glucose entry (Rowlands et al., 2014). A second important component, the *PGC1* (peroxisome proliferator-activated receptor γ coactivator-1α) gene, has also been found to respond positively to exercise in ways that benefit glucose usage (Santos, Tewari, & Benite-Ribeiro, 2014). This gene is a master regulator of mitochondrial activity, which is key to energy production. Its expression is essential for proper glucose disposal and is subject to epigenetic modification by high-energy diets and reduced physical activity. The resultant decreased expression of the *PGC1* gene contributes to insulin resistance. Exercise appears to attenuate the epigenetic effects, thereby increasing expression of this gene and reducing insulin resistance. In this way exercise's effects on *PGC1* expression can help to prevent the development of insulin resistance-related chronic conditions such as metabolic syndrome and Type 2 diabetes and more effectively manage existing disease.

In spite of the well-documented benefits of regular exercise, physical activity is not routinely prescribed within the health care system (Dacey, Kennedy, Phillips, & Polak, 2014; Virmani et al., 2013). The Healthy People 2020 guidelines include a strong statement of the need for increased physical activity among Americans, based on the discovery that greater than 80% of adults do not meet current guidelines for aerobic and muscle-strengthening activities and greater than 80% of adolescents do not meet the youth guidelines (www.healthypeople.gov/2020/topicsobjectives2020/overview.aspx?topicid=33).

Given the well-documented health benefits of physical activity, a significant contribution could be made through effective behavioral change therapy.

The American College of Sports Medicine (Garber et al., 2011) recommends prescribing exercise interventions and promoting their adoption and adherence by combining behavioral change therapy, the inclusion of an experienced fitness instructor, and a focus on activities that are enjoyable to the participant.

LIFESTYLE DOMAIN: *THOUGHTS AND EMOTIONS*

This lifestyle domain is particularly important to behavioral change. Mindfulness-based positive psychology works by targeting neural growth in the parts of the neo-mammalian brain associated with emotional regulation, cognitive flexibility, and perception (Keyworth et al., 2014). There is a growing body of literature that supports a mindfulness-based approach to working with thoughts and emotions (Kashdan & Ciarrochi, 2013). A meta-analysis of 39 studies and over 6,000 participants exposed to positive psychological interventions found that these strategies were impactful in increasing subjective well-being and psychological well-being, and reducing depressive symptoms (Bolier et al., 2013). A mindfulness-based, positive psychological approach teaches skills for working with painful, maladaptive cognitions and feelings and trains the mind in developing a positive, flexible, open, self-controlled, receptive, and goal-directed stance toward life (Hanson, 2009). Cheung, De Ridder, Gillebaart, and Kroese (2014) have demonstrated that those skilled in mindful meditation practices can accelerate the growth of neural substrates associated with greater trait self-control, which positively correlates with experiencing greater life satisfaction and happiness. Promising findings by Kaliman et al. (2014) suggest that mindfulness-based lifestyle interventions may impact inflammatory processes known to underlie chronic disease through the epigenetic regulation of pro-inflammatory gene expression.

LIFESTYLE DOMAIN: *RELATIONSHIPS WITH SELF AND OTHERS*

This domain focuses on the influence on health of developing positive relationships with oneself and with others and of having a spiritual sense of meaning and purpose in one's life. Cultivating self-compassion, self-appreciation, self-acceptance, insight, and an awareness of one's strengths appears to enhance health and well-being. It has been documented that self-affirmation improves psychological functioning and that self-compassion is a potential stimulator for self-affirming beliefs that appear to enhance pro-social, relational behaviors (Lindsay & Creswell, 2014). In fact, pro-social behaviors in adolescents have been correlated with decreasing inflammatory indicators, such as overweight and obesity, proinflammatory cytokine levels, and cholesterol levels (Schreier, Schonert-Reichl, & Chen, 2013). These results are encouraging because inflammation is a common promoter of chronic disease. In contrast, there is strong evidence suggesting that socially isolated individuals have significantly increased indicators for stress and chronic inflammation (Copertaro et al., 2014).

Researchers find that focusing attention on positive traits in oneself and others and increasing the attention one pays to things for which one is grateful can yield positive health outcomes (Emmons & McCullough, 2003; Lyubomirsky, Sousa, & Dickerhoof, 2006). There are robust data that the brain is powerfully charged to create neural connections wherever focused attention is placed (Hanson, 2013). There is strong evidence that focusing on positive traits correlates with positive chronic disease outcomes by changing negative perceptions that drive underlying inflammatory processes (Meyerson, Grant, Carter, & Kilmer, 2011). Furthermore, focusing on positive traits potentially modulates neuroendocrine and neuroimmune processes involved in the development and management of chronic disease (Antoni et al., 2009). It is suggested that those who routinely train their mind to see, value, and appreciate pleasant daily events (i.e., helping others, creating, interacting, playing, learning, spiritual activity, nature) experience greater heartfelt positivity and physical well-being as well as an enhanced capacity for mindfulness (Catalino & Frederickson, 2011).

LIFESTYLE DOMAIN: *SLEEP AND RELAXATION*

Sleep plays a restorative role for the brain and for the body in general. Currently the sleep period is estimated to have decreased by approximately 2 hours per day over the past 50 years (Lucassen, Rother, & Cizza, 2012; Misra & Khurana, 2008). Numerous studies have demonstrated that insufficient quality or quantity of sleep can lead to a variety of behavioral, neurochemical, endocrine, immune, cellular, molecular, and metabolic changes throughout the body (Anafi et al., 2013; Buxton et al., 2012; Chrousos, 2009; Cizza, Lucassen, & Rother, 2012; Hanlon & Van Cauter, 2011; Knutson, Ryden, Mander, & Van Cauter, 2006; Kurien, Chong, Ptáček, & Fu, 2013; Van Cauter, 2011). Irwin (2015) provides a good overview of the importance of sleep on health.

Exactly how an impaired sleep/wake cycle compromises health is not yet understood but promising research over the past decade suggests there are complex interactions among environmental cues (such as chronic stress), the sleep/wake cycle, and gene expression (Archer et al., 2014; Orozco-Solis & Sassone-Corsi, 2014).

Humans have a 24-hour circadian rhythm and this internal clock mechanism is important to our personal sleep pattern. The circadian clock mechanism is a key component of homeostasis and controls the timing and quality of both sleep and wakefulness (Franken, 2013). Anxiety, depression, and cognitive dysfunction, all conditions frequently seen in the primary care clinic, have been linked to disruption of circadian rhythms (Chrousos, 2009).

Several of the genes that encode components of the human biological clock have been identified, and epigenetic markings have been detected. When the clock mechanism is impaired, whether through genetic mutations or metabolic cues that affect epigenetic control of gene expression, circadian rhythms are impaired and promote the development of many of today's chronic disorders (Aguilar-Arnal & Sassone-Corsi, 2013; Garcia-Rios et al., 2014).

To date, mindfulness and the relaxation response have been primary approaches used to counter the negative influence of chronic stress on healthy sleep patterns (Bhasin et al., 2013). In a recent randomized controlled trial of 54 adults with chronic insomnia, mindfulness was found to be effective in improving sleep (Ong et al., 2014). Gross et al. (2011) found mindfulness to be more effective than pharmacotherapy for insomnia. In a meta-analysis, Winbush, Gross, and Kreitzer (2007) found that mindfulness techniques were associated with improved sleep patterns and that mindfulness-based stress reduction was especially helpful in reducing worry and other cognitive processes that interfered with quality sleep.

A SYSTEMS APPROACH TO HEALTH AND WELL-BEING FACILITATED THROUGH MINDFULNESS TRAINING: THE MINDFULNESS-BASED THERAPEUTIC LIFESTYLE CHANGE (MBTLC) PROGRAM

As BHSs, the salient question then is how can we best teach and guide patients to regain control of their own health and well-being? The first step is to use the behavioral aspects of systems medicine to deliver an effective behavioral change program for chronic disease. Such a program would focus on the key external factors that communicate with our cells and influence our molecular, biochemical, and physiological responses: nutrition, physical activity, thoughts and emotions, relationships, and sleep and relaxation. Using mindfulness training as the foundation for effective lifestyle interventions, the behavioral health specialist can educate patients on which lifestyle choices are appropriate for each modifiable lifestyle domain and facilitate their developing the skills that will allow them to make needed behavioral changes that can be sustained for the long-term. The following is a case example illustrating the application of this approach for a patient with chronic medical and psychiatric illness.

Case Example

The patient is a 42-year-old never-married African American woman with multiple medical and psychiatric complaints. Her diagnoses include hypertension, major depression, hyperlipidemia, morbid obesity, diabetes, vitamin D deficiency, fatigue, insomnia, and constipation. She is compliant with her medications. She complains of worsening extreme fatigue leading to vocational absenteeism/social isolation/heightened frustration with coworkers/friends/family. She experiences an increase in weight and a lack of motivation for self-care. She lacks exercise and motivation for physical activity of any kind. She experienced early childhood trauma and abuse. She has been treated for dysthymic depression with various serotonin-specific reuptake inhibitors and serotonin-norepinephrine reuptake inhibitors for 13 years and has been in behavioral therapy for 3 years.

The treatment plan for this patient targeted the appropriate medical/pharmacological and lifestyle aspects of care:

Medical

- Depression: slowly reduce psychiatric medications, continue mental health counseling
- Hypertension: diet and lifestyle therapy, continue medication until blood pressure improves

- Hyperlipidemia: lifestyle therapy
- Morbid obesity: lifestyle therapy
- Diabetes: lifestyle therapy
- Vitamin D deficiency: 2,000 IU vitamin D_3 daily
- Fatigue: lifestyle therapy; vitamin B_{12} testing
- Insomnia: lifestyle therapy; continue trazodone 50 mg daily, PRN
- Constipation: lifestyle therapy

Lifestyle Therapy

- Nutrition: nutrition counseling; cardiometabolic food plan (addresses weight, hypertension, diabetes, hyperlipidemia, constipation); log of foods, quantity, and emotional state while eating; 1,000-mg mixed essential fatty acids twice daily
- Physical activity: walking program with an ultimate goal of 10,000 steps per day self-monitored using a pedometer and recorded on an activity log; engage in resistance and stretching exercises; home yoga program
- Thoughts and emotions: participate in mental health counseling, daily mindfulness practice to improve self-acceptance, positive outlook, self-esteem, optimism, courage, self-appreciation, perseverance
- Relationships with self and others: participate in mental health counseling, resume church activities, and personal friendships as health improves
- Sleep and relaxation: commitment to adequate hours of sleep; improve sleep hygiene to improve quality, relaxation through deep breathing training

Outcome measures targeted by this treatment program included:

Biomarkers

- Reduction in blood pressure
- Reduced weight and body fat
- Constipation resolved
- Decreased fasting glucose
- Decreased total cholesterol, LDL cholesterol, and triglycerides
- Medication reduction: discontinuation/reduction of medications for hypertension, diabetes, depression, and insomnia

Lifestyle Parameters

- Changes in nutrition, physical activity, thoughts and emotions, relationships with self and others, sleep
- Dietary supplementation: vitamin D_3 at 1,000 IU/day, essential fatty acids at 2,000 mg/day, phosphorylated B-complex at 1 capsule per day
- Quality of life assessment: improvements in overall health, increased energy level, reductions in anxiety and emotional reactivity, improved ability to work and carry out daily activities, feeling of calm and peaceful

Systems approaches, such as Mindfulness-Based Therapeutic Lifestyle Change (MBTLC) model and functional medicine, are seen as important advances in mapping the future of prevention and health promotion through root cause analysis that leads to integrated treatment strategy. Dr. Harvey Fineberg, President of the Institute of Medicine, astutely addresses the need for comprehensive, systems science applied to chronic disease (Fineberg, 2013). In his 2013 commentary in the *Journal of the American Medical Association*, Dr. Fineberg writes:

> Risk factor analyses will become more useful over time as epidemiologists, statisticians, biologists, and other scientists are able to map the several layers of causal factors onto the expression of illness and its consequences. In this way, genetic, metabolic, physiologic, behavioral, environmental, and social factors will be traced through defined pathways to disease and premature mortality. This is a huge undertaking, the epidemiologic equivalent of the grand unified theory of forces in particle physics. Even partial elucidation of these epidemiologic interactions promises to reveal powerful ways to prevent disease and premature mortality. Importantly, this integrative research objective requires lines of inquiry at both the social and biological levels. *Trying to understand the causation of disease using only one of these lines of research is like trying to clap with one hand* [emphasis added]. (p. 586)

REFERENCES

Aguilar-Arnal, L., & Sassone-Corsi, P. (2013). The circadian epigenome: How metabolism talks to chromatin remodeling. *Current Opinion in Cell Biology*, *25*(2), 170–176.

Aldana, S. G., Whitmer, W. R., Greenlaw, R., Avins, A. L., Salberg, A., Barnhurst, M., ... Lipsenthal L. (2003). Cardiovascular risk reductions associated with aggressive lifestyle modification and cardiac rehabilitation. *Heart Lung*, *32*(6), 374–382.

American Diabetes Association. (2013). Economic costs of diabetes in the U.S. in 2012. *Diabetes Care*, *36*(4), 1033–1046.

Anafi, R. C., Pellegrino, R., Schokley, K. R., Romer, M., Tufik, S., & Pack, A. I. (2013). Sleep is not just for the brain: Transcriptional responses to sleep in peripheral tissues. *BMC Genomics*, *14*, 362.

Antoni, M. H., Lechner, S., Diaz, A., Vargas, S. Holley, H., Phillips, K., ... Blomberg, B. (2009). Cognitive behavioral stress management effects on psychosocial and physiological adaptation in women undergoing treatment for breast cancer. *Brain, Behavior and Immunity*, *23*(5), 580–591.

Archer, S. N., Laing, E. E., Möller-Levet, C. S., van der Veen, D. R., Bucca, G., Lazar, A. S., ... Dijk, D. J. (2014). Mistimed sleep disrupts circadian regulation of the human transcriptome. *Proceedings of the National Academy of Sciences of the United States of America*, *111*(6), 682–691.

Bacalini, M. G., Friso, S., Olivieri, F., Pirazzini, C., Giuliani, C., Capri, M., ... Garagnani, P. (2014). Present and future of anti-ageing epigenetic diets. *Mechanisms of Ageing and Development*, *136–137*, 101–115.

Baer, R. A., Carmody, J., & Hunsinger, M. (2012). Weekly change in mindfulness and mindfulness-perceived stress in a mindfulness-based stress reduction program. *Journal of Clinical Psychology*, *68*(7), 755–765.

Baer, R. A., Smith, G. T., Hopkins, J., Krietemeyer, J., & Toney, L. (2006). Using self-report assessment methods to explore facets of mindfulness. *Assessment*, *13*(1), 27–45.

Barlow, C. E., Defina, L. F., Radford, N. B., Berry, J. D., Cooper, K. H., Haskell, W. L., ... Lakoski, S. G. (2012). Cardiorespiratory fitness and long-term survival in "low-risk" adults. *Journal of the American Heart Association*, *1*(4), 001354.

Bellavance, M. A., & Rivest, S. (2014). The HPA–immune axis and the immunomodulatory actions of glucocorticoids in the brain. *Frontiers in Immunology*, *31*(5), 136.

Ben-Shahar, T. (2014). *Choose the life you want: The mindful way to happiness*. New York, NY: The Experiment, LLC.

Benson, H., Bhasin, M. K., Chang, B. H., Denninger, J. W., Dusek, J. A., Fricchione, G. L., & Libermann, T. A. (2013). Relaxation response induces temporal transcriptome changes in energy metabolism, insulin secretion and inflammatory pathways. *PLoS One*, *8*(5), 62817.

Bhasin, M. K., Dusek, J. A., Chang, B. H., Joseph, M. G., Denninger, J. W., Fricchione, G. L., . . . Libermann T. A. (2013). Relaxation response induces temporal transcriptome changes in energy metabolism, insulin secretion and inflammatory pathways. *PLoS One*, *8*(5), 62817.

Black, D. S., Cole, S. W., Irwin, M. R., Breen, E., St. Cyr, N. M., Nazarian, N., ... Lavretsky, H. (2013). Yogic meditation reverses NF-kB and IRF-related transcriptome dynamics in leukocytes of family dementia caregivers in a randomized controlled trial. *Psychoneuroendocrinology*, *38*(3), 348–355.

Bolier, L., Haverman, M., Westerhof, G. J., Riper, H., Smit, F., & Bohlmeijer, E. (2013). Positive psychology interventions: A meta-analysis of randomized controlled studies. *BMC Public Health*, *8*(13), 119.

Bower, J. E., Greendale, G., Crosswell, A. D., Garet, D., Sternlieb, B., Ganz, P. A., ... Cole, S. W. (2014).Yoga reduces inflammatory signaling in fatigued breast cancer survivors: A randomized controlled trial. *Psychoneuroendocrinology*, *43*, 20–29.

Buxton, O. M., Cain, S. W., O'Connor, S. P., Porter, J. H., Duffy, J. F., Wang, W., ... Shea, S. A. (2012). Adverse metabolic consequences in humans of prolonged sleep restriction combined with circadian disruption. *Science Translational Medicine*, *4*(129), 129–143.

Catalino, L. I., & Fredrickson, B. A. (2011). A Tuesday in the life of a flourisher: The role of positive emotional reactivity in optimal mental health. *Emotion*, *11*(4), 938–950.

Cayoun, B. A. (2005). *From co-emergence dynamics to human perceptual evolution: The role of neuroplasticity during mindfulness training*. Keynote address presented at the 2005 National Conference of the New Zealand Psychological Society, Otago University, Dunedin, New Zealand.

Cheung, T. T., De Ridder, D., Gillebaart, M., & Kroese, F. (2014). Why are people with high self-control happier? The effect of trait self-control on happiness as mediated by regulatory focus. *Frontiers in Psychology*, *5*, 722.

Chrousos, G. P. (2009). Stress and disorders of the stress system. *Nature Review Endocrinology*, *5*(7), 374–381.

Cizza, G., Lucassen, E. A., & Rother, K. I. (2012). Interacting epidemics? Sleep curtailment, insulin resistance, and obesity. *Annals of New York Academy of Sciences*, *1264*, 110–134.

Cooney, C. A. (2006). Germ cells carry the epigenetic benefits of grandmother's diet. *Proceedings of the National Academy of Sciences of the United States of America*, *103*(46), 17071–17072.

Copertaro, A., Bracci, M., Manzella, N., Barbaresi, M., Copertaro B., & Santarelli, L. L. (2014). Low perceived social support is associated with CD8+CD57+ lymphocyte expansion and increased TNF-α levels. *Biomed Research International*, *2014*, 635784.

Creswell J. D., Irwin M. R., Burklund, L. J., Lieberman, M. D., Arevalo, J. M., Ma, J., Breen, E. C., & Cole, S. W. (2012). Mindfulness-based stress reduction training reduces loneliness and pro-inflammatory gene expression in older adults: A small randomized controlled trial. *Brain Behavior and Immunity*, *26*(7), 1095–1101.

Dacey, M. L., Kennedy, M. A., Phillips, E. M., & Polak, R. (2014). Physical activity counseling in medical school education: A systematic review. *Medical Education Online*, *19*, 24325.

Davidson, R. J., Jackson, D. C., & Kalin, N. H. (2000). Emotion, plasticity, context, and regulation: Perspectives from affective neuroscience. *Psychological Bulletin*, *126*, 890–909.

Davidson, R. J., Kabat-Zinn, J., Schumacher, J., Rosenkrantz, M., Muller, D., Santorelli, S. F., & Sheridan, J. F. (2003). Alterations in brain and immune function produced by mindfulness meditation. *Psychosomatic Medicine*, *65*(4), 564–570.

Davidson, R. J., & McEwen, B. S. (2012). Social influences on neuroplasticity: Stress and interventions to promote well-being. *Nature Neuroscience*, *15*(5), 689–695.

Dod, H. S., Bhardwaj, R., Salia, V., Weidner, G., Hobbs, G. R., Konat, G. W., ... Jain, A. C. (2010). Effect of intensive lifestyle changes on endothelial function and on inflammatory markers of atherosclerosis. *American Journal of Cardiology*, *105*(3), 362–367.

Emmons, R. A., & McCullough, M. E. (2003). Counting blessings versus burdens: An experimental investigation of gratitude and subjective well-being in daily life. *Journal of Personality and Social Psychology*, *84*(2), 377–389.

Espeland, M. A., Glick, H. A., Bertoni, A., Brancati, F. L., Bray, G. A., Clark, J. M., ... Look AHEAD Research Group. (2014). Impact of an intensive lifestyle intervention on use and cost of medical services among overweight and obese adults with type 2 diabetes: The action for health in diabetes. *Diabetes Care*, *37*(9), 2548–2556.

Fenech, M. F. (2014). Nutriomes and personalised nutrition for DNA damage prevention, telomere integrity maintenance and cancer growth control. *Cancer Treatment and Research*, *159*, 427–441.

Fineberg, H. V. (2013). The state of health in the United States. *Journal of the American Medical Association*, *310*(6), 585–586.

FitzGerald, M. J. T., & Folan-Curran, J. (2002). *Clinical neuroanatomy and related neurosciences* (4th ed.). London: Saunders.

Fraga, M. F., Ballestar, E., Paz, M. F., Ropero, S., Setien, F., Ballestar, M. L., ... Esteller, M. (2005). Epigenetic differences arise during the lifetime of monozygotic twins. *Proceedings of the National Academy of Sciences of the United States of America*, *102*(30), 10604–10609.

Franken, P. (2013). A role for clock genes in sleep homeostasis. *Current Opinions in Neurobiology*, 23(5), 864–872.

Frattaroli, J., Weidner, G., Dnistrian, A. M., Kemp, C., Daubenmier, J. J., Marlin, R. O., ... Ornish, D. (2008). Clinical events in prostate cancer lifestyle trial: Results from two years of follow-up. *Urology*, 72(6), 1319–1323.

Garber, C. E., Blissmer, B., Deschenes, M. R., Franklin, B. A., Lamonte, M. J., Lee, I. M., Nieman, D. C., ... American College of Sports Medicine. (2011). Quantity and quality of exercise for developing and maintaining cardiorespiratory, musculoskeletal, and neuromotor fitness in apparently healthy adults: Guidance for prescribing exercise. *Medicine and Science of Sports and Exercise*, *43*(7), 1334–1359.

Garcia-Rios, A., Gomez-Delgado, F. J., Garaulet, M., Alcala-Diaz, J. F., Delgado-Lista, F. J., Marin, C., ... Perez-Martinez, P. (2014). Beneficial effect of CLOCK gene polymorphism rs1801260 in combination with low-fat diet on insulin metabolism in the patients with metabolic syndrome. *Chronobiology International*, *31*(3), 401–406.

Gard, T., Hölzel, B. K., Sack, A. T., Hempel, H., Lazar, S. W., Vaitl, D., & Ott, U. (2012). Pain attenuation through mindfulness is associated with decreased cognitive control and increased sensory processing in the brain. *Cerebral Cortex*, 22(11), 2692–2702.

Gary, R. A., & Brunn, K. (2014). Aerobic exercise as an adjunct therapy for improving cognitive function in heart failure. *Cardiology Research and Practice*, 157508.

Go, A. S., Mozaffarian, D., Roger, V. L., Benjamin, E. J., Berry, J. D., Blaha M. J., ... American Heart Association Statistics Committee and Stroke Statistics Subcommittee. (2014). Executive summary: Heart disease and stroke statistics—2014 update: A report from the American Heart Association. *Circulation*, *129*(3), 399–410.

Gothe, N. P., Kramer, A. F., & McAuley, E. (2014). The effects of an 8-week hatha yoga intervention on executive function in older adults. *Journals of Gerontology: Series A, Biological Sciences and Medical Sciences*, *69*(9), 1109–1116.

Gross, C. R., Kreitzer, M. J., Reilly-Spong, M., Wall, M., Winbush, N. Y., Patterson, R., ... Cramer-Bornemann M. (2011). Mindfulness-based stress reduction versus pharmacotherapy for chronic primary insomnia: A randomized controlled clinical trial. *Explore* (NY). 7(2), 76–87.

Guintivano, J., & Kaminsky, Z. A. (2014). Role of epigenetic factors in the development of mental illness throughout life. *Neuroscience Research*, doi:10.1016/j.neures.2014.08.003. [Epub ahead of print].

Gupta, S., Rohatgi, A., Ayers, C. R., Willis, B. L., Haskell, W. L., Khera, A., ... Berry, J. D. (2011). Cardiorespiratory fitness and classification of risk of cardiovascular disease mortality. *Circulation*, *123*(13), 1377–1383.

Hanlon, E. C., & Van Cauter, E. (2011). Quantification of sleep behavior and of its impact on the cross-talk between the brain and peripheral metabolism. *Proceedings of the National Academy of Sciences of the United States of America*, *108*(3), 15609–15616.

Hanson, R. (2009). *Buddha's brain: The practical neuroscience of happiness, love, and wisdom*. Oakland, CA: New Harbinger Publication.

Hanson, R. (2013). *Hardwiring happiness*. New York, NY: Random House.

Hebb, D. O. (1949). *Organization of behavior*. New York, NY: Wiley.

Henning, S. M., Wang, P., Carpenter, C. L., & Heber, D. (2013). Epigenetic effects of green tea polyphenols in cancer. *Epigenomics*, *5*(6), 729–741.

Hing, B., Gardner, C., & Potash, J. B. (2014). Effects of negative stressors on DNA methylation in the brain: Implications for mood and anxiety disorders. *American Journal of Medical Genetics. Part B, Neuropsychiatric Genetics*, *165B*(7), 541–554.

Hölzel, B. K., Carmody, J., Vangel, M., Congleton, C., Yerramsetti, S. M., Gard, T., & Lazar, S. W. (2011). Mindfulness practice leads to increases in regional brain gray matter density. *Psychiatry Research*, *191*(1), 36–43.

Hötting, K., & Röder, B. (2013). Beneficial effects of physical exercise on neuroplasticity and cognition. *Neuroscience and Biobehavioral Reviews*, *37*(9 Pt B), 2243–2257.

Irwin, M. R. (2008). Human psychoneuroimmunology: 20 years of discovery. *Brain, Behavior, and Immunity*, *22*(2), 129–139.

Irwin, M. R. (2015). Why sleep is important for health: A psychoneuroimmunology perspective. *Annual Reviews of Psychology*, *66*, 143–172.

Jang, H., & Serra, C. (2014). Nutrition, epigenetics, and diseases. *Clinical Nutrition Research*, *3*(1), 1–8.

Jiménez-Chillarón, J. C., Díaz, R., Martínez, D., Pentinat, T., Ramón-Krauel, M., Ribó, S., & Plösch T. (2012). The role of nutrition on epigenetic modifications and their implications on health. *Biochimie*, *94*(11), 2242–2263.

Joven, J., Micol, V., Segura-Carretero, A., Alonso-Villaverde, C., Menéndez, J. A., & Bioactive Food Components Platform. (2014). Polyphenols and the modulation of gene expression pathways: Can we eat our way out of the danger of chronic disease? *Critical Reviews in Food Science and Nutrition*, *54*(8), 985–1001.

Kabat-Zinn, J. (1982). An outpatient program in behavioural medicine for chronic pain patients based on the practice of mindfulness meditation: Theoretical considerations and preliminary results. *General Hospital Psychiatry*, *4*, 33–47.

Kabat-Zinn, J. (2003). Mindfulness-based interventions in context: Past, present, and future. *Clinical Psychology: Science and Practice*, *10*(2), 144–156.

Kabat-Zinn, J., Massion, A. O., Kristeller, J., Peterson, L. G., Fletcher, K. E., Pbert, L., ... Santorelli, S. F. (1992). Effectiveness of a meditation-based stress reduction program in the treatment of anxiety disorders. *American Journal of Psychiatry*, *149*(7), 936–943.

Kaliman, P., Alvarez-López, M. J., Cosín-Tomás, M., Rosenkranz, M. A., Lutz, A., & Davidson, R. J. (2014). Rapid changes in histone deacetylases and inflammatory gene expression in expert meditators. *Psychoneuroendocrinology*, *40*, 96–107.

Kashdan, T. B., & Ciarrochi, J. V. (Eds.). (2013). *Mindfulness, acceptance, and positive psychology*. Oakland, CA: New Harbinger Publications.

Keyworth, C., Knopp, J., Roughley, K., Dickens, C., Bold, S., Coventry, P. (2014). A mixed-methods pilot study of the acceptability and effectiveness of a brief meditation and mindfulness intervention for people with diabetes and coronary heart disease. *Behavioral Medicine*, *40*(2), 53–64.

Knutson, K. L., Ryden, A. M., Mander, B. A., & Van Cauter, E. (2006). Role of sleep duration and quality in the risk and severity of type 2 diabetes mellitus. *Archives of Internal Medicine*, *166*(16), 1768–1774.

Konner, M., & Eaton, S. B. (2010). Paleolithic nutrition: Twenty-five years later. *Nutrition in Clinical Practice*, *25*(6), 594–602.

Kristeller, J., & Hallett, C. (1999). An exploratory study of a meditation-based intervention for binge eating disorder. *Journal of Health Psychology*, *4*(3), 357–363.

Kurien, P. A., Chong, S. Y., Ptáček, L. J., & Fu, Y. H. (2013). Sick and tired: How molecular regulators of human sleep schedules and duration impact immune function. *Current Opinions in Neurobiology*, *23*(5), 873–879.

Layous, K., Chancellor, J., & Lyubomirsky, S. (2014). Positive activities as protective factors against mental health conditions. *Journal of Abnormal Psychology*, *123*, 3–12.

Layous, K., & Lyubomirsky, S. (2014). The how, why, what, when, and who of happiness: Mechanisms underlying the success of positive interventions. In J. Gruber & J. Moscowitz (Eds.), *Positive emotion: Integrating the light sides and dark sides* (pp. 473–495). New York, NY: Oxford University Press.

Lindsay, E. K., & Creswell, J. D. (2014). Helping the self help others: Self-affirmation increases self-compassion and pro-social behaviors. *Frontiers in Psychology*, *5*, 421.

Lucassen, E. A., Rother, K. I., & Cizza, G. (2012). Interacting epidemics? Sleep curtailment, insulin resistance, and obesity. *Annals of the New York Academy of Sciences*, *1264*(1), 110–134.

Lyubomirsky, S., Sheldon, K. M., & Schkade, D. (2005). Pursuing happiness: The architecture of sustainable change. *Review of General Psychology*, *9*, 111–131.

Lyubomirsky, S., Sousa, L., & Dickerhoof, R. (2006). The costs and benefits of writing, talking, and thinking about life's triumphs and defeats. *Journal of Personality and Social Psychology*, *90*, 692–708.

MacLean, P. D. (1990). *The triune brain in evolution: Role in paleocerebral functions*. New York, NY: Plenum Press.

Marchand, W. R. (2014). Neural mechanisms of mindfulness and meditation: Evidence from neuroimaging studies. *World Journal of Radiology*, *6*(7), 471–479.

McEwen, B. S., & Getz, L. (2013). Lifetime experiences, the brain and personalized medicine: An integrative perspective. *Metabolism*, *62*(Suppl 1), S20–S26.

Meyerson, D. A., Grant, K. E., Carter, J. S., & Kilmer, R. P. (2011). Posttraumatic growth among children and adolescents: A systematic review. *Clinical Psychology Reviews*, *31*(6), 949–964.

Miceli, M., Bontempo, P., Nebbioso, A., & Altucci, L. (2014). Natural compounds in epigenetics: A current view. *Food and Chemical Toxicology*, *73*, 71–83.

Micha, R., Kalantarian, S., Wirojratana, P., Byers, T., Danaei, G., Elmadfa, I., & Global Burden of Diseases, Nutrition and Chronic Disease Expert Group. (2012). Estimating the global and regional burden of suboptimal nutrition on chronic disease: Methods and inputs to the analysis. *European Journal of Clinical Nutrition*, *66*(1), 119–129.

Milenkovic, D., Berghe, W. V., Boby, C., Leroux, C., Declerck, K., Szarc vel Szic, K., ... Weseler, A. R., (2014). Dietary flavanols modulate the transcription of genes associated with cardiovascular pathology without changes in their DNA methylation state. *PLoS One*, *9*(4), e95527.

Miller, C. K., Kristeller, J. L., Headings, A., Nagaraja, H., & Miser, W. F. (2012). Comparative effectiveness of a mindful eating intervention to a diabetes self-management intervention among adults with type 2 diabetes: A pilot study. *Journal of the Academy of Nutrition and Dietetics*, *112*(11), 1835–1842.

Misra, A., & Khurana, L. (2008). Obesity and the metabolic syndrome in developing countries. *Journal of Clinical Endocrinology and Metabolism*. *93*(11 Suppl 1), S9–S30.

Morgan, N., Irwin, M. R., Chung, M., & Wang, C. (2014). The effects of mind-body therapies on the immune system: Meta-analysis. *PLoS One*, *9*(7), e100903.

National Cancer Institute. (2013). Cancer prevalence and cost of care projections web site. Retrieved on January 23, 2015, from http://costprojections.cancer.gov/

Neylan, T. C. (1998). Hans Selye and the field of stress research. *Neuropsychiatry Classics*, *10*(2), 230, 231.

Nieuwenhuys, R., Voogd, J., & van Huijzen, C. (2007). *The human central nervous system* (4th ed.). Berlin-Heidelberg: Springer Science + Business Media.

Ong, J. C., Manber, R., Segal, Z., Xia, Y., Shapiro, S., & Wyatt, J. K. (2014). A messaging system diagram, 5 domains, 10.29.14 randomized controlled trial of mindfulness meditation for chronic insomnia. *Sleep*, *37*(9), 1553–1563.

Ornish, D., Lin, J., Chan, J. M., Epel, E., Kemp, C., Weidner, G., ... Blackburn, E. H. (2013). Effect of comprehensive lifestyle changes on telomerase activity and telomere length in men with biopsy-proven low-risk prostate cancer: 5-year follow-up of a descriptive pilot study. *Lancet Oncology*, *14*(11), 1112–1120.

Ornish, D., Lin, J., Daubenmier, J., Weidner, G., Epel, E., Kemp, C., ... Blackburn, E. H. (2008a). Increased telomerase activity and comprehensive lifestyle changes: A pilot study. *Lancet Oncology*, *9*(11), 1048–1057. Erratum in: *Lancet Oncology*, *9*(12), 1124.

Ornish, D., Magbanua, M. J., Weidner, G., Weinberg, V., Kemp, C., Green, C., ... Carroll P. R. (2008b). Changes in prostate gene expression in men undergoing an intensive nutrition and lifestyle intervention. *Proceedings of the National Academy of Sciences of the United States of America, 105*(24), 8369–8374.

Ornish, D., Scherwitz, L. W., Doody, R. S., Kesten, D., McLanahan, S. M., Brown, S. E., ... Gotto, A. M., Jr. (1983). Effects of stress management training and dietary changes in treating ischemic heart disease. *Journal of the American Medical Association, 249*(1), 54–59.

Orozco-Solis, R., & Sassone-Corsi, P. (2014). Epigenetic control and the circadian clock: Linking metabolism to neuronal responses. *Neuroscience, 264*, 76–87.

Park, S. H., Han, K. S., & Kang, C. B. (2014). Effects of exercise programs on depressive symptoms, quality of life and self-esteem in older people: A systematic review of randomized controlled trials. *Applied Nursing Research, 27*(4), 219–226.

Pate, J. L., & Buono, M. J. (2014). The physiological responses to Bikram yoga in novice and experienced practitioners. *Alternative Therapies in Health and Medicine, 20*(4), 12–18.

Patel, N. K., Newstead, A. H., & Ferrer, R. L. (2012). The effects of yoga on physical functioning and health related quality of life in older adults: A systematic review and meta-analysis. *Journal of Alternative and Complementary Medicine, 18*(10), 902–917.

Paulson, S., Davidson, R., Jha, A., & Kabat-Zinn, J. (2013). Becoming conscious: The science of mindfulness. *Annals of the New York Academy of Sciences, 1303*, 87–104.

Remely, M., Lovrecic, L., de la Garza, A. L., Migliore, L., Peterlin, B., Milagro, F. I., ... Haslberger, A. G. (2014). Therapeutic perspectives of epigenetically active nutrients. British Journal of Pharmacology. doi: 10.1111/bph.12854. [Epub ahead of print].

Reul, J. M. (2014). Making memories of stressful events: A journey along epigenetic, gene transcription, and signaling pathways. *Frontiers of Psychiatry, 5*, 5.

Richter, E. A., & Hargreaves, M. (2013). Exercise, GLUT4, and skeletal muscle glucose uptake. *Physiological Reviews, 93*(3), 993–1017.

Rosenbloom, C. A., Lacey, K. P., & Stang, J., for the Academy Positions Committee Workgroup. (2013). Practice paper of the Academy of Nutrition and Dietetics: The role of nutrition in health promotion and chronic disease prevention. *Journal of the Academy of Nutrition and Dietetics, 113*, 983–993.

Rowlands, D. S., Page, R. A., Sukala, W. R., Giri, M., Ghimbovschi, S. D., Hayat, I., ... Hoffman, E. P. (2014). Multi-omic integrated networks connect DNA methylation and miRNA with skeletal muscle plasticity to chronic exercise in type 2 diabetic obesity. *Physiological Genomics, 46*(20), 747–765.

Sales, N. M., Pelegrini, P. B., & Goersch, M. C. (2014). Nutrigenomics: Definitions and advances of this new science. *Journal of Nutrition and Metabolism, 2014*, 202759.

Santos, J. M., Tewari, S., & Benite-Ribeiro, S. A. (2014). The effect of exercise on epigenetic modifications of PGC1: The impact on type 2 diabetes. *Medical Hypotheses, 82*(6), 748–753.

Schreier, H. M., Schonert-Reichl, K. A., & Chen, E. (2013). Effect of volunteering on risk factors for cardiovascular disease in adolescents: A randomized controlled trial. *Journal of the American Medical Association: Pediatrics, 167*(4), 327–332.

Schwartz, J. M. (1997). *Brain lock: Free yourself from obsessive behavior.* New York, NY: Harper Collins.

Schwartz, J. M., & Gladding, R. (2012). *You are not your brain: The 4-step solution for changing bad habits, ending unhealthy thinking, and taking control of your life.* New York, NY: Penguin.

Segal, Z. V., Williams, J. M. G., & Teasdale, J. D. (2002). *Mindfulness-based cognitive therapy for depression: A new approach to preventing relapse.* New York, NY: Guilford Press.

Siegel, D. J. (2012). *Pocket guide to interpersonal neurobiology: An integrative handbook of the mind.* New York, NY: W. W. Norton.

Siegel, D. J. (2007). *The mindful brain: Reflection and attunement in the cultivation of well-being.* New York, NY: W. W. Norton.

Silberman, A., Banthia, R., Estay, I. S., Kemp, C., Studley, J., Hareras, D., & Ornish, D. (2010). The effectiveness and efficacy of an intensive cardiac rehabilitation program in 24 sites. *American Journal of Health Promotion, 24*(4), 260–266.

Slawson, D. L., Fitzgerald, N., & Morgan, K. T. (2013). Position of the Academy of Nutrition and Dietetics: The role of nutrition in health promotion and chronic disease prevention. *Journal of the Academy of Nutrition and Dietetics, 113*, 972–979.

Stankiewicz, A. M., Swiergiel, A. H., & Lisowski, P. (2013). Epigenetics of stress adaptations in the brain. *Brain Research Bulletin, 98*, 76–92.

Strasser, B., & Pesta, D. (2013). Resistance training for diabetes prevention and therapy: Experimental findings and molecular mechanisms. *Biomed Research International, 2013*, 805217.

Tammen, S. A., Friso, S., & Choi, S. W. (2013). Epigenetics: The link between nature and nurture. *Molecular Aspects of Medicine, 34*(4), 753–764.

Van Cauter, E. (2011). Sleep disturbances and insulin resistance. *Diabetic Medicine, 28*(12), 1455–1462.

Vedhara, K., Fox, J., & Wang, E. (2013). The measurement of stress-related immune dysfunction in psychoneuroimmunology. *Neuroscience and Biobehavioral Reviews*, 23, 699–715.

Vickers, M. H. (2014). Early life nutrition, epigenetics and programming of later life disease. *Nutrients, 6*(6), 2165–2178.

Virmani, A., Pinto, L., Binienda, Z., & Ali, S. (2013). Food, nutrigenomics, and neurodegeneration—neuroprotection by what you eat! *Molecular Neurobiology, 48*(2), 353–362.

Waterland, R. A., Dolinoy, D. C., Lin, J. R., Smith, C. A., Shi, X., & Tahiliani, K. G. (2006). Maternal methyl supplements increase offspring DNA methylation at Axin Fused. *Genesis, 44*, 401–406.

Waterland, R. A., & Jirtle, R. L. (2003). Transposable elements: Targets for early nutritional effects on epigenetic gene regulation. *Molecular and Cellular Biology*, 23(15), 5293–5300.

Winbush, N. Y., Gross, C. R., & Kreitzer, M. J. (2007). The effects of mindfulness-based stress reduction on sleep disturbance: A systematic review. *Explore* (NY), 3(6), 585–591.

Wolff, G. L., Kodell, R. L., Moore, S. R., & Cooney, C. A. (1998). Maternal epigenetics and methyl supplements affect agouti gene expression in Avy/a mice. *Federation of American Societies for Experimental Biology Journal, 11*, 949–957.

Zannas, A. S., & West, A. E. (2014). Epigenetics and the regulation of stress vulnerability and resilience. *Neuroscience, 264*, 157–170.

INDEX

Printed in the United States
By Bookmasters